Male Pelvic Imaging

Editors

KARTIK S. JHAVERI
MUKESH G. HARISINGHANI

RADIOLOGIC CLINICS
OF NORTH AMERICA

www.radiologic.theclinics.com

Consulting Editor
FRANK H. MILLER

November 2012 • Volume 50 • Number 6

ELSEVIER

1600 John F. Kennedy Boulevard • Suite 1800 • Philadelphia, Pennsylvania 19103-2899

http://www.theclinics.com

RADIOLOGIC CLINICS OF NORTH AMERICA Volume 50, Number 6
November 2012 ISSN 0033-8389, ISBN 13: 978-1-4557-5827-2

Editor: Adrianne Brigido
Developmental Editor: Donald Mumford

Radiologic Clinics of North America (ISSN 0033-8389) is published bimonthly by Elsevier Inc., 360 Park Avenue South, New York, NY 10010-1710. Months of issue are January, March, May, July, September, and November. Periodicals postage paid at New York, NY and additional mailing offices. Subscription prices are USD 421 per year for US individuals, USD 659 per year for US institutions, USD 202 per year for US students and residents, USD 491 per year for Canadian individuals, USD 827 per year for Canadian institutions, USD 606 per year for international individuals, USD 827 per year for international institutions, and USD 290 per year for Canadian and foreign students/residents. To receive student and resident rate, orders must be accompanied by name of affiliated institution, date of term and the signature of program/residency coordinatior on institution letterhead. Orders will be billed at individual rate until proof of status is received. Foreign air speed delivery is included in all *Clinics* subscription prices. All prices are subject to change without notice. **POSTMASTER:** Send address changes to *Radiologic Clinics of North America*, Elsevier Health Sciences Division, Subscription Customer Service, 3251 Riverport Lane, Maryland Heights, MO63043. **Customer Service: Telephone: 1-800-654-2452** (U.S. and Canada); **1-314-447-8871** (outside U.S. and Canada). **Fax: 1-314-447-8029. E-mail: journalscustomerservice-usa@ elsevier.com** (for print support); **journalsonlinesupport-usa@elsevier.com** (for online support).

Reprints. For copies of 100 or more of articles in this publication, please contact the Commercial Reprints Department, Elsevier Inc., 360 Park Avenue South, New York, New York 10010-1710. Tel.: (+1) 212-633-3812; Fax: (+1) 212-462-1935; E-mail: reprints@elsevier.com.

Radiologic Clinics of North America also published in Greek Paschalidis Medical Publications, Athens, Greece.

Radiologic Clinics of North America is covered in *MEDLINE/PubMed (Index Medicus), EMBASE/Excerpta Medica, Current Contents/Life Sciences, Current Contents/Clinical Medicine, RSNA Index to Imaging Literature, BIOSIS, Science Citation Index,* and *ISI/BIOMED.*

Printed in the United States of America.

Contributors

CONSULTING EDITOR

FRANK H. MILLER, MD
Professor of Radiology; Chief, Body Imaging
Section and Fellowship Program and GI
Radiology; Medical Director MRI, Department
of Radiology, Feinberg School of Medicine,
Northwestern University, Chicago, Illinois

GUEST EDITORS

KARTIK S. JHAVERI, MD
Associate Professor, Department of Medical
Imaging, University of Toronto; Staff
Radiologist, Abdominal Imaging, University
Health Network, Mt. Sinai and Women's
College Hospital, Toronto, Ontario, Canada

MUKESH G. HARISINGHANI, MD
Associate Professor, Harvard Medical
School; Director of Abdominal MRI,
Massachusetts General Hospital, Boston,
Massachusetts

AUTHORS

LEJLA AGANOVIC, MD
Assistant Clinical Professor of Radiology,
Department of Radiology, VA Hospital,
University of California San Diego, San Diego,
California

LAURA L. AVERY, MD
Division of Emergency Radiology, Department
of Radiology, Massachusetts General Hospital,
Harvard Medical School, Boston,
Massachusetts

FIONA CASSIDY, MD
Assistant Clinical Professor of Radiology,
Department of Radiology, VA Hospital,
University of California San Diego, San Diego,
California

AZADEH ELMI, MD
Division of Abdominal Imaging and
Intervention, Massachusetts General
Hospital, Harvard Medical School, Boston,
Massachusetts

JURGEN J. FÜTTERER, MD, PhD
Department of Radiology, Radboud University
Nijmegen Medical Centre, Nijmegen,
The Netherlands; MIRA Institute for Biomedical
Technology and Technical Medicine,
University of Twente, Enschede,
The Netherlands

SANGEET GHAI, MD, FRCR
Assistant Professor, University of Toronto;
Joint Department of Medical Imaging,
University Health Network, Mount Sinai
Hospital, Women's College Hospital, Toronto,
Ontario, Canada

ALPANA M. HARISINGHANI, MD
Medical Research Associate, Perceptive
Informatics, Billerica, Massachusetts

MUKESH G. HARISINGHANI, MD
Associate Professor, Harvard Medical
School; Director of Abdominal MRI,
Massachusetts General Hospital, Boston,
Massachusetts

SANDEEP S. HEDGIRE, MD
Division of Abdominal Imaging and
Intervention, Massachusetts General Hospital,
Harvard Medical School, Boston,
Massachusetts

KARTIK S. JHAVERI MD
Associate Professor, Department of Medical
Imaging, University of Toronto; Staff
Radiologist, Abdominal Imaging, University
Health Network, Mt. Sinai and Women's
College Hospital, Toronto, Ontario, Canada

ADAM J. JUNG, MD, PhD
Assistant Professor, Department of Radiology
and Biomedical Imaging, University of
California San Francisco, San Francisco,
California

DOW-MU KOH, MD, MRCP, FRCR
Consultant Radiologist in Functional Imaging,
Department of Radiology, Royal Marsden
Hospital, Royal Marsden NHS Foundation
Trust, Sutton, United Kingdom

VIVEK K. PARGAONKAR, MD
Division of Abdominal Imaging and
Intervention, Massachusetts General Hospital,
Harvard Medical School, Boston,
Massachusetts

ROCIO PEREZ-JOHNSTON, MD
Fellow in Abdominal Imaging and Interventional
Radiology, Department of Radiology, Division
of Abdominal Imaging, Massachusetts General
Hospital, Boston, Massachusetts

MARK A. PRESTON, MD
Department of Urology, Massachusetts
General Hospital, Harvard Medical School,
Boston, Massachusetts

SYED ARSALAN RAZA, MBBS, FRCR
Clinical Fellow, Department of Medical
Imaging, University of Toronto; Abdominal
Imaging, University Health Network, Mt. Sinai
and Women's College Hospital, Toronto,
Ontario, Canada; Staff Radiologist,
Department of Diagnostic Imaging,
Cape Breton Regional Hospital, Sydney,
Nova Scotia, Canada

MEIR H. SCHEINFELD, MD, PhD
Division of Emergency Radiology, Montefiore
Medical Center, Albert Einstein College of
Medicine, Bronx, New York

ANURADHA SHENOY-BHANGLE, MD
Fellow in Abdominal Imaging and Interventional
Radiology, Department of Radiology, Division
of Abdominal Imaging, Massachusetts General
Hospital, Boston, Massachusetts

AJAY SINGH, MD
Associate Director, Night Imaging Services,
Department of Radiology, Division of
Abdominal Imaging, Massachusetts General
Hospital, Boston, Massachusetts

ASLAM SOHAIB, MRCP, FRCR
Consultant Radiologist, Department of
Radiology, Royal Marsden Hospital, Royal
Marsden NHS Foundation Trust, Sutton,
United Kingdom

SHAHIN TABATABAEI, MD
Department of Urology, Massachusetts
General Hospital, Harvard Medical School,
Boston, Massachusetts

SAMAN SHAFAAT TALAB, MD
Department of Urology, Massachusetts
General Hospital, Harvard Medical School,
Boston, Massachusetts

ANTS TOI, MD, FRCPC, FAIUM
Professor, Radiology, University of Toronto;
Professor, Obstetrics and Gynecology,
University of Toronto; Joint Department of
Medical Imaging, University Health Network,
Mount Sinai Hospital, Women's College
Hospital, Toronto, Ontario, Canada

ANTONIO C. WESTPHALEN, MD, MAS
Associate Professor, Department of Radiology
and Biomedical Imaging, University of
California San Francisco, San Francisco,
California

Contents

> No consensus exists at present regarding the use of imaging for the evaluation of prostate cancer. Ultrasonography is mainly used for biopsy guidance and magnetic resonance imaging is the mainstay in evaluating the extent of local tumor. Computed tomography and radionuclide bone scanning are mainly reserved for assessment of advanced disease. Positron emission tomography is gaining acceptance in the evaluation of treatment response and recurrence. The combination of anatomic, functional, and metabolic imaging modalities has promise to improve treatment. This article reviews current imaging techniques and touches on the evolving technologies being used for detection and follow-up of prostate cancer.

> This article reviews the anatomy of the prostate gland, magnetic resonance (MR) imaging techniques, and the role MR imaging in the setting of prostate cancer. Sequences discussed include T2-weighted MR imaging, proton (^{1}H) MR spectroscopic imaging, diffusion-weighted MR imaging, and dynamic contrast-enhanced MR imaging. MR imaging can be applied as an adjuvant tool to establish the diagnosis, localize, determine the extent, and estimate the aggressiveness of prostate cancers. The role of transrectal ultrasonography, computed tomography, and radionuclide scans is also briefly discussed.

> Transrectal ultrasound and ultrasound guided prostate biopsy is the current standard for detecting prostate cancer. Newer techniques such as elastography and contrast enhanced ultrasound may help in lesion detection and monitoring. Advances are occurring in several areas including multiparametric MRI, understanding of the nature of prostate cancer and new therapies including focal therapy and active surveillance. These changes are creating an increasing role for targeted biopsies following MRI and for use of MRI for treatment monitoring.

> Approximately 30% of patients who underwent radical prostatectomy or radiation therapy will develop biochemical recurrent disease. Biochemical recurrent disease is defined as an increase in the serum value of prostate-specific antigen (PSA) after reaching the nadir. Prostate recurrence can present as PSA-only relapse, local recurrent disease, distant metastases, or a combination of local and distant recurrence. In this review, the role of magnetic resonance imaging in the work-up of recurrent prostate cancer is discussed.

penile fractures, MR imaging should be performed with the patient in the erect position to avoid kinking between the pendulous and fixed parts and thus enable better demonstration of the site of tunica albuginea disruption for surgical planning. MR imaging is better than ultrasound in delineating primary penile malignancies and demonstrating lymph nodal involvement.

This article presents a radiologic perspective of male infertility. Basic embryologic, anatomic, and physiologic concepts underpinning male reproduction are explained. Common and uncommon abnormalities related to male infertility and subfertility are described, with emphasis on imaging findings and management strategies.

Prompt imaging plays an important role in the evaluation of male pelvic soft tissue trauma. Using appropriate imaging modalities, with optimization of contrast administration when appropriate, is essential for accurate diagnosis. Traumatic bladder rupture, either extraperitoneal or intraperitoneal, is diagnosed with high accuracy using computed tomography cystography. Suspicion of urethral injury warrants evaluation with retrograde urethrography to evaluate for the presence of injury and injury location. Early identification of laceration of the testicular tunica albuginea is essential. Understanding both normal penile anatomy and the imaging appearance of corpus rupture (as opposed to a hematoma) is imperative for proper diagnosis and management.

GOAL STATEMENT

The goal of the *Radiologic Clinics of North America* is to keep practicing radiologists and radiology residents up to date with current clinical practice in radiology by providing timely articles reviewing the state of the art in patient care.

ACCREDITATION

The *Radiologic Clinics of North America* is planned and implemented in accordance with the Essential Areas and Policies of the Accreditation Council for Continuing Medical Education (ACCME) through the joint sponsorship of the University of Virginia School of Medicine and Elsevier. The University of Virginia School of Medicine is accredited by the ACCME to provide continuing medical education for physicians.

The University of Virginia School of Medicine designates this enduring material activity for a maximum of 15 *AMA PRA Category 1 Credit*(s)™ for each issue, 90 credits per year. Physicians should only claim credit commensurate with the extent of their participation in the activity.

The American Medical Association has determined that physicians not licensed in the US who participate in this CME enduring material activity are eligible for a maximum of 15 *AMA PRA Category 1 Credit*(s)™ for each issue, 90 credits per year.

Credit can be earned by reading the text material, taking the CME examination online at http://www.theclinics.com/home/cme, and completing the evaluation. After taking the test, you will be required to review any and all incorrect answers. Following completion of the test and evaluation, your credit will be awarded and you may print your certificate.

FACULTY DISCLOSURE/CONFLICT OF INTEREST

The University of Virginia School of Medicine, as an ACCME accredited provider, endorses and strives to comply with the Accreditation Council for Continuing Medical Education (ACCME) Standards of Commercial Support, Commonwealth of Virginia statutes, University of Virginia policies and procedures, and associated federal and private regulations and guidelines on the need for disclosure and monitoring of proprietary and financial interests that may affect the scientific integrity and balance of content delivered in continuing medical education activities under our auspices.

The University of Virginia School of Medicine requires that all CME activities accredited through this institution be developed independently and be scientifically rigorous, balanced and objective in the presentation/discussion of its content, theories and practices.

All authors/editors participating in an accredited CME activity are expected to disclose to the readers relevant financial relationships with commercial entities occurring within the past 12 months (such as grants or research support, employee, consultant, stock holder, member of speakers bureau, etc.). The University of Virginia School of Medicine will employ appropriate mechanisms to resolve potential conflicts of interest to maintain the standards of fair and balanced education to the reader. Questions about specific strategies can be directed to the Office of Continuing Medical Education, University of Virginia School of Medicine, Charlottesville, Virginia.

The faculty and staff of the University of Virginia Office of Continuing Medical Education have no financial affiliations to disclose.

The authors/editors listed below have identified no financial or professional relationships for themselves or their spouse/partner:

Lejla Aganovic, MD; Laura L. Avery, MD; Adrianne Brigido, (Acquisitions Editor); Fiona Cassidy, MD; Azadeh Elmi, MD; Jurgen J. Fütterer, MD, PhD; Sangeet Ghai, MD, FRCR; Alpana M. Harisinghani, MD; Mukesh G. Harisinghani, MD (Guest Editor); Sandeep S. Hedgire, MD; Adam J. Jung, MD, PhD; Dow-Mu Koh, MD, MRCP, FRCR; Frank H. Miller, MD (Consulting Editor); Vivek K. Paragaonkar, MD; Rocio Perez-Johnston, MD; Mark A. Preston, MD; Syed Arsalan Raza, MBBS, FRCR; Meir H. Scheinfeld, MD, Phd; Anuradha Shenoy-Bhangle, MD; Ajay Singh, MD; Aslam Sohaib, MRCP, FRCR; Saman Shafaat Talab, MD; Ants Toi, MD, FRCPC; and Antonio C. Westphalen, MD, MAS.

The authors/editors listed below have identified the following financial or professional relationships for themselves or their spouse/partner:

Klaus D. Hagspiel, MD (Test Author) is an industry funded research/investigator for Siemens Medical Solutions.
Kartik S. Jhaveri, MD (Guest Editor) receives research support from Bayer.
Shahin Tabatabaei, MD is on the Advisory Board for Taris and American Medical Systems, is a consultant for Smith & Nephew, receives research support from Ethicon.

Disclosure of Discussion of Non-FDA Approved Uses for Pharmaceutical Products and/or Medical Devices.
The University of Virginia School of Medicine, as an ACCME provider, requires that all faculty presenters identify and disclose any off-label uses for pharmaceutical and medical device products. The University of Virginia School of Medicine recommends that each physician fully review all the available data on new products or procedures prior to clinical use.

TO ENROLL

To enroll in the Radiologic Clinics of North America Continuing Medical Education program, call customer service at 1-800-654-2452 or sign up online at http://www.theclinics.com/home/cme. The CME program is available to subscribers for an additional annual fee USD 245.

RADIOLOGIC CLINICS OF NORTH AMERICA

Guest Editors

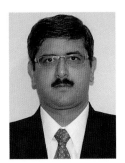

Kartik S. Jhaveri, MD

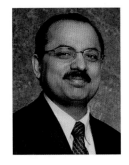

Mukesh G. Harisinghani, MD

Dr Kartik Jhaveri is an Associate Professor at the University of Toronto, Faculty Abdominal Radiologist in the Joint Department of Medical Imaging of the University Health Network, Mount Sinai Hospital and Women's College Hospital. He has served as an Assistant Editor (Genitourinary Section) of the *American Journal of Roentgenology*. He has many peer-reviewed publications, book chapters, and scientific presentations to his credit. He has lectured internationally on Abdominal MRI and Genitourinary topics including at the RSNA and ISMRM. He leads multiple research initiatives in body MRI.

Dr Mukesh Harisinghani is the Director of Abdominal MRI, Director of Clinical Discovery Program Center for Molecular Imaging Research, and Associate Professor of Radiology at Massachusetts General Hospital and Harvard Medical School. He is also the Genitourinary Section Editor for the *American Journal of Roentgenology*. Dr Harisinghani has been practicing in the field of Radiology since 1995, and his research interests include MRI applications in body imaging, genitourinary radiology, and translational molecular imaging. His clinical expertise is in MR applications within the abdomen and pelvis.

Radiol Clin N Am 50 (2012) xi
http://dx.doi.org/10.1016/j.rcl.2012.10.006
0033-8389/12/$ – see front matter © 2012 Published by Elsevier Inc.

radiologic.theclinics.com

Prostate Cancer Imaging
What the Urologist Wants to Know

Saman Shafaat Talab, MD[a], Mark A. Preston, MD[a],
Azadeh Elmi, MD[b], Shahin Tabatabaei, MD[a],*

KEYWORDS

- Prostate cancer • Transrectal ultrasonography • Magnetic resonance imaging • Diagnosis
- Staging • Follow-up

KEY POINTS

- Ultrasound-guided biopsy is still the mainstay of diagnosis; however, contrast-enhanced ultrasonography, sonoelastography, and magnetic resonance (MR) imaging–directed biopsy are changing the diagnostic approach to prostate cancer, with improving biopsy yield.
- Multiparametric MR imaging is an acceptable imaging modality for the diagnosis and staging of prostate cancer, and has been shown to increase accuracy in the detection of recurrence of prostate cancer.
- MR imaging has shown promising diagnostic performance as a potential adjunct to improve the selection of patients who can be safely managed with active surveillance.
- Radionucleotide bone scanning and computed tomography (CT) scanning supplement clinical and biochemical evaluation for suspected metastasis to bones, lymph nodes, and other organs.
- Positron emission tomography/CT has an emerging role in prostate cancer imaging, as it is a noninvasive whole-body examination that allows evaluation of local and distant disease in one step.
- Whole-body MR imaging is promising in the early detection of metastases to lymph nodes and/or bone.

INTRODUCTION

Prostate cancer is the second leading cause of cancer death among men in the United States, and continues to present an enormous health care burden.[1] The last 3 decades have witnessed a remarkable stage shift in the presentation of prostate cancer. Optimal imaging is a key component of staging and treatment planning and, because of its steady progress in accuracy, the morbidity of treatments has diminished while treatment outcomes have improved. Although the introduction of prostate-specific antigen (PSA) screening is considered an important breakthrough, the role of imaging in diagnosis and management of prostate cancer cannot be overemphasized. As conventional diagnostic techniques such as random ultrasound-guided biopsy are limited by high false-negative rates, new imaging techniques are necessary to allow tumor visualization to improve cancer detection rates. Emerging functional imaging techniques including diffusion-weighted magnetic resonance (DW-MR) imaging, dynamic contrast-enhanced MR (DCE-MR) imaging, MR spectroscopy, and positron emission tomography (PET) have demonstrated promise in surmounting these limitations and may have significant implications in the future.

Disclosure: The authors have nothing to disclose.
a Department of Urology, Harvard Medical School, Massachusetts General Hospital, 55 Fruit Street, GRB-1102, Boston, MA 02114, USA; b Division of Abdominal Imaging and Interventional Radiology, Massachusetts General Hospital, Harvard Medical School, 55 Fruit Street, White 270, Boston, MA 02114, USA
* Corresponding author. Department of Urology, Harvard Medical School, Massachusetts General Hospital, 55 Fruit Street, GRB-1102, Boston, MA 02114.
E-mail address: stabatabaei@partners.org

Radiol Clin N Am 50 (2012) 1015–1041
http://dx.doi.org/10.1016/j.rcl.2012.08.004

ANATOMY

The prostate gland is located in the subperitoneal compartment between the pelvic diaphragm and the peritoneal cavity. The normal prostate in adult males weighs about 18 g. It measures 3 cm in length, 4 cm in width, and 2 cm in depth, and surrounds the prostatic urethra. Although ovoid, the prostate is referred to as having anterior, posterior, and lateral surfaces, with a narrowed apex inferiorly and a broad base superiorly that is contiguous with the base of the bladder. The apex of the prostate is continuous with the striated urethral sphincter. A capsule composed of collagen, elastin, and abundant smooth muscle encloses the prostate.

The prostate is divided into 3 zones with different embryologic origins: the central zone, the transition zone, and the peripheral zone. These zones can be distinguished based on their histology, anatomic landmarks, biological functions, and susceptibility to pathologic disorders.[2] Seventy percent of adenocarcinomas arise in the peripheral zone, 20% arise in the transition zone, and only 10% arise in the central zone.

Clinically the prostate is divided to 2 lateral lobes, separated by a central sulcus that is palpable on rectal examination, and a middle lobe, which may project into the bladder in older men. These lobes do not correspond to histologically defined structures in the normal prostate, but are usually related to pathologic enlargement of the transition zone laterally and the periurethral glands centrally.[3]

The prostate gland grows in size throughout life, mainly through the formation of benign hyperplastic nodules in the transition zone, starting in the third decade of life. Benign prostate hyperplasia (BPH) leads to a significant prostate size and contour variation among men, which has remarkable implications on prostate imaging and treatment options for prostate cancer.

DIAGNOSIS OF PROSTATE CANCER

The widespread use of serum PSA assay has led to a dramatic downstaging of prostate cancer at diagnosis. A lesser volume of cancer at presentation makes the cancer imaging more challenging. This section highlights the diagnostic performance of imaging modalities in evaluating patients with prostate cancer showing an increase in PSA or a positive digital rectal examination (DRE). **Table 1** summarizes sensitivity, specificity, and predictive values for each technique.

Transrectal Ultrasonography

Initially described by Watanabe and colleagues[31] in 1968, transrectal ultrasonography (TRUS) plays a crucial role in the diagnosis and management of prostate cancer. At present, TRUS is the most commonly used modality for imaging the prostate gland and is predominantly used for determining prostate size (useful for calculating PSA density), zonal anatomy, and guiding prostate biopsies. In the initial evaluation for suspicion of prostate cancer, TRUS also provides information regarding the existence and location of cancer foci. Prostate cancer is typically visualized as a hypoechoic lesion in the peripheral zone (**Fig. 1**A, B), and may be accompanied by asymmetry or protrusion into the prostatic capsule. In advanced disease, asymmetry between the seminal vesicles may also be seen through TRUS.[32] However, the reliability of the findings is operator dependent, and TRUS suffers from poor test characteristics for the diagnosis of prostate cancer, with a positive predictive value of 45% to 91%, a negative predictive value of 11% to 79%, and an overall accuracy of only up to 62%.[6–8,33,34] Of importance is that more than 40% of cancers are isoechoic and therefore not visible with conventional ultrasound methods.[34] Accordingly, various novel ultrasound techniques have been developed during the last decade to boost the sensitivity of TRUS-guided prostate biopsy by enhancing accuracy of biopsy target detection, without the need to increase the number of biopsy cores.

Color Doppler and Power Doppler Ultrasonography

Color Doppler ultrasonography (CD-US) is an adjunct technique to traditional gray-scale imaging. It is designed to help clinicians better identify areas of increased vascularity that may be associated with tumor (**Fig. 1**C). Prostate cancer, like many other neoplasms, demonstrates neovascularity and increased microvessel density with inherent prognostic implications.[35] Application of CD-US may increase sensitivity and specificity of the detection of prostate cancer and may improve the accuracy of targeted biopsy. Malignant lesions are characterized by asymmetrically increased flow patterns, particularly in higher-grade (Gleason score of 8, 9, or 10) prostate cancers. In some reports, it has been shown that CD-US correlates positively with the grade and stage, as well as biochemical recurrence of prostate cancer, after initial treatment.[36] However, the published data show mixed results regarding CD-US for targeted biopsy of prostate lesions. In 2009, Eisenberg and colleagues[8] compared preoperative gray-scale and power Doppler findings with pathologic analysis of 620 radical prostatectomy specimens, and reported that power Doppler imaging improved

Table 1
Imaging modalities for the diagnosis of prostate cancer

Imaging Modality	Reference	Year of Publication	No. of Patients	Sensitivity (%)	Specificity (%)	PPV (%)	NPV (%)
Transrectal Ultrasonography							
Gray-scale							
	4	1999	166	39.4	81.5	83.3	36.4
	5	2000	251	44.1	73.6	—	—
	6	2000	47	50	82	84	47
	7	2003	282	87.9	57.6	72.3	79.1
	8	2010	620	59	47	91	11
Color Doppler							
	7	2003	282	92.4	72	80.6	88.2
	9	2007	137	29	80	18	88
	8	2009	620	40	35	88	6
	10	2011	100	23	68	—	—
Contrast-enhanced							
	11	1999	18	85	80	92	67
	12	2003	85	93	87	88	93
	10	2011	100	54	42	—	—
	13	2012	150	73.1	87.3	66.4	90.4
Elastography							
	14	2002	100	51	83	—	—
	15	2008	492	86	72	—	—
	16	2008	109	75.4	76.6	87.8	59
	17	2012	353	60.8	68.4	32.4	87.8
MR imaging							
Anatomic MR imaging							
	18	1994	71	91	27	91	27
	19	2007	70	84	50	76	63
	20	2007	40	43	81	—	—
	21	2007	49	54	91	79	77
	22	2008	40	51	91	79	73
DW-MR imaging							
	21	2007	49	81	84	76	88
	23	2007	42	93.3	57.4	—	—
	22	2008	40	57	90	79	75
	24	2009	52	78–88	88–89	—	—
DCE-MR imaging							
	25	1997	57	73	81	—	—
	26	2005	53	96	82	82	96
	27	2006	34	95	88	72	98
	22	2008	40	46	93	81	72
	28	2011	42	90	77	—	—
MR spectroscopic imaging							
	6	2000	47	76	57	76	56
	27	2006	34	80	87	68	93
	29	2006	39	75	89	88	74
	30	2011	50	92	85	—	—

Abbreviations: NPV, negative predictive value; PPV, positive predictive value.

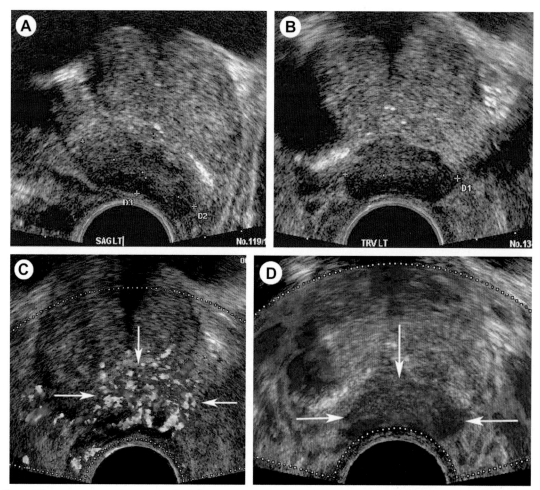

Fig. 1. Gleason 8 prostate cancer in the left mid-gland to apex. (*A*) Sagittal gray-scale demonstrates a hypoechoic mass lesion extending from the left mid-gland to apex (calipers). (*B*) Transverse image confirms the mass. (*C*) Transverse color Doppler image demonstrates marked hyperemia associated with the mass (*arrows*). (*D*) Transverse elastogram demonstrates increased tissue stiffness in the mass as blue color (*arrows*). (*Reprinted from Linden RA, Halpern EJ. Advances in transrectal ultrasound imaging of the prostate. Semin Ultrasound CT MR 2007;28(4):252; Copyright 2012, Elsevier; with permission.*)

the specificity of TRUS but did not improve the overall accuracy or sensitivity. On the other hand, Sauvain and colleagues[7] reported that in 282 patients with serum PSA of greater than 4 ng/mL, the overall sensitivity of power Doppler sonography for detection of prostatic cancer reached 92.4% along with specificity, positive predictive value (PPV) and negative predictive value (NPV) of 72%, 80.6%, and 88.2%, respectively.

The wide range of reported data regarding the accuracy of Doppler imaging in prostate cancer detection might suggest operator dependency and subjective interpretation of images, which is the inherent nature of all ultrasound imaging techniques. Furthermore, false-positive results may be associated with hypervascular prostate tissue in patients with benign prostatic hyperplasia

or prostatitis. The other issue is the lower sensitivity of CD-US in detecting intermediate-grade cancers (Gleason scores of 5, 6, and 7), owing to their lower rate of neoangiogenesis.[33,37]

Contrast-Enhanced Ultrasonography

Contrast-enhanced ultrasonography (CE-US) is the application of ultrasound contrast medium to traditional medical sonography. Several studies have demonstrated its value in the evaluation of the macro- and microvascularization of various organs including the liver, spleen, kidney, and intestine.[38] The currently used ultrasound contrast agents consist of a solution of gas-filled microbubbles with a diameter of 1 to 10 μm that are stabilized with a shell. The contrast agents are administered intravenously and provide enhanced visualization of blood flow within the microvasculature. This process effectively increases the sensitivity for detecting low flow in small vessels, which are not usually visualized by conventional Doppler ultrasonography (**Fig. 2**). The advantages of CE-US in comparison with other imaging modalities include the absence of ionizing radiation, the widespread availability, and the absence of nephrotoxicity.[39,40] An increasing body of data demonstrates applicability of CE-US in the detection of prostate cancer. Sedelaar and colleagues[41] studied the correlation between microvessel density in radical prostatectomy specimens and preoperative CE-US findings, and found that CE-US–enhanced areas had a 1.93-times higher microvessel density compared with the nonenhanced areas.

The detection of augmented vasculature of tumor tissue provided by this technique appears helpful for targeted prostate biopsy. It has been reported that CE-US–targeted biopsy is 2 to 3 times (11%–32.6% vs 5.3%–17.9%, respectively) more likely to be positive compared with conventional systematic biopsy in patients with cancer. However, in the majority of studies, the overall cancer detection rate is similar between systematic biopsy and CE-US–targeted biopsy.[10,42–45] In 2007, Mitterberger and colleagues[45] prospectively compared ultrasound-guided systematic biopsy versus CE-US–targeted biopsy in 690 patients. The overall cancer detection rate was 32%, including 26% by targeted biopsy and 24% by random systematic biopsy. The investigators also reported a significantly higher Gleason score in targeted biopsy (6 or higher, mean 6.8) in comparison with systematic biopsy (4–6, mean 5.4). This finding suggests a potential role for CE-US in the identification of more aggressive high-grade cancers that are accompanied by enhanced neovascularization (**Fig. 3**).

Sonoelastography

Elastography is a form of signal processing applied to TRUS that evaluates the stiffness of tissue (**Fig. 1**D).[46] The increased cellular density associated with prostate adenocarcinoma results in areas with limited elasticity or compressibility within the prostate gland that can be identified by elastography. Elastograms are obtained in real time through slight compression and decompression of the gland during TRUS examination, and may potentially enhance the accuracy of targeted prostate biopsy (**Fig. 4**).

Pallwein and colleagues[47] reported that elastography-targeted biopsy detected more cases of prostate cancer than did systematic biopsy, with fewer than half the number of biopsy cores. In another study from the same group, in 94 patients with serum PSA of 1.25 to 4 ng/mL, the cancer detection rate per core was 4.7-fold greater for elastography-targeted than for systematic biopsy.[48] In a recently published prospective study in 353 patients, it was shown that the detection rate of prostate cancer was significantly higher using elastography-guided systematic biopsy (51.1%) in comparison with gray-scale ultrasonography (39.4%), with sensitivity, specificity, PPV, and NPV of 60.8%, 68.4%, 32.4%, and 87.8%, respectively.[17] These investigators also observed an increase in sensitivity of elastography-guided biopsy from the gland base toward the apex that probably is due to a smaller volume of prostate tissue at the apex. The sensitivity of elastography is limited by large prostate volume, or small size and deep location of tumor.

Magnetic Resonance Imaging

Sonographic-guided prostate biopsy is prone to undersampling and fails to diagnose prostate cancer in 23% of patients after initial biopsy.

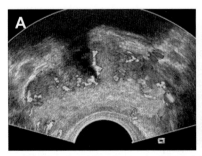
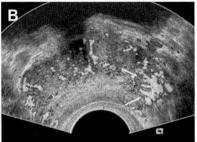
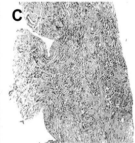

Fig. 2. Color Doppler ultrasonography (*A*) versus contrast-enhanced color Doppler (*B*) in a 49-year-old man with biopsy-proven prostate cancer. Three positive biopsy cores were obtained from left mid-gland only on contrast-enhanced color Doppler. Corresponding histopathology reveals Gleason score 9 prostate cancer (*C*). (*Reprinted from* Mitterberger M, Pinggera GM, Horninger W, et al. Comparison of contrast enhanced color Doppler targeted biopsy to conventional systematic biopsy: impact on Gleason score. J Urol 2007;178(2):466; Copyright 2012, Elsevier; with permission.)

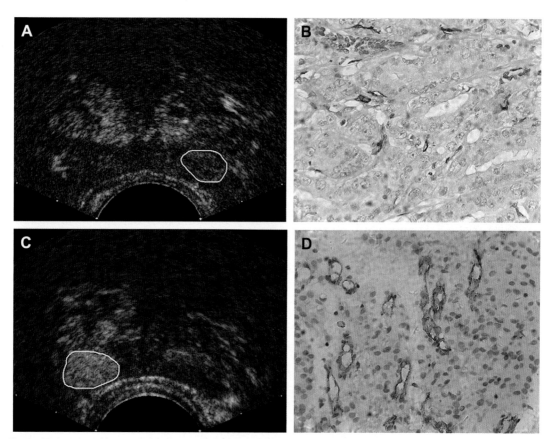

Fig. 3. (*Upper panels*) Contrast-enhanced TRUS showing a focal area of prostate cancer in a 76-year-old man with a Gleason score of 3 + 3 and a PSA level of 5.87 ng/mL. (*A*) Contrast image presents a poorly enhanced region in the left peripheral zone, and the peak intensity (PI) of the lesion was only 7.29 dB. (*B*) Pathologic examination demonstrated that there were a few microvessels (stained in brown) in the lesion, and the microvessel density (MVD) was 57 (anti-CD31 antibody, original magnification ×400). (*Lower panels*) Contrast-enhanced TRUS showing a focal area of prostate cancer in an 85-year-old man with a Gleason score of 4 + 5 and a PSA level of 14.27 ng/mL. (*C*) Contrast image presents a marked enhanced region in the right peripheral zone, and the PI of the lesion was 12.19 dB. (*D*) Pathologic examination demonstrated that there were rich microvessels (stained in brown) in the lesion, and the MVD was 90 (anti-CD31 antibody, original magnification ×400). (*Reprinted from* Jiang J, Chen Y, Zhu Y, et al. Contrast-enhanced ultrasonography for the detection and characterization of prostate cancer: correlation with microvessel density and Gleason score. Clin Radiol 2011;66(8):735–6; Copyright 2012, Elsevier; with permission.)

Thus repeat biopsies, with their inherent risks, are required for accurate diagnosis of prostate cancer.[49] These limitations often lead to delay in diagnosis and inaccurate risk assessments. MR imaging, with its excellent soft-tissue resolution, can provide functional and anatomic tissue information and is the most sensitive modality available for the detection and local staging of prostate cancer. A time interval of 8 to 10 weeks between the biopsy procedure and MR imaging have been recommended to ensure resolution of hemorrhage; however, this may lead to a delay in therapy.[50]

Anatomic MR imaging

Conventional MR imaging is performed using endorectal and pelvic phased-array coils on a magnet that is at least 1.5 T. Morphologic information are obtained on T1-weighted and T2-weighted high-resolution images for accurate localization and staging of prostate cancer.[51] The prostate is best assessed on T2-weighted MR imaging whereby the peripheral zone is differentiated from the central zone by displaying an intermediate to high signal intensity.[52] Prostate cancer typically displays as an area of low signal intensity within a bright peripheral zone on T2-weighted MR images (**Figs. 5** and **6**). However, the differential diagnosis for an area of low signal intensity is extensive and includes postbiopsy hemorrhage, prostatitis, benign prostatic hyperplasia, hormone or radiation therapy effects, calcification, or fibromuscular hyperplasia.[52,53]

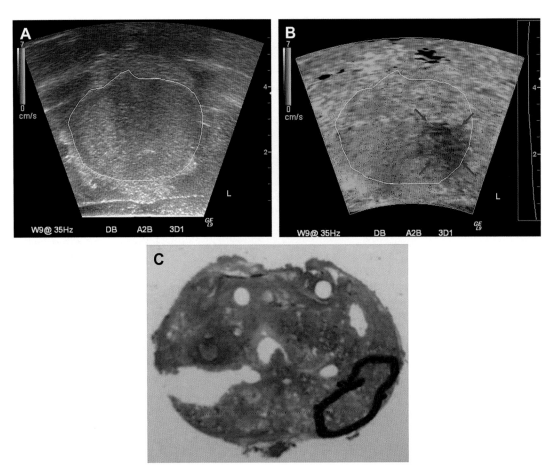

Fig. 4. (A) B-mode ultrasound, (B) sonoelastographic, and (C) histologic images. A deficit in the sonoelastogram (*red arrows*) was verified as a cancerous mass by histology (*blue outline*). Note that sonoelastographic regions where the vibration amplitude is low are shown as dark green and regions with high vibration are depicted as bright green. (*Reprinted from* Hoyt K, Castaneda B, Zhang M, et al. Tissue elasticity properties as biomarkers for prostate cancer. Cancer Biomark 2008;4(4–5):213–25; Copyright 2012, IOS Press; with permission.)

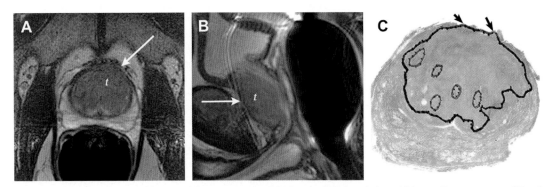

Fig. 5. Images of a 54-year-old man with preoperative PSA level of 12.6 ng/mL and biopsy Gleason score of 3 + 3. Prostate was normal (stage T1c) at clinical examination. Unenhanced (A) transverse and (B) sagittal T2-weighted fast spin-echo (5000/96 [effective]) MR images show large tumor (t) in the transition zone and tumor bulging with interruption of very low signal intensity anterior fibromuscular stroma by tumor of slightly higher signal intensity, suggestive of anterior extracapsular extension (ECE) (*arrow*). (C) Transverse gross pathologic whole-mount specimen. Outer linear margin defines border of tumor predominantly Gleason grade 3 with established anterior ECE (*arrows*), stage pT3a. Internal smaller marked regions define Gleason grade 4 components (hematoxylin-eosin stain). (*Reprinted from* Hricak H, Choyke PL, Eberhardt SC, et al. Imaging prostate cancer: a multidisciplinary perspective. Radiology 2007;243(1):34; Copyright 2012, Radiology Society of North America; with permission.)

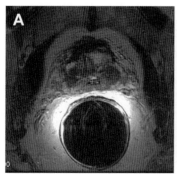 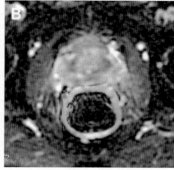 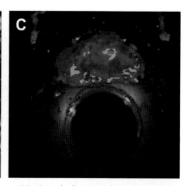

Fig. 6. MR images of a 55-year-old man. (*A*) Axial T2-weighted image shows T2 signal abnormality throughout the prostate gland without correlating diffusion or perfusion abnormality, suggestive of diffuse involvement of the gland with low-grade tumor (*B*) and (*C*). There is no evidence of extracapsular extension. Pathologic evaluation reveled Gleason score 3 + 3, bilateral, involving all 4 quadrants, confined to the gland.

T1-weighted images are useful in detecting lymph nodes, bone metastasis, and postbiopsy hemorrhage (which can mimic tumor on T2-weighted images), whereas T2-weighted images provide depiction of the zonal anatomy of the prostate gland. The pseudocapsule that separates the central from the peripheral zone appears hypointense. Malignancy usually arises in the peripheral zone and appears as foci of low signal intensity on T2-weighted images. Anatomic MR imaging is considered to have sensitivity and specificity of 43% to 91% and 27% to 91%, respectively, for detection of prostate cancer.[18–22] Nonetheless, gland atrophy, benign hyperplasia, prostatitis, and posttreatment changes can mimic malignancy on T2-weighted images. One important drawback in anatomic imaging of prostate cancer occurs with tumors located in the central gland. The signal-intensity characteristics of the central gland, especially when hypertrophied, may overlap with tumor tissue. In addition, T2-weighted imaging has limited accuracy for tumor localization early after transrectal ultrasound-guided biopsy. The low T2 signal from postbiopsy hemorrhage may cause an overestimation of tumor presence.[54,55] To overcome these challenges and improve diagnostic accuracy, functional MR imaging techniques such as DW-MR imaging, DCE-MR imaging, and MR spectroscopy have been developed to add value to anatomic MR imaging.

Diffusion-weighted imaging

In this technique, proton diffusion properties within water are used to acquire image contrast. Cancerous tissue has a higher cellular density than normal glandular prostate tissue; therefore, the movement of water molecules is restricted, resulting in lower apparent diffusion coefficient (ADC) values than are found in healthy prostate tissue.[56] In the evaluation of prostate cancers, both DW-MR imaging and ADC maps have shown improved sensitivity and specificity.[57–59] Several studies have reported improvement in sensitivity for localizing prostate cancer ranging from 81% to 84% when combining DW-MR imaging and T2-weighted images, compared with anatomic MR imaging alone.[21,60] Nevertheless, detection of tumors smaller than 5 mm, as well as tumors in the transitional zone, is still challenging.[59] Hemorrhage into prostate gland may decrease ADC values, affecting the tissue contrast on diffusion images for distinguishing benign mass from malignant tissues. Nonetheless, DW-MR imaging remains more sensitive than anatomic MR imaging for detecting a tumor within areas of hemorrhage. Rosenkrantz and colleagues[61] showed significantly lower ADC values in peripheral-zone tumors when compared with postbiopsy hemorrhage, and also reported a weak, but significant, correlation between ADC and Gleason score and tumor size. The role of DW-MR imaging in localizing prostate cancer in cases with a previous failed TRUS biopsy, in the presence of persistently elevated PSA, has been demonstrated. The practical implication of such findings might be decreasing the number of repeat biopsies necessary in patients with a high risk of cancer when DW-MR imaging is performed before a repeat biopsy.[62] In the future, parametric MR imaging maps may be fused with real-time TRUS images for targeted biopsy of suspect lesions.[63] The potential for predicting tumor aggressiveness is one of the most exciting roles of DW-MR imaging in prostate cancer. Correlation between Gleason score and ADC values has been demonstrated in several studies, and a significant difference in ADC values of patients with low versus intermediate risk has been reported.[64] Pretreatment ADC value has been proposed to be an independent imaging biomarker for predicting biochemical relapse after radical prostatectomy in multivariate analysis.[65] Although DW-MR imaging is rapidly evolving, it has the disadvantage of being vulnerable to motion and susceptibility artifacts.

Dynamic contrast-enhanced MR imaging

DCE-MR imaging enables noninvasive character-ization of tumor tissue vascularity. This vascularity is an integral feature of tumors that is detected based on sequential acquisition of rapid MR sequences, before and during the infusion of a contrast agent, to track the entrance of diffusible contrast agents into the prostatic tissue over time. This technique enables detection of leaky vessels within the prostate tumors, which produce different enhancement patterns to those shown with benign tissues. DCE-MR imaging is a powerful imaging technique for the depiction of angiogen-esis and vasculogenesis. In prostate cancer spe-cifically, DCE-MR imaging contributes to the

multiparametric data to better detect, localize, and characterize tumors. An additional advantage of this method is that it enables noninvasive differ-entiation of high-grade from low-grade tumors and benign prostatic hyperplasia. Abnormal enhancement patterns are seen in both tumor foci and benign nodules, while the distinctive feature of malignancy is that the tumors show early enhancement and early washout (**Fig. 7**). This pattern is highly predictive of prostate cancer, but is not pathognomonic. A sensitivity and specificity of 73% and 81% have been re-ported for this technique in the detection of organ-confined prostate cancer, which is higher than those of T2-weighted images.[25] The practical point is that the sensitivity and specificity dramat-ically increase to 90% and 88% for lesions larger than 0.5 mL. This fact has the potential to prefer-entially diagnose clinically significant cancers, because studies suggest that 80% of tumors of less than 0.5 mL in volume will probably not be significant during the patient's lifetime.[66–69]

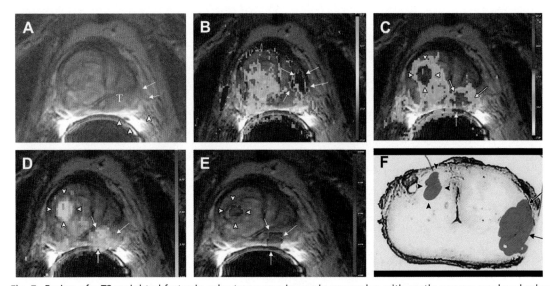

Fig. 7. Fusion of a T2-weighted fast spin-echo transverse image in gray value with partly opaque rendered color overlay of 4 contrast-enhancement parameters. (*A*) Transverse T2-weighted fast spin-echo image obtained through the prostate demonstrates a lesion of low signal intensity (T) in the left peripheral zone with bulging (*arrows*) and obliteration (*arrowheads*) of the rectoprostatic angle. (*B*) The start-of-enhancement parameter demonstrates an earlier enhancement in part of the low-signal-intensity lesion (*arrows*) compared with the right peripheral zone (red vs green). (*C*) Fast time to peak (red) is present in the left peripheral zone (*arrows*) and right central gland (*arrowheads*). (*D*) Peak enhancement is increased markedly in the center of the lesion in the left peripheral zone (*arrows*) and right central gland (*arrowheads*). (*E*) A negative washout area (red) is seen in the left peripheral zone (*arrows*) and right central gland (*arrowheads*). (*F*) Photomicrograph shows stage T3a disease with prostate capsule penetration in the left peripheral zone (*arrows*) and a prostate tumor lesion (red) in the right central gland (*arrowheads*). (*Reprinted from* Fütterer JJ, Engelbrecht MR, Huisman HJ, et al. Staging prostate cancer with dynamic contrast-enhanced endorectal MR imaging prior to radical prostatectomy: experienced versus less experienced readers. Radiology 2005;237(2):545; Copyright 2012, Radiology Society of North America; with permission.)

MR spectroscopic imaging

MR spectroscopy suppresses water and fat signals, enabling assessment of intracellular metabolic information that are characteristic for specific tissues.[70] MR spectroscopy provides detailed information about cellular metabolism in the prostate by displaying relative concentrations of substances such as citrate, choline, and creatine. Prostate cancer displays a higher choline level because of its increased cell turnover, and a decreased level of citrate, when compared with normal prostate tissue (**Fig. 8**).[71] In prostate tissue, the resonances for the prostate metabolites such as choline, creatine, polyamines, and citrate occur at distinct frequencies. The changes in these concentrations can be used to identify malignant processes. It is suggested that one of the characteristics of prostate cancer is a higher choline plus creatine-to-citrate ratio.[72] However, prostatitis and postbiopsy changes may also show the same trend. As MR spectroscopy is usually performed after anatomic MR imaging, overlaying

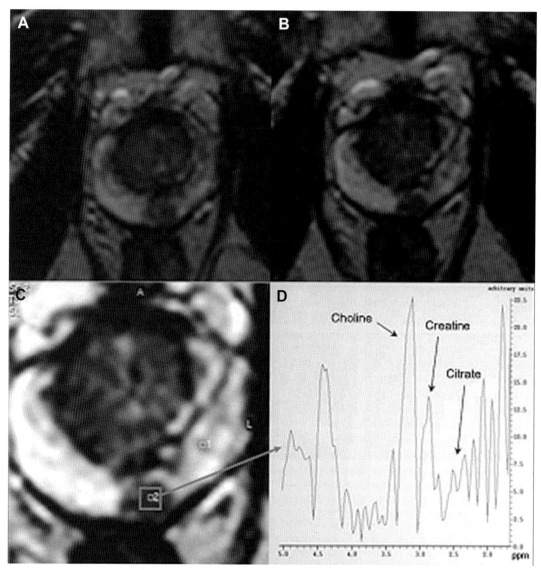

Fig. 8. (*A–D*) MR spectroscopic imaging. Focal low-intensity area in the peripheral left median portion on axial T2-weighted images. The spectrum obtained from the area with altered signal intensity showed increased choline and reduced citrate, a pattern consistent with cancer (*D*). The histopathologic analysis confirmed the neoplastic nature of the lesion. (*Reprinted from* Manenti G, Squillaci E, Carlani M, et al. Magnetic resonance imaging of the prostate with spectroscopic imaging using a surface coil. Initial clinical experience. Radiol Med 2006;111(1):29; Copyright 2012, Springer; with permission.)

the spectral data on the T2-weighted images can be helpful for localizing the tumor. A sensitivity, specificity, and diagnostic accuracy of 70%, 89%, and 79%, respectively, has been reported for combined MR imaging/MR spectroscopy in the diagnosis of prostate cancer.[29] In addition, MR spectroscopy has shown promise in predicting tumor volume, extracapsular extension, and estimation of the aggressiveness of cancer and treatment response.[71] A multi-institutional study led by the American College of Radiology Imaging Network demonstrated similar modest accuracy for both anatomic MR imaging and MR imaging combined with MR spectroscopy in the sextant localization of peripheral-zone prostate cancer. On the other hand, Yuen and colleagues[73] reported an increase in cancer detection in high-risk patients using the same combination of modalities when tumor is rising from the transitional zone or anterior peripheral zone, which are the parts of the prostate that are not easily palpable and targeted during biopsy. Another potential application of MR spectroscopy is to rule out the presence of prostate cancer in patients with a persistently rising PSA value and negative prostate biopsies. MR spectroscopy is technically challenging, and requires a longer acquisition time and more expertise than other functional MR imaging techniques. Artifacts from postbiopsy hemorrhage and difficulty in obtaining optimal shimming for each patient are key limitations.

Multiparametric MR imaging

Multiparametric MR imaging is an imaging modality for the diagnosis and staging of prostate cancer that has been shown to increase accuracy from 64% to 79% in the detection of prostate cancer in the transitional zone.[74] The suggested protocol for prostate cancer currently includes T1-weighted and T2-weighted MR imaging in combination with DW-MR imaging and DCE-MR imaging. High specificity of the multiparametric approach would prevent the unnecessary performance of systematic random biopsies and delay in diagnosis and treatment. A recent study by Turkbey and colleagues[75] indicated that multiparametric MR imaging facilitates accurate tumor detection with a PPV of 98% in the overall prostate. These investigators reported T2-weighted images along with ADC maps and DCE-MR imaging as the most helpful approach for tumor detection in the central gland, which is a location with significant overlap between malignancy and benign hyperplasia. In addition, they defined a combination of DW-MR imaging and DCE-MR imaging as the most sensitive technique for anterior peripheral-zone tumors.

STAGING OF PROSTATE CANCER

Cancer staging is typically the most important predictor of survival, and often dictates the cancer treatment options that need to be considered. The TNM staging system is widely used to stage prostate cancer using a combination of DRE, PSA testing, prostate biopsy findings, and imaging studies (according to National Comprehensive Cancer Network [NCCN] guidelines). Imaging for the purpose of staging prostate cancer has become increasingly more utilized and important, as new technology and techniques have rapidly developed. Staging of prostate cancer with imaging (CT, MR imaging, bone scan) is generally not recommended in men with low-risk disease (Gleason ≤6, PSA <10, clinical stage T1c) because the positive yield is exceptionally low.[76] Imaging can provide additional useful information, thus enabling patients and clinicians to make educated decisions regarding risk-adjusted patient-specific therapy. Patients can now choose management options ranging from active surveillance to radiation therapy, radical prostatectomy, hormonal therapy, or even focal therapy. It is imperative all tools available are used to accurately stage patients so that cancer is controlled while limiting complications.

Radical prostatectomy is well established as a definitive treatment option in the management of localized prostate cancer. The goals of this procedure are to achieve excellent oncologic control with negative surgical margins while preserving urinary continence and erectile function, whenever possible. A nerve-sparing radical prostatectomy preserves the neurovascular bundle running along the posterior-lateral aspect of the prostate. This procedure is the standard of care for men with a low preoperative risk of extraprostatic diseases who wish to retain erectile function, and is also associated with improved urinary continence.[77–82] The primary risk of nerve sparing is a positive surgical margin in a patient with organ-confined or extraprostatic extension.[83,84] Positive margins subsequently confer an increased risk of biochemical recurrence, local recurrence and, potentially, systemic progression.[84–88] As such, accurate preoperative staging is of great importance for guiding treatment, and imaging techniques could provide a significant contribution.

This section reviews imaging modalities for prostate cancer staging that are currently widely used, as well as newer modalities coming into the mainstream. **Table 2** summarizes sensitivity, specificity, and predictive values for each technique.

Table 2
Imaging modalities in the staging of prostate cancer

Imaging Modality	Reference	Year of Publication	No. of Patients	Extracapsular Extension				Seminal Vesicle Invasion			
				Sensitivity	Specificity	PPV	NPV	Sensitivity	Specificity	PPV	NPV
Transrectal Ultrasonography											
	89	1994	117	91	—	79	—	—	—	—	—
	90	1999	114	32.6	68.4	45.5	—	42.2	42.2	36.8	—
	91	2004	171	11.8	96	—	88	9.8	99	—	—
	92 [a]	69	82	94	96	79	88	97	88	97	—
	93	2011	620	31	92	58	80	4	99.8	67	93
CT scan											
	94	1987	32	75	60	—	—	33	60	—	—
	95	1992	160	2.5	92	—	—	5.8	99	—	—
	96	1996	30	13	89	57	—	19	97	83	—
MR imaging											
Anatomic MR imaging	97	1996	56	22	84	40	70	23	93	50	80
	98	2002	336	38	94	—	—	34	99	—	—
	99	2006	356	—	—	—	—	63	97	—	—
	100	2007	54	71	73	—	—	75	92	—	—
	101	2012	65	66.7	95.7	66.7	95.7	62.5	97.5	62.5	97.5
DCE-MR imaging	66	2001	38	33	94	50	88	NA	97	NA	100
	102 [b]	2005	124	74	94	86	87	71	100	—	—
MR spectroscopic imaging	103	1999	53	50	91	63	86	—	—	—	—

Abbreviation: NA, no data available.
[a] 3-dimensional transrectal ultrasonography.
[b] Dynamic contrast-enhanced MR images in conjunction with the T2-weighted MR; maximal values from 2 groups of readers were included.

Staging Local Disease (T-Staging)

Transrectal ultrasonography

Studies conducted in the pre-PSA era, when cancers were more commonly locally advanced and palpable, reported a sensitivity of approximately 80% for detecting extracapsular extension (ECE) and seminal vesicle invasion (SVI) on TRUS.[104] Thus TRUS has limited benefit in the staging of prostate cancer, as typically it can only detect ECE or SVI when there is gross extension of disease.[105–107] ECE is visualized as a bulging or contour irregularity of the capsular adjacent to a hypoechoic lesion, and can be accompanied by loss of the rectoprostatic angle.[92,105,108] For the diagnosis of ECE on TRUS, sensitivities range from 11.8% to 91% and specificities range from 68.4% to 96%.[89,91,109–111] Seminal-vesicle invasion can be seen as a hypoechoic solid lesion within the normally cystic seminal vesicle or as extension of a hypoechoic lesion at the base of the prostate into the seminal vesicle. Sensitivities range from 4% to 88%, with specificity of up to 99.8% for the diagnosis of SVI via TRUS.[93,110,112,113]

Newer techniques using color or power Doppler modes to identify regions of hypervascularity have been shown to improve detection of prostate cancer.[7,106,114] Unfortunately, this has not yet translated into improved accuracy of staging. CE-US has also shown potential for improved diagnosis of prostate cancer but with limited additional benefit in staging.[115,116]

Ultrasonography will continue to be used predominantly for aiding prostate biopsy in the foreseeable future, with the potential for improvements in diagnostic ability. Its use in staging will likely be minimal, because of operator dependency, subjective interpretation of images, and the vastly superior imaging characteristics of MR imaging.

Computed tomography

Despite recent advancements in technology and the use of contrast enhancement, CT imaging lacks the soft-tissue resolution required to distinguish prostate anatomy from adjacent structures, and thus diagnose and stage prostate cancer effectively.[94,106,117] However, because of its wide dissemination, relatively small cost, and ease of use, its use remains widespread.

When imaging clinically apparent, grossly advanced disease with marked ECE or SVI, the specificity of CT is quite high, ranging from 80% to 89%.[96,117,118] However, because of the poor ability of CT to differentiate cancerous tissue from normal tissue, the sensitivity is very low, ranging from 26% to 29%.[95,96,117,118] As such,

the role of CT scanning in the local staging of prostate cancer is limited. A recent study which has been done at Massachusetts General Hospital (accepted to be published) highlighted the clinical relevance of incidental findings on initial staging CT in patients with prostate cancer. A considerable prevalence of incidental synchronous cancers and vascular events with kidney cancers was shown to be the most common synchronous malignancy. The investigators demonstrated an incremental value of CT in prostate cancer staging, with emphasis on focused evaluation of the kidneys.

MR imaging

Up to 40% of clinically localized disease (cT1, cT2) will have extraprostatic extension at the time of diagnosis.[83] Subsequently, MR imaging is increasingly being used for staging prostate cancer because it is noninvasive, has no ionizing radiation, and provides the highest spatial resolution among imaging modalities. Indications for MR imaging in prostate cancer, albeit controversial, include staging of intermediate and high-risk cases to evaluate for visibility of tumor, extraprostatic extension, and involvement of seminal vesicles or lymph nodes.[119–121] The NCCN guidelines recommend "pelvic CT or MR imaging if T3, T4 or T1-T2 and nomogram indicated probability of lymph node involvement >20%."

The staging performance of MR imaging is influenced by several factors including publication year, sample size, histologic gold standard, number of imaging planes, turbo spin echo, endorectal coil, and contrast agent used.[122] Furthermore, MR imaging of the prostate has a steep learning curve, and may be inaccurate and unreliable when performed by a less experienced practitioner.[123] Two meta-analyses have been conducted to assess the performance and accuracy of MR imaging for staging prostate cancer across studies.[122,124] Sonnad and colleagues[124] first reported that the summary receiver-operating characteristic (ROC) curve for MR imaging in staging of prostate cancer has a joint maximum sensitivity and specificity of 74%. The larger, more recent meta-analysis found the joint maximum sensitivity and specificity to be similar, at 71%.[122] These results are based on anatomic MR imaging techniques and may improve with further development of functional MR imaging studies. These factors should all be taken into account when determining an operative plan based on staging with MR imaging.

Anatomic MR imaging The strength of MR imaging in staging prostate cancer is its ability to detect ECE and SVI. On T2-weighted imaging, ECE is visualized as direct extension of tumor into periprostatic fat or an interruption in the contour of the prostatic capsule.[125] Further findings include asymmetry of the neurovascular bundle, tumor envelopment of the neurovascular bundle, an angulated, retracted, or irregular contour, obliteration of the rectoprostatic angle, or a tumor-capsule interface of greater than 1 cm.[103,106,125–129] The reported sensitivity (22%–71%) and specificity (73%–95.7%) for detection of ECE by MR imaging varies quite widely, but likely has improved with development of better techniques in recent years (**Fig. 9**A).[97–101] For example, prostate imaging can be obtained with higher signal-to-noise ratio and higher spatial resolution using 3-T MR imaging with an endorectal coil, in comparison with 1.5 T.[130,131]

SVI is typically visualized as extension of tumor from the base of the prostate and the presence of focal mass of low signal intensity within the seminal vesicle (**Fig. 10**). Further features seen are a disruption of normal architecture of the seminal vesicle, enlarged low-signal intensity ejaculatory ducts, and obliteration of the angle between the prostate and the seminal vesicle as seen on sagittal images.[99] The sensitivity and specificity of detection of SVI by MR imaging has been reported as 23% to 75% and 92% to 99%, respectively.[97–101]

Dynamic contrast-enhanced MR imaging DCE-MR imaging shows promise in improved staging for prostate cancer and potentially in identifying high-grade disease.[122] Prostate cancer appears heterogeneous because of the more permeable vessels, and show early, rapid enhancement with early washout on DCE-MR imaging. A recent study using DCE-MR imaging combined with T2-weighted 3-T assessed the value of this modality for determining ECE.[130] MR imaging staging results were compared with radical prostatectomy

pathology specimens. The overall sensitivity, specificity, PPV, and NPV for ECE were 75%, 92%, 79%, and 91%, respectively. Futterer and colleagues[102] demonstrated that the use of multisection DCE-MR imaging in staging prostate cancer may improve staging performance for the less experienced readers but had no benefit for the experienced reader. Ogura and colleagues[66] demonstrated an accuracy rate of 97% for SVI detection on DCE-MR imaging, and interpreted early enhancement in the seminal vesicles on dynamic T1-weighted images as SVI (see **Fig. 10**C). Multiparametric MR imaging constitutes a selection of the aforementioned techniques with much versatility in prostate imaging. Multiparametric MR imaging is arguably the best currently available imaging technique in localizing, staging, and determining the aggressiveness and volume of prostate cancer. The optimal technical approach (field strength, sequence, endorectal coil usage) and combination of multiparametric MR imaging techniques is still unclear, but the potential for aiding the management of prostate cancer is evident.

MR spectroscopy MR spectroscopy has been shown to contribute significant incremental value to staging nomograms in predicting organ-confined prostate cancer, and especially in intermediate-risk and high-risk groups ($P<.01$).[132] Furthermore, MR spectroscopy may provide information regarding prostate cancer aggressiveness, as studies have shown that the (choline + creatine)/citrate ratio in a lesion correlates with Gleason grade.[129,133] A well-recognized problem in MR staging of prostate cancer is the wide variation in accuracy, potentially attributable to interobserver variability and a lack of standardized diagnostic criteria. MR spectroscopy has the potential to improve this, as documented in a study that found MR spectroscopy improved accuracy for the less

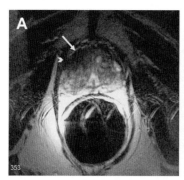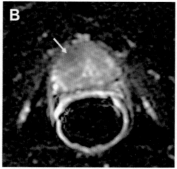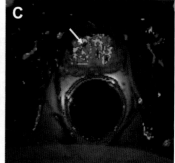

Fig. 9. MR images of a 65-year-old man. (*A*) Axial T2-weighted image shows a focal region of low T2 signal in the right transitional zone in the mid-gland (*arrow*). There is extracapsular extension (*arrowhead*). (*B*) The tumor shows restricted diffusion and low apparent diffusion coefficient (ADC) (*arrow*). (*C*) DCE-MR imaging with quantitative color-coded map of reverse flow of contrast medium (Kep) shows elevated values within the tumor focus (*arrow*). Pathologic examination confirmed the diagnosis (Gleason score 3 + 4).

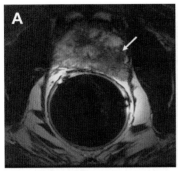 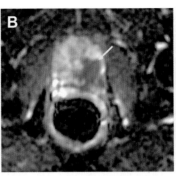 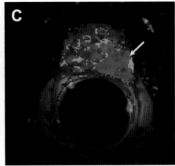

Fig. 10. MR images of a 60-year-old man. (*A*) Axial T2-weighted image shows a nodular mass in the left postero-lateral aspect of the prostate with extracapsular extension (*arrow*) and seminal vesicle invasion. (*B*) The tumor shows restricted diffusion and low ADC (*arrow*). (*C*) DCE-MR imaging with quantitative color-coded map of reverse flow of contrast medium (Kep) shows elevated values within the tumor focus (*arrow*). Pathologic examination confirmed the diagnosis (Gleason score 4 + 5).

experienced reader when compared with MR imaging (area under the ROC curve increased from 0.62 to 0.75, *P*<.05).[103] Functional MR imaging techniques display a tremendous amount of potential for the improved accuracy of staging of prostate cancer, and will only improve with additional technological advancement and refinement of techniques.

Staging of Metastatic Nodal Disease (N-Staging)

The knowledge of lymph node metastases, when present, is important, as it commonly guides treatment and is a strong predictor of disease recurrence and progression. Both CT and MR imaging are commonly used to detect lymph node metastases as recommended in the NCCN guidelines (ie, pelvic CT or MR imaging if T3, T4, or T1-T2 and nomogram indicated probability of lymph node involvement >20%). There are validated nomograms that provide risk stratification for lymph node involvement using PSA level, Gleason grade, and clinical stage that can be used to guide imaging studies.

CT and MR imaging are forms of cross-sectional imaging, both of which are widely used and employ a lymph node size of greater than 10 mm to indicate suspicion of lymph node metastases. However, both are subsequently limited because of their inability to detect metastases in lymph nodes smaller than 10 mm. The reported sensitivity and specificity for CT detection of lymph node metastases range from 5% to 77% and 75% to 100%, respectively.[134] This range is similar to the reported sensitivity and specificity for detection by MR imaging of lymph node metastases, from 6% to 68% and 78% to 97%, respectively.[134]

A technique that has shown significant promise, but has been limited in uptake, is high-resolution

MR imaging with lymphotropic superparamagnetic nanoparticles. This technique allows the detection of occult lymph node metastases, as it is not dependent on nodal size. Ultrasmall superparamagnetic particles of iron oxide (USPIO) are administered intravenously and migrate to lymph nodes where they are phagocytosed by macrophages. In malignant nodal infiltration there is an absence of macrophage activity, leading to signal modification, as affected lymph nodes will appear hyperintense on T2-weighted MR imaging.[135] Harisinghani and colleagues[136] reported that MR imaging with lymphotropic nanoparticles had a significantly higher sensitivity than conventional MR imaging in the detection of metastases on a node-by-node basis (90.5% vs 35.4%, *P*<.001), and a sensitivity of 100% and a specificity of 95.7% in detecting nodal metastases on a per-patient basis (**Fig. 11**). Despite these findings, the technique is limited by its time-consuming nature, high level of expertise required, and limited sensitivity in small lymph nodes (<0.5 mm).[117,137]

Staging of Metastatic Bone Disease (M-Staging)

Bone is the most common location for prostate cancer metastases, accounting for approximately 80% of all metastases.[68] Radionucleotide (^{99m}Tc methylene diphosphonate) bone scintigraphy is the most commonly used imaging modality for detecting bone metastases in prostate cancer. The NCCN guidelines recommend a "bone scan if T1 and PSA >20 or T2 and PSA >10 or Gleason score ≥8 or T3, T4 or symptomatic." Nevertheless, they are frequently used in low-risk patients despite the positive yield ranging from 1% to 13% in patients with a PSA less than 20 ng/mL and a Gleason score of less than 8.[69–73]

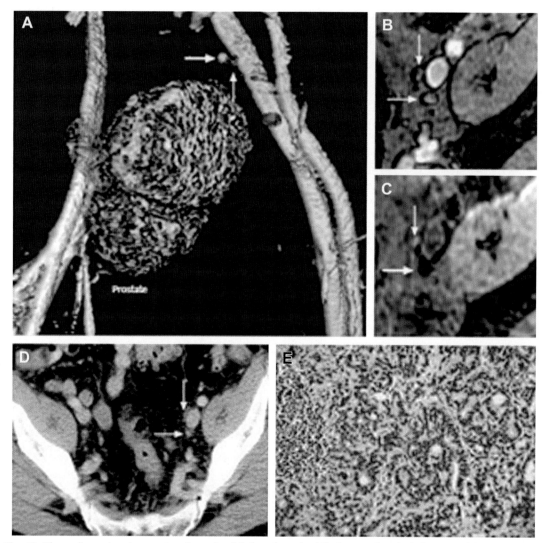

Fig. 11. Three-dimensional reconstruction of pelvic lymph nodes (*A*), Conventional MR imaging (*B*), MR imaging with lymphotropic superparamagnetic nanoparticles (*C*), abdominal CT (*D*), and histopathological findings (*E*). Panel *A* shows a 3-dimensional reconstruction of the prostate, iliac vessels, and metastatic (red) and nonmetastatic (green) lymph nodes, to assist in the planning of surgery and radiotherapy. There is a malignant node (*thick arrow*) immediately adjacent to the normal node (*thin arrow*) posteromedial to the iliac vessels. In panel *B*, conventional MR imaging shows that the signal intensity is identical in the 2 nodes (*arrows*). In panel *C*, MR imaging with lymphotropic superparamagnetic nanoparticles shows that the signal in the normal node is decreased (*thick arrow*) but that it is high in the metastatic node (*thin arrow*). In panel *D*, abdominal CT fails to differentiate between the 2 lymph nodes (*arrows*). In Panel *E*, histopathological examination of the malignant lymph node reveals sheaths of carcinoma cells (hematoxylin-eosin, original magnification ×200). (*Reprinted from* Harisinghani MG, Barentsz J, Hahn PF, et al. Noninvasive detection of clinically occult lymph node metastases in prostate cancer. N Engl J Med 2003;348(25):2497; Copyright 2012, Massachusetts Medical Society; with permission.)

A bone scan can detect bone metastases up to 18 months before evidence on plain film.[74] Unfortunately, because a bone scan images the secondary effects of prostate cancer on bone, false positives from degenerative change, inflammation, Paget disease, or trauma occur frequently.[73] This limitation in specificity often leads to subsequent confirmatory imaging with modalities such as plain radiography, CT, MR imaging, or PET/CT scan.

MR imaging appears to be superior to bone scan, as it is sensitive to early changes in bone marrow that precede the osteoblastic response in the bone matrix.[73] Bone metastases lead to a lengthened T1 relaxation time and signal loss, which contrasts with the surrounding high-signal marrow fat.[73] MR imaging has been shown to detect bone metastases in 37.5% of patients with a negative or inconclusive bone scan and plain films, and has a reported sensitivity and specificity of 100% and 88%, respectively.[73,75] MR imaging lacks whole-body coverage but can assess the spine and pelvis, where most metastases arise, and with new technology can be conducted in minutes.

ROLE OF IMAGING MODALITIES IN ACTIVE SURVEILLANCE

According to the NCCN definition, active surveillance of prostate cancer involves actively monitoring the course of disease with the expectation to intervene with curative intent if the cancer progresses. Multiple studies have shown that low-risk prostate cancer can be safely managed on active surveillance with a very small risk of developing metastatic or lethal disease.[138–141] However, a key concern is that some patients selected for inclusion based on favorable low-risk characteristics will have been undersampled on TRUS biopsy and will actually have more aggressive disease. Commonly it is anterior-zone or transitional-zone tumors that may not be adequately sampled on TRUS biopsy, owing their location. MR imaging is currently the best imaging modality for detecting and staging prostate cancer, and thus is being investigated as a potential adjunct to improve selection of patients who can be safely managed with active surveillance.

One prospective study investigated the MR imaging findings among 60 men with low-risk prostate cancer before active surveillance.[142] A multiparametric combination of T2-weighted, echo-planar, DW-, and multi- and DCE-MR imaging was used. MR imaging appeared to have a high yield for predicting reclassification of disease on repeat prostate biopsy. The PPV and NPV for MR imaging predicting reclassification were 83% (95% confidence interval [CI] 73–93) and 81% (95% CI 71–91), respectively.[142] Of detected lesions larger than 1 cm, 55% were located in the anterior zone, 27% in the transitional zone, and 27% in the peripheral zone. Further research is required to solidify inclusion criteria and indicators for timely intervention for patients on active surveillance, but it is likely that MR imaging will have an important role to play.

RECURRENCE OF PROSTATE CANCER

Diagnosis of recurrence of prostate cancer is challenging by imaging, at least in the early stages. At present, serial serum PSA measurement plays the main role in the assessment of recurrence and progression of prostate cancer following initial radical treatment[143]; however, definition of biochemical failure is a topic of debate.

The current consensus considers a PSA increase over a threshold of 0.2 ng/mL as the cutoff that necessitates further evaluation.[70] The leading role of imaging would be in identifying the patients with local recurrence who would potentially benefit from salvage radiotherapy. Detecting the site of recurrence is difficult, mainly because of the absence of any signs or symptoms.[144] A critical diagnostic dilemma for the evaluation of patients with biochemical failure is to differentiate between patients who only have local recurrence and those who have metastatic spread. At this point, diagnostic imaging strategies are able to provide crucial information toward differentiating local recurrence versus metastatic spread and in helping plan further therapeutic interventions. On the other hand, with the increasing success rate of early salvage therapy, detection of tumor recurrence at the earliest possible stage has a significant impact on patients' mortality and morbidity.

Commonly used imaging modalities in this setting include TRUS-guided biopsy (from prostatic fossa or irradiated prostate for local recurrence), CT scan, and endorectal coil MR imaging, as well as bone scan to identify metastatic lesions. However, in the early phase of relapse with a low PSA level (<5 ng/mL), all these modalities are not satisfactory and are limited by poor sensitivity.[145,146] Meanwhile, depicting the local recurrence after radiotherapy is challenging, considering the radiation-induced tissue changes and fibrosis.

The current vignette focused on newer imaging modalities, which mainly represent functional characteristics of tissue, with potentially higher sensitivity and specificity in the detection of tumor tissue when compared with conventional imaging techniques.

Identification of Local Recurrence

After radical prostatectomy

As many as 30% of patients with biochemical failure after radical prostatectomy have local recurrence, and evaluation of the prostatic bed seems beneficial in this setting.[147] The vesicourethral anastomosis is the most frequent location of recurrence in patients undergoing radical prostatectomy, with the retrovesical space being another common site.[148,149]

Application of CT in the evaluation of local recurrence has shown a sensitivity of 36% for detection of lesions.[150] On the other hand, endorectal MR imaging has shown increased diagnostic performance for this purpose in patients with an increasing PSA level but no palpable tumor in the prostatic fossa. Low signal intensity on both T1-weighted and T2-weighted images may be seen in the vesicourethral anastomosis, indicating normal postoperative scarring. It is important that granulation tissue may occasionally be present in the surgical bed, mimicking tumor recurrence.[151] Retained seminal vesicles have been reported on MR imaging in as many as 20% of patients after radical prostatectomy, so this finding should be identified to avoid misinterpreting it as a recurrence.[152] Some investigators have reported a high sensitivity and specificity for evaluation of local recurrence using anatomic MR imaging[151,153] Others have reported sensitivities and specificities ranging from 48% to 100% and 52% to 100%, respectively.[151,154] Application of intravenous contrast would be helpful, as the residual tumor tissue would enhance earlier than the fibrotic tissue. Two recent studies demonstrated significant improvement in sensitivity and specificity when using DCE-MR imaging alone or in combination with anatomic MR imaging.[154,155] In addition, ADC values may be useful as a biomarker for monitoring treatment response and predicting local recurrence of prostate cancer. In a recent report, DW-MR imaging was shown to be capable of identifying local recurrence after radical prostatectomy in patients for whom conventional cross-sectional imaging, such as CT and anatomic MR imaging, had failed to demonstrate a recurrence.[156]

In another study,[157] the accuracy of MR spectroscopy and DCE-MR imaging in the depiction of local recurrence of prostate cancer in 70 patients with biochemical progression after radical prostatectomy was evaluated. MR spectroscopy analysis alone showed sensitivity of 84% and specificity of 88% when compared with anastomotic biopsy as the gold standard; DCE-MR imaging analysis alone, sensitivity of 71% and specificity of 94%; and combined MR spectroscopy/DCE-MR imaging, sensitivity of 87% and specificity of 94%. The investigators concluded that combined MR spectroscopy and DCE-MR imaging is an accurate method to identify local recurrence of prostate cancer in patients with biochemical failure.[157] Recent studies recommend MR imaging (in particular DCE-MR imaging) for localization of recurrence early, in patients with PSA levels of less than 2 ng/mL. In these studies the highest diagnostic performance was found when the multiparametric approach was applied. The role of choline PET/CT scans in detecting recurring prostate cancer has been evaluated widely. Choline is a new tracer that has been most commonly used to study prostate cancer with PET/CT (Fig. 12). Castellucci and colleagues[158] reported sensitivity of 73% and specificity of 69% for the prediction of choline PET/CT in terms of positive recurrence results in 190 patients previously treated with radical prostatectomy and with PSA failure.

A recent meta-analysis on PET/CT predictive values for recurrence or progression of prostate cancer after radical prostatectomy demonstrated sensitivity between 60% and 95%, specificity between 36% and 93%, PPV between 60% and 92%, NPV between 61% and 96%, and accuracy between 78% and 89%.[159] The investigators concluded that PET/CT has not shown significant yield in terms of detection rate for local recurrence in patients with a low level of PSA, but multiparametric MR imaging is promising in patients with low PSA and with small-diameter lesions. It is worth mentioning that at present most important urologic societies do not consider these modalities in the follow-up of patients with suspected local recurrence after radical prostatectomy.[70,160,161]

After radiation therapy

One important point that should be considered when assessing a possible recurrence in the prostate after radiation therapy is that recurrence tends to occur at the site of the primary tumor. Posttreatment changes appear diffusely hypoechoic at TRUS, making identification of recurrence inaccurate with sensitivity close to that of DRE.[162] On the other hand, the T2 images would demonstrate a decrease in signal intensity in the entire prostate and the seminal vesicles, leading to decreased contrast between the prostate tissue and the recurring tumor.[163] Another challenge would be the presence of a focal hypointense region on T2 images that may represent the persistence of the original tumor rather than a recurrence. One good candidate in this situation is DCE-MR imaging. The slow and low enhancement of the fibrotic tissue would allow an acceptable contrast with that of the recurring tumor with high vascularity. Accordingly, Tamada and colleagues[164] reported high specificity and accuracy (95% and 91%, respectively) for DCE-MR imaging in detecting local recurrence after brachytherapy despite the relatively low sensitivity (68%). This technique has been also shown to improve the detection of recurrence after radiotherapy in other studies by showing early arterial enhancement of tumor nodules and early washout.[163,165] Kim and colleagues[166] evaluated the incremental value of 3-T DW-MR imaging in patients with biochemical failure after radiation therapy. These investigators demonstrated an increase in diagnostic

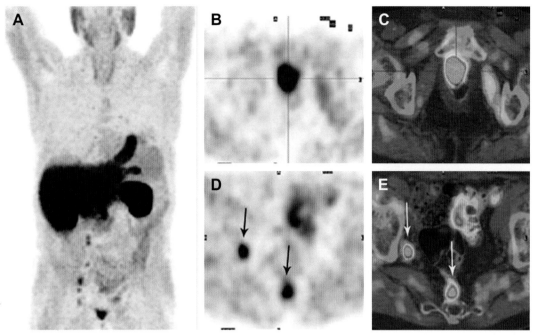

Fig. 12. (*A*) A 77-year-old man with PSA 8.5 ng/mL and previous radical prostatectomy. Positron emission tomography (PET) maximum-intensity projection image shows multiple areas of pathologic ^{18}F-choline uptake. (*B–E*) PET and fused axial views (*B, C*) show pathologic uptake at the level of the prostate bed and in the pelvic lymph nodes (*D, E*) (*arrows*). (*Reprinted from* Pelosi E, Arena V, Skanjeti A, et al. Role of whole-body ^{18}F-choline PET/CT in disease detection in patients with biochemical relapse after radical treatment for prostate cancer. Radiol Med 2008;113(6):899; Copyright 2012, Springer; with permission.)

performance for predicting locally recurrent prostate cancer after radiation therapy using combined T2-weighted images and DWI-MR imaging (sensitivity and specificities of 62% and 97% vs 25% and 92%) (**Fig. 13**). Studies on MR spectroscopy have documented good correlation between spectroscopic data and tissue findings[167,168]; however, the specificity is limited owing to high false positives, as some benign glands have high levels of choline after radiation therapy. Another

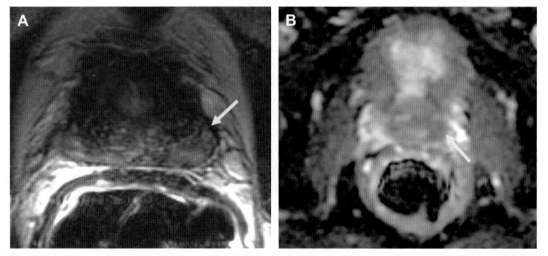

Fig. 13. MR images of a 64 year-old man with a PSA level of 9.63 ng/mL, 2 years after radiation therapy. (*A*) Axial T2-weighted image shows focal area of T2 signal abnormality (*arrow*) in the left base peripheral gland with corresponding restricted diffusion on ADC map (*B*). Pathologic examination confirmed tumor recurrence (*arrow*).

merging modality in this field is choline and acetate PET/CT, which has shown good visual interpretation for local recurrence. The poor spatial resolution would be undesirable, as it cannot allow precise location of the recurrence within the prostate and would thus be a limitation in treatment planning of the recurring tumor.[169]

Identification of Metastases

The standard workup to identify distant metastases, including abdominal and pelvic CT and bone scan, has low diagnostic yield in asymptomatic patients with biochemical failure.[170,171] At present, imaging modalities such as whole-body MR imaging and fluoride, choline, or acetate PET/CT have been promising in the early detection of metastatic lymph nodes and bone metastases with pathologic fracture.[172,173] In a large study of 358 patients with biochemical recurrence after radical prostatectomy, investigators reported an overall sensitivity of 85%, specificity 93%, PPV 91%, and NPV 87% for choline PET/CT, with a statistically significant correlation between PSA levels and PET/CT results. A PSA cutoff value of 1.4 ng/mL could best discriminate PPV and NPV for choline PET/CT.[174] Reviewing the currently available data on different PSA cutoff levels for recommending PET/CT in assessing recurrence of prostate cancer shows that the routine use of this modality was not recommended for PSA values less than 1 ng/mL.[161] Patients with equivocal findings on a bone scan warrant additional imaging studies. ^{18}F-Fluorodeoxyglucose PET is the modality of choice in this setting, at least in patients with aggressive disease. CT is usually used for assessment of advanced lytic lesions suspicious for pathologic fracture. Scattoni and colleagues[175] have prospectively evaluated the accuracy of choline PET/CT in the diagnosis of lymph node recurrence in 25 patients with prostate cancer who had PSA failure after surgery. A lesion-based analysis showed that sensitivity, specificity,

Table 3
Pearls and pitfalls of imaging in prostate cancer

Pearls	Potential Pitfalls
Ultrasonography	
Widely available	Operator dependent
Lower cost	Large number of cancers are not associated with
Prostate dimensions and volume	sonographic abnormalities
Facilitating systematically directed biopsies	40% of cancers are isoechoic and are not visible on conventional ultrasonography
MR Imaging	
High soft-tissue resolution	Expensive
Prostate dimensions and volume	The need for endorectal coil
Detection of asymmetry in prostate contour	Limited accuracy of conventional MR imaging for
Seminal vesicle involvement	tumor localization after transrectal
Involvement of pelvic or periaortic lymph nodes	ultrasound-guided biopsy due to postbiopsy
Typical appearances of recurrence after radical prostatectomy	hemorrhage
Functional MR imaging techniques improves overall imaging performance in the detection of tumor recurrence	Susceptibility to motion (motion artifacts)
	Residual seminal vesicles may mimic tissue recurrence
	Metallic clip may interfere with interpretation after prostatectomy
	After radiotherapy the recurring tumor may not be apparent on anatomic imaging
PET/CT	
Whole-body tomography imaging	High costs
Ability to evaluate metabolic functions	Uses ionizing radiation
Enables distinguishing neoplastic tissue from fibrosis and necrosis	The poor spatial resolution would be undesirable for precise localization
Detection of metastatic lymph node and bony metastasis	Limitation of FDG-PET in prostate cancer due to the low glycolytic activity of this tumor
Potential for detection of early lesions using new tracers	Need for on-site cyclotron

Abbreviation: FDG, ^{18}F-labeled fluorodeoxyglucose.

PPV, NPV, and accuracy were 64%, 90%, 86%, 72%, and 77%, respectively. The reported low NPV was attributed to the limited capability of choline PET/CT to detect microscopic nodes.

PEARLS AND PITFALLS

The development of imaging techniques with high diagnostic performance in diagnosis and follow-up of patients with prostate cancer is challenging. The soft-tissue planes of the prostate are difficult to visualize on anatomic imaging. Another factor could be biology of the development and progression of prostate cancer. The selection of an imaging modality should be based on the questions that need to be answered for a particular patient as well as the diagnostic profile of the imaging techniques. Such important considerations are summarized in **Table 3**.

SUMMARY

The selection of imaging techniques in prostate cancer depends on the disease status of the patients as well as the clinical application of the provided information. Ultrasound-guided biopsy is still the mainstay of diagnosis; however, CE-US and MR imaging–directed biopsy are changing the diagnostic approach to prostate cancer, with improving biopsy yield. Multiparametric MR imaging has improved sensitivity and specificity of imaging for detecting and localizing primary and recurrent prostate cancer, especially in patients who have risk factors for ECE. Lymphotropic nanoparticle MR imaging and PET/CT have emerging roles in the noninvasive evaluation of metastatic lymph nodes.

REFERENCES

1. Jemal A, Siegel R, Ward E, et al. Cancer statistics, 2009. CA Cancer J Clin 2009;59(4):225–49.
2. Lee CH, Akin-Olugbade O, Kirschenbaum A. Overview of prostate anatomy, histology, and pathology. Endocrinol Metab Clin North Am 2011;40(3):565–75, viii–ix.
3. Brooks JD. Anatomy. In: Wein AJ, editor. Campbell-Walsh urology. 9th edition. Philadelphia: Saunders Elsevier; 2007.
4. Salomon L, Colombel M, Patard JJ, et al. Value of ultrasound-guided systematic sextant biopsies in prostate tumor mapping. Eur Urol 1999;35(4):289–93.
5. Halpern EJ, Strup SE. Using gray-scale and color and power Doppler sonography to detect prostatic cancer. AJR Am J Roentgenol 2000;174(3):623–7.
6. Wefer AE, Hricak H, Vigneron DB, et al. Sextant localization of prostate cancer: comparison of sextant biopsy, magnetic resonance imaging and magnetic resonance spectroscopic imaging with step section histology. J Urol 2000;164(2):400–4.
7. Sauvain JL, Palascak P, Bourscheid D, et al. Value of power Doppler and 3D vascular sonography as a method for diagnosis and staging of prostate cancer. Eur Urol 2003;44(1):21–30 [discussion: 30–1].
8. Eisenberg ML, Cowan JE, Carroll PR, et al. The adjunctive use of power Doppler imaging in the preoperative assessment of prostate cancer. BJU Int 2010;105(9):1237–41.
9. Nelson ED, Slotoroff CB, Gomella LG, et al. Targeted biopsy of the prostate: the impact of color Doppler imaging and elastography on prostate cancer detection and Gleason score. Urology 2007;70(6):1136–40.
10. Taverna G, Morandi G, Seveso M, et al. Colour Doppler and microbubble contrast agent ultrasonography do not improve cancer detection rate in transrectal systematic prostate biopsy sampling. BJU Int 2011;108(11):1723–7.
11. Bogers HA, Sedelaar JP, Beerlage HP, et al. Contrast-enhanced three-dimensional power Doppler angiography of the human prostate: correlation with biopsy outcome. Urology 1999;54(1):97–104.
12. Roy C, Buy X, Lang H, et al. Contrast enhanced color Doppler endorectal sonography of prostate: efficiency for detecting peripheral zone tumors and role for biopsy procedure. J Urol 2003;170(1):69–72.
13. Xie SW, Li HL, Du J, et al. Contrast-enhanced ultrasonography with contrast-tuned imaging technology for the detection of prostate cancer: comparison with conventional ultrasonography. BJU Int 2012;109(11):1620–6.
14. Cochlin DL, Ganatra RH, Griffiths DF. Elastography in the detection of prostatic cancer. Clin Radiol 2002;57(11):1014–20.
15. Pallwein L, Mitterberger M, Pinggera G, et al. Sonoelastography of the prostate: comparison with systematic biopsy findings in 492 patients. Eur J Radiol 2008;65(2):304–10.
16. Salomon G, Kollerman J, Thederan I, et al. Evaluation of prostate cancer detection with ultrasound real-time elastography: a comparison with step section pathological analysis after radical prostatectomy. Eur Urol 2008;54(6):1354–62.
17. Brock M, von Bodman C, Palisaar RJ, et al. The Impact of real-time elastography guiding a systematic prostate biopsy to improve cancer detection rate: a prospective study of 353 patients. J Urol 2012;187(6):2039–43.
18. Hricak H, White S, Vigneron D, et al. Carcinoma of the prostate gland: MR imaging with pelvic phased-array coils versus integrated endorectal-pelvic phased-array coils. Radiology 1994;193(3):703–9.

19. Casciani E, Polettini E, Bertini L, et al. Contribution of the MR spectroscopic imaging in the diagnosis of prostate cancer in the peripheral zone. Abdom Imaging 2007;32(6):796–802.

20. Costouros NG, Coakley FV, Westphalen AC, et al. Diagnosis of prostate cancer in patients with an elevated prostate-specific antigen level: role of endorectal MRI and MR spectroscopic imaging. AJR Am J Roentgenol 2007;188(3):812–6.

21. Haider MA, van der Kwast TH, Tanguay J, et al. Combined T2-weighted and diffusion-weighted MRI for localization of prostate cancer. AJR Am J Roentgenol 2007;189(2):323–8.

22. Tamada T, Sone T, Jo Y, et al. Prostate cancer: relationships between postbiopsy hemorrhage and tumor detectability at MR diagnosis. Radiology 2008;248(2):531–9.

23. Reinsberg SA, Payne GS, Riches SF, et al. Combined use of diffusion-weighted MRI and 1H MR spectroscopy to increase accuracy in prostate cancer detection. AJR Am J Roentgenol 2007; 188(1):91–8.

24. Lim HK, Kim JK, Kim KA, et al. Prostate cancer: apparent diffusion coefficient map with T2-weighted images for detection—a multireader study. Radiology 2009;250(1):145–51.

25. Jager GJ, Ruijter ET, van de Kaa CA, et al. Dynamic TurboFLASH subtraction technique for contrast-enhanced MR imaging of the prostate: correlation with histopathologic results. Radiology 1997;203(3):645–52.

26. Kim JK, Hong SS, Choi YJ, et al. Wash-in rate on the basis of dynamic contrast-enhanced MRI: usefulness for prostate cancer detection and localization. J Magn Reson Imaging 2005;22(5):639–46.

27. Futterer JJ, Heijmink SW, Scheenen TW, et al. Prostate cancer localization with dynamic contrast-enhanced MR imaging and proton MR spectroscopic imaging. Radiology 2006;241(2):449–58.

28. Sung YS, Kwon HJ, Park BW, et al. Prostate cancer detection on dynamic contrast-enhanced MRI: computer-aided diagnosis versus single perfusion parameter maps. AJR Am J Roentgenol 2011; 197(5):1122–9.

29. Manenti G, Squillaci E, Carlani M, et al. Magnetic resonance imaging of the prostate with spectroscopic imaging using a surface coil. Initial clinical experience. Radiol Med 2006;111(1):22–32.

30. Yamamura J, Salomon G, Buchert R, et al. MR imaging of prostate cancer: diffusion weighted imaging and (3D) hydrogen 1 (H) MR spectroscopy in comparison with histology. Radiol Res Pract 2011;2011:616852.

31. Watanabe H, Kato H, Kato T, et al. Diagnostic application of ultrasonotomography to the prostate. Nihon Hinyokika Gakkai Zasshi 1968;59(4):273–9 [in Japanese].

32. Tabatabaei S, Saylor PJ, Coen J, et al. Prostate cancer imaging: what surgeons, radiation oncologists, and medical oncologists want to know. AJR Am J Roentgenol 2011;196(6):1263–6.

33. Ross R, Harisinghani M. Prostate cancer imaging—what the urologic oncologist needs to know. Radiol Clin North Am 2006;44(5):711–22, viii.

34. Heijmink SW, Futterer JJ, Strum SS, et al. State-of-the-art uroradiologic imaging in the diagnosis of prostate cancer. Acta Oncol 2011;50(Suppl 1): 25–38.

35. Brawer MK. Quantitative microvessel density. A staging and prognostic marker for human prostatic carcinoma. Cancer 1996;78(2):345–9.

36. Ismail M, Petersen RO, Alexander AA, et al. Color Doppler imaging in predicting the biologic behavior of prostate cancer: correlation with disease-free survival. Urology 1997;50(6):906–12.

37. Linden RA, Halpern EJ. Advances in transrectal ultrasound imaging of the prostate. Semin Ultrasound CT MR 2007;28(4):249–57.

38. Nicolau C, Ripolles T. Contrast-enhanced ultrasound in abdominal imaging. Abdom Imaging 2012;37(1):1–19.

39. Claudon M, Cosgrove D, Albrecht T, et al. Guidelines and good clinical practice recommendations for contrast enhanced ultrasound (CEUS)—update 2008. Ultraschall Med 2008;29(1):28–44.

40. Wilson SR, Greenbaum LD, Goldberg BB. Contrast-enhanced ultrasound: what is the evidence and what are the obstacles? AJR Am J Roentgenol 2009;193(1):55–60.

41. Sedelaar JP, van Leenders GJ, Hulsbergen-van de Kaa CA, et al. Microvessel density: correlation between contrast ultrasonography and histology of prostate cancer. Eur Urol 2001;40(3):285–93.

42. Pelzer A, Bektic J, Berger AP, et al. Prostate cancer detection in men with prostate specific antigen 4 to 10 ng/ml using a combined approach of contrast enhanced color Doppler targeted and systematic biopsy. J Urol 2005;173(6):1926–9.

43. Halpern EJ, Ramey JR, Strup SE, et al. Detection of prostate carcinoma with contrast-enhanced sonography using intermittent harmonic imaging. Cancer 2005;104(11):2373–83.

44. Frauscher F, Klauser A, Volgger H, et al. Comparison of contrast enhanced color Doppler targeted biopsy with conventional systematic biopsy: impact on prostate cancer detection. J Urol 2002; 167(4):1648–52.

45. Mitterberger M, Pinggera GM, Horninger W, et al. Comparison of contrast enhanced color Doppler targeted biopsy to conventional systematic biopsy: impact on Gleason score. J Urol 2007;178(2):464–8 [discussion: 468].

46. Ophir J, Cespedes I, Ponnekanti H, et al. Elastography: a quantitative method for imaging the

elasticity of biological tissues. Ultrason Imaging 1991;13(2):111–34.

47. Pallwein L, Mitterberger M, Struve P, et al. Comparison of sonoelastography guided biopsy with systematic biopsy: impact on prostate cancer detection. Eur Radiol 2007;17(9):2278–85.

48. Aigner F, Pallwein L, Junker D, et al. Value of real-time elastography targeted biopsy for prostate cancer detection in men with prostate specific antigen 1.25 ng/ml or greater and 4.00 ng/ml or less. J Urol 2010;184(3):913–7.

49. Roehl KA, Antenor JA, Catalona WJ. Serial biopsy results in prostate cancer screening study. J Urol 2002;167(6):2435–9.

50. Qayyum A, Coakley FV, Lu Y, et al. Organ-confined prostate cancer: effect of prior transrectal biopsy on endorectal MRI and MR spectroscopic imaging. AJR Am J Roentgenol 2004;183(4):1079–83.

51. Heijmink SW, Futterer JJ, Hambrock T, et al. Prostate cancer: body-array versus endorectal coil MR imaging at 3 T—comparison of image quality, localization, and staging performance. Radiology 2007;244(1):184–95.

52. Futterer JJ. MR imaging in local staging of prostate cancer. Eur J Radiol 2007;63(3):328–34.

53. Schiebler ML, Schnall MD, Pollack HM, et al. Current role of MR imaging in the staging of adenocarcinoma of the prostate. Radiology 1993;189(2):339–52.

54. White S, Hricak H, Forstner R, et al. Prostate cancer: effect of postbiopsy hemorrhage on interpretation of MR images. Radiology 1995;195(2):385–90.

55. Ocak I, Bernardo M, Metzger G, et al. Dynamic contrast-enhanced MRI of prostate cancer at 3 T: a study of pharmacokinetic parameters. AJR Am J Roentgenol 2007;189(4):849.

56. Somford DM, Futterer JJ, Hambrock T, et al. Diffusion and perfusion MR imaging of the prostate. Magn Reson Imaging Clin N Am 2008;16(4):685–95, ix.

57. Haider MA, Amoozadeh Y, Jhaveri KS. DW-MRI for disease characterization in the pelvis. In: Koh DM, Thoeny HC, editors. Diffusion-weighted MR imaging: applications in the body. Berlin: Springer; 2010. p. 143–56.

58. Zelhof B, Pickles M, Liney G, et al. Correlation of diffusion-weighted magnetic resonance data with cellularity in prostate cancer. BJU Int 2009;103(7):883–8.

59. Yoshimitsu K, Kiyoshima K, Irie H, et al. Usefulness of apparent diffusion coefficient map in diagnosing prostate carcinoma: correlation with stepwise histopathology. J Magn Reson Imaging 2008;27(1):132–9.

60. Tanimoto A, Nakashima J, Kohno H, et al. Prostate cancer screening: the clinical value of diffusion-weighted imaging and dynamic MR imaging in combination with T2-weighted imaging. J Magn Reson Imaging 2007;25(1):146–52.

61. Rosenkrantz AB, Kopec M, Kong X, et al. Prostate cancer vs. post-biopsy hemorrhage: diagnosis with T2- and diffusion-weighted imaging. J Magn Reson Imaging 2010;31(6):1387–94.

62. Park BK, Lee HM, Kim CK, et al. Lesion localization in patients with a previous negative transrectal ultrasound biopsy and persistently elevated prostate specific antigen level using diffusion-weighted imaging at three Tesla before rebiopsy. Invest Radiol 2008;43(11):789–93.

63. Xu S, Kruecker J, Turkbey B, et al. Real-time MRI-TRUS fusion for guidance of targeted prostate biopsies. Comput Aided Surg 2008;13(5):255–64.

64. deSouza NM, Riches SF, Vanas NJ, et al. Diffusion-weighted magnetic resonance imaging: a potential non-invasive marker of tumour aggressiveness in localized prostate cancer. Clin Radiol 2008;63(7):774–82.

65. Park SY, Kim CK, Park BK, et al. Prediction of biochemical recurrence following radical prostatectomy in men with prostate cancer by diffusion-weighted magnetic resonance imaging: initial results. Eur Radiol 2011;21(5):1111–8.

66. Ogura K, Maekawa S, Okubo K, et al. Dynamic endorectal magnetic resonance imaging for local staging and detection of neurovascular bundle involvement of prostate cancer: correlation with histopathologic results. Urology 2001;57(4):721–6.

67. Namimoto T, Morishita S, Saitoh R, et al. The value of dynamic MR imaging for hypointensity lesions of the peripheral zone of the prostate. Comput Med Imaging Graph 1998;22(3):239–45.

68. Mirowitz SA, Brown JJ, Heiken JP. Evaluation of the prostate and prostatic carcinoma with gadolinium-enhanced endorectal coil MR imaging. Radiology 1993;186(1):153–7.

69. Brown G, Macvicar DA, Ayton V, et al. The role of intravenous contrast enhancement in magnetic resonance imaging of prostatic carcinoma. Clin Radiol 1995;50(9):601–6.

70. Heidenreich A, Aus G, Bolla M, et al. EAU guidelines on prostate cancer. Eur Urol 2008;53(1):68–80.

71. Sciarra A, Panebianco V, Salciccia S, et al. Modern role of magnetic resonance and spectroscopy in the imaging of prostate cancer. Urol Oncol 2011;29(1):12–20.

72. Fuchsjager M, Akin O, Shukla-Dave A, et al. The role of MRI and MRSI in diagnosis, treatment selection, and post-treatment follow-up for prostate cancer. Clin Adv Hematol Oncol 2009;7(3):193–202.

73. Yuen JS, Thng CH, Tan PH, et al. Endorectal magnetic resonance imaging and spectroscopy for the detection of tumor foci in men with prior

negative transrectal ultrasound prostate biopsy. J Urol 2004;171(4):1482–6.

74. Yoshizako T, Wada A, Hayashi T, et al. Usefulness of diffusion-weighted imaging and dynamic contrast-enhanced magnetic resonance imaging in the diagnosis of prostate transition-zone cancer. Acta Radiol 2008;49(10):1207–13.

75. Turkbey B, Mani H, Shah V, et al. Multiparametric 3T prostate magnetic resonance imaging to detect cancer: histopathological correlation using prostatectomy specimens processed in customized magnetic resonance imaging based molds. J Urol 2011;186(5):1818–24.

76. Lavery HJ, Brajtbord JS, Levinson AW, et al. Unnecessary imaging for the staging of low-risk prostate cancer is common. Urology 2011;77(2):274–8.

77. Oefelein MG. Prospective predictors of urinary continence after anatomical radical retropubic prostatectomy: a multivariate analysis. World J Urol 2004;22(4):267–71.

78. Burkhard FC, Kessler TM, Fleischmann A, et al. Nerve sparing open radical retropubic prostatectomy—does it have an impact on urinary continence? J Urol 2006;176(1):189–95.

79. Kundu SD, Roehl KA, Eggener SE, et al. Potency, continence and complications in 3,477 consecutive radical retropubic prostatectomies. J Urol 2004; 172(6 Pt 1):2227–31.

80. Dubbelman YD, Dohle GR, Schroder FH. Sexual function before and after radical retropubic prostatectomy: a systematic review of prognostic indicators for a successful outcome. Eur Urol 2006;50(4): 711–8 [discussion: 718–20].

81. Hollabaugh RS Jr, Dmochowski RR, Kneib TG, et al. Preservation of putative continence nerves during radical retropubic prostatectomy leads to more rapid return of urinary continence. Urology 1998;51(6):960–7.

82. Walz J, Burnett AL, Costello AJ, et al. A critical analysis of the current knowledge of surgical anatomy related to optimization of cancer control and preservation of continence and erection in candidates for radical prostatectomy. Eur Urol 2010;57(2):179–92.

83. Hull GW, Rabbani F, Abbas F, et al. Cancer control with radical prostatectomy alone in 1,000 consecutive patients. J Urol 2002;167(2 Pt 1):528–34.

84. Grossfeld GD, Chang JJ, Broering JM, et al. Impact of positive surgical margins on prostate cancer recurrence and the use of secondary cancer treatment: data from the CaPSURE database. J Urol 2000;163(4):1171–7 [quiz: 1295].

85. Han M, Partin AW, Pound CR, et al. Long-term biochemical disease-free and cancer-specific survival following anatomic radical retropubic prostatectomy. The 15-year Johns Hopkins experience. Urol Clin North Am 2001;28(3):555–65.

86. Yossepowitch O, Bjartell A, Eastham JA, et al. Positive surgical margins in radical prostatectomy: outlining the problem and its long-term consequences. Eur Urol 2009;55(1):87–99.

87. Chuang AY, Nielsen ME, Hernandez DJ, et al. The significance of positive surgical margin in areas of capsular incision in otherwise organ confined disease at radical prostatectomy. J Urol 2007; 178(4 Pt 1):1306–10.

88. Preston MA, Carriere M, Raju G, et al. The prognostic significance of capsular incision into tumor during radical prostatectomy. Eur Urol 2011;59(4):613–8.

89. Ohori M, Egawa S, Shinohara K, et al. Detection of microscopic extracapsular extension prior to radical prostatectomy for clinically localized prostate cancer. Br J Urol 1994;74(1):72–9.

90. Colombo T, Schips L, Augustin H, et al. Value of transrectal ultrasound in preoperative staging of prostate cancer. Minerva Urol Nefrol 1999;51(1):1–4.

91. Ozgur A, Onol FF, Turkeri LN. Important preoperative prognostic factors for extracapsular extension, seminal vesicle invasion and lymph node involvement in cases with radical retropubic prostatectomy. Int Urol Nephrol 2004;36(3):369–73.

92. Mitterberger M, Pinggera GM, Pallwein L, et al. The value of three-dimensional transrectal ultrasonography in staging prostate cancer. BJU Int 2007; 100(1):47–50.

93. Eisenberg ML, Cowan JE, Davies BJ, et al. The importance of tumor palpability and transrectal ultrasonographic appearance in the contemporary clinical staging of prostate cancer. Urol Oncol 2011;29(2):171–6.

94. Platt JF, Bree RL, Schwab RE. The accuracy of CT in the staging of carcinoma of the prostate. AJR Am J Roentgenol 1987;149(2):315–8.

95. Engeler CE, Wasserman NF, Zhang G. Preoperative assessment of prostatic carcinoma by computerized tomography. Weaknesses and new perspectives. Urology 1992;40(4):346–50.

96. Tarcan T, Turkeri L, Biren T, et al. The effectiveness of imaging modalities in clinical staging of localized prostatic carcinoma. Int Urol Nephrol 1996;28(6): 773–9.

97. Perrotti M, Kaufman RP Jr, Jennings TA, et al. Endo-rectal coil magnetic resonance imaging in clinically localized prostate cancer: is it accurate? J Urol 1996;156(1):106–9.

98. Cornud F, Flam T, Chauveinc L, et al. Extraprostatic spread of clinically localized prostate cancer: factors predictive of pT3 tumor and of positive endorectal MR imaging examination results. Radiology 2002;224(1):203–10.

99. Sala E, Akin O, Moskowitz CS, et al. Endorectal MR imaging in the evaluation of seminal vesicle invasion: diagnostic accuracy and multivariate feature analysis. Radiology 2006;238(3):929–37.

100. Park BK, Kim B, Kim CK, et al. Comparison of phased-array 3.0-T and endorectal 1.5-T magnetic resonance imaging in the evaluation of local staging accuracy for prostate cancer. J Comput Assist Tomogr 2007;31(4):534–8.

101. Baccos A, Schiavina R, Zukerman Z, et al. Accuracy of endorectal magnetic resonance imaging (MRI) and dynamic contrast enhanced-MRI (DCE-MRI) in the preoperative local staging of prostate cancer. Urologia 2012;79(2):116–22 [in Italian].

102. Futterer JJ, Engelbrecht MR, Huisman HJ, et al. Staging prostate cancer with dynamic contrast-enhanced endorectal MR imaging prior to radical prostatectomy: experienced versus less experienced readers. Radiology 2005;237(2):541–9.

103. Yu KK, Scheidler J, Hricak H, et al. Prostate cancer: prediction of extracapsular extension with endorectal MR imaging and three-dimensional proton MR spectroscopic imaging. Radiology 1999;213(2):481–8.

104. Futterer JJ, Barentsz J, Heijmijnk ST. Imaging modalities for prostate cancer. Expert Rev Anticancer Ther 2009;9(7):923–37.

105. Ukimura O, Troncoso P, Ramirez EI, et al. Prostate cancer staging: correlation between ultrasound determined tumor contact length and pathologically confirmed extraprostatic extension. J Urol 1998;159(4):1251–9.

106. Ravizzini G, Turkbey B, Kurdziel K, et al. New horizons in prostate cancer imaging. Eur J Radiol 2009;70(2):212–26.

107. Turkbey B, Albert PS, Kurdziel K, et al. Imaging localized prostate cancer: current approaches and new developments. AJR Am J Roentgenol 2009;192(6):1471–80.

108. Hricak H, Choyke PL, Eberhardt SC, et al. Imaging prostate cancer: a multidisciplinary perspective. Radiology 2007;243(1):28–53.

109. Lorentzen T, Nerstrom H, Iversen P, et al. Local staging of prostate cancer with transrectal ultrasound: a literature review. Prostate Suppl 1992;4:11–6.

110. Rifkin MD, Zerhouni EA, Gatsonis CA, et al. Comparison of magnetic resonance imaging and ultrasonography in staging early prostate cancer. Results of a multi-institutional cooperative trial. N Engl J Med 1990;323(10):621–6.

111. Smith JA Jr. Transrectal ultrasonography for the detection and staging of carcinoma of the prostate. J Clin Ultrasound 1996;24(8):455–61.

112. Hardeman SW, Causey JQ, Hickey DP, et al. Transrectal ultrasound for staging prior to radical prostatectomy. Urology 1989;34(4):175–80.

113. Akin O, Hricak H. Imaging of prostate cancer. Radiol Clin North Am 2007;45(1):207–22.

114. Cornud F, Hamida K, Flam T, et al. Endorectal color Doppler sonography and endorectal MR imaging features of nonpalpable prostate cancer: correlation with radical prostatectomy findings. AJR Am J Roentgenol 2000;175(4):1161–8.

115. Aigner F, Mitterberger M, Rehder P, et al. Status of transrectal ultrasound imaging of the prostate. J Endourol 2010;24(5):685–91.

116. Halpern EJ, Rosenberg M, Gomella LG. Prostate cancer: contrast-enhanced us for detection. Radiology 2001;219(1):219–25.

117. Pinto F, Totaro A, Palermo G, et al. Imaging in prostate cancer staging: present role and future perspectives. Urol Int 2012;88(2):125–36.

118. Yu KK, Hricak H. Imaging prostate cancer. Radiol Clin North Am 2000;38(1):59–85, viii.

119. Choi S. The role of magnetic resonance imaging in the detection of prostate cancer. J Urol 2011;186(4):1181–2.

120. Brown JA, Rodin DM, Harisinghani M, et al. Impact of preoperative endorectal MRI stage classification on neurovascular bundle sparing aggressiveness and the radical prostatectomy positive margin rate. Urol Oncol 2009;27(2):174–9.

121. Choi WW, Williams SB, Gu X, et al. Overuse of imaging for staging low risk prostate cancer. J Urol 2011;185(5):1645–9.

122. Engelbrecht MR, Jager GJ, Laheij RJ, et al. Local staging of prostate cancer using magnetic resonance imaging: a meta-analysis. Eur Radiol 2002;12(9):2294–302.

123. Harris RD, Schned AR, Heaney JA. Staging of prostate cancer with endorectal MR imaging: lessons from a learning curve. Radiographics 1995;15(4):813–29 [discussion: 829–32].

124. Sonnad SS, Langlotz CP, Schwartz JS. Accuracy of MR imaging for staging prostate cancer: a meta-analysis to examine the effect of technologic change. Acad Radiol 2001;8(2):149–57.

125. Wang L, Akin O, Mazaheri Y, et al. Are histopathological features of prostate cancer lesions associated with identification of extracapsular extension on magnetic resonance imaging? BJU Int 2010;106(9):1303–8.

126. Outwater EK, Petersen RO, Siegelman ES, et al. Prostate carcinoma: assessment of diagnostic criteria for capsular penetration on endorectal coil MR images. Radiology 1994;193(2):333–9.

127. Yu KK, Hricak H, Alagappan R, et al. Detection of extracapsular extension of prostate carcinoma with endorectal and phased-array coil MR imaging: multivariate feature analysis. Radiology 1997;202(3):697–702.

128. Wang L, Mullerad M, Chen HN, et al. Prostate cancer: incremental value of endorectal MR imaging findings for prediction of extracapsular extension. Radiology 2004;232(1):133–9.

129. Claus FG, Hricak H, Hattery RR. Pretreatment evaluation of prostate cancer: role of MR imaging and

1H MR spectroscopy. Radiographics 2004; 24(Suppl 1):S167–80.

130. Bloch BN, Genega EM, Costa DN, et al. Prediction of prostate cancer extracapsular extension with high spatial resolution dynamic contrast-enhanced 3-T MRI. Eur Radiol 2012. [Epub ahead of print].

131. Futterer JJ, Barentsz JO, Heijmink SW. Value of 3-T magnetic resonance imaging in local staging of prostate cancer. Top Magn Reson Imaging 2008; 19(6):285–9.

132. Wang L, Hricak H, Kattan MW, et al. Prediction of organ-confined prostate cancer: incremental value of MR imaging and MR spectroscopic imaging to staging nomograms. Radiology 2006; 238(2):597–603.

133. Hricak H. MR imaging and MR spectroscopic imaging in the pre-treatment evaluation of prostate cancer. Br J Radiol 2005;78(Spec No 2):S103–11.

134. Hovels AM, Heesakkers RA, Adang EM, et al. The diagnostic accuracy of CT and MRI in the staging of pelvic lymph nodes in patients with prostate cancer: a meta-analysis. Clin Radiol 2008;63(4):387–95.

135. Heesakkers RA, Hovels AM, Jager GJ, et al. MRI with a lymph-node-specific contrast agent as an alternative to CT scan and lymph-node dissection in patients with prostate cancer: a prospective multicohort study. Lancet Oncol 2008;9(9):850–6.

136. Harisinghani MG, Barentsz J, Hahn PF, et al. Noninvasive detection of clinically occult lymph-node metastases in prostate cancer. N Engl J Med 2003;348(25):2491–9.

137. Lutje S, Boerman OC, van Rij CM, et al. Prospects in radionuclide imaging of prostate cancer. Prostate 2012;72(11):1262–72.

138. Tosoian JJ, Trock BJ, Landis P, et al. Active surveillance program for prostate cancer: an update of the Johns Hopkins experience. J Clin Oncol 2011;29(16):2185–90.

139. Klotz L, Zhang L, Lam A, et al. Clinical results of long-term follow-up of a large, active surveillance cohort with localized prostate cancer. J Clin Oncol 2010;28(1):126–31.

140. Dall'Era MA, Konety BR, Cowan JE, et al. Active surveillance for the management of prostate cancer in a contemporary cohort. Cancer 2008; 112(12):2664–70.

141. Soloway MS, Soloway CT, Eldefrawy A, et al. Careful selection and close monitoring of low-risk prostate cancer patients on active surveillance minimizes the need for treatment. Eur Urol 2010; 58(6):831–5.

142. Margel D, Yap SA, Lawrentschuk N, et al. Impact of multiparametric endorectal coil prostate magnetic resonance imaging on disease reclassification among active surveillance candidates: a prospective cohort study. J Urol 2012;187(4):1247–52.

143. Sakai I, Harada K, Kurahashi T, et al. Usefulness of the nadir value of serum prostate-specific antigen measured by an ultrasensitive assay as a predictor of biochemical recurrence after radical prostatectomy for clinically localized prostate cancer. Urol Int 2006;76(3):227–31.

144. Salomon CG, Flisak ME, Olson MC, et al. Radical prostatectomy: transrectal sonographic evaluation to assess for local recurrence. Radiology 1993; 189(3):713–9.

145. Hricak H, Schoder H, Pucar D, et al. Advances in imaging in the postoperative patient with a rising prostate-specific antigen level. Semin Oncol 2003;30(5):616–34.

146. Saleem MD, Sanders H, Abu El Naser M, et al. Factors predicting cancer detection in biopsy of the prostatic fossa after radical prostatectomy. Urology 1998;51(2):283–6.

147. Naito S. Evaluation and management of prostate-specific antigen recurrence after radical prostatectomy for localized prostate cancer. Jpn J Clin Oncol 2005;35(7):365–74.

148. Cirillo S, Petracchini M, D'Urso L, et al. Endorectal magnetic resonance imaging and magnetic resonance spectroscopy to monitor the prostate for residual disease or local cancer recurrence after transrectal high-intensity focused ultrasound. BJU Int 2008;102(4):452–8.

149. Sala E, Eberhardt SC, Akin O, et al. Endorectal MR imaging before salvage prostatectomy: tumor localization and staging. Radiology 2006;238(1):176–83.

150. Kramer S, Gorich J, Gottfried HW, et al. Sensitivity of computed tomography in detecting local recurrence of prostatic carcinoma following radical prostatectomy. Br J Radiol 1997;70(838):995–9.

151. Sella T, Schwartz LH, Swindle PW, et al. Suspected local recurrence after radical prostatectomy: endorectal coil MR imaging. Radiology 2004;231(2): 379–85.

152. Sella T, Schwartz LH, Hricak H. Retained seminal vesicles after radical prostatectomy: frequency, MRI characteristics, and clinical relevance. AJR Am J Roentgenol 2006;186(2):539–46.

153. Silverman JM, Krebs TL. MR imaging evaluation with a transrectal surface coil of local recurrence of prostatic cancer in men who have undergone radical prostatectomy. AJR Am J Roentgenol 1997;168(2):379–85.

154. Cirillo S, Petracchini M, Scotti L, et al. Endorectal magnetic resonance imaging at 1.5 Tesla to assess local recurrence following radical prostatectomy using T2-weighted and contrast-enhanced imaging. Eur Radiol 2009;19(3):761–9.

155. Casciani E, Polettini E, Carmenini E, et al. Endorectal and dynamic contrast-enhanced MRI for detection of local recurrence after radical prostatectomy. AJR Am J Roentgenol 2008;190(5):1187–92.

156. Giannarini G, Nguyen DP, Thalmann GN, et al. Diffusion-weighted magnetic resonance imaging detects local recurrence after radical prostatectomy: initial experience. Eur Urol 2012;61(3): 616–20.

157. Sciarra A, Panebianco V, Salciccia S, et al. Role of dynamic contrast-enhanced magnetic resonance (MR) imaging and proton MR spectroscopic imaging in the detection of local recurrence after radical prostatectomy for prostate cancer. Eur Urol 2008;54(3):589–600.

158. Castellucci P, Fuccio C, Nanni C, et al. Influence of trigger PSA and PSA kinetics on 11C-Choline PET/CT detection rate in patients with biochemical relapse after radical prostatectomy. J Nucl Med 2009;50(9):1394–400.

159. Alfarone A, Panebianco V, Schillaci O, et al. Comparative analysis of multiparametric magnetic resonance and PET-CT in the management of local recurrence after radical prostatectomy for prostate cancer. Crit Rev Oncol Hematol 2012. [Epub ahead of print].

160. Krause BJ, Souvatzoglou M, Tuncel M, et al. The detection rate of [11C] choline-PET/CT depends on the serum PSA-value in patients with biochemical recurrence of prostate cancer. Eur J Nucl Med Mol Imaging 2008;35(1):18–23.

161. Heidenreich A, Bellmunt J, Bolla M, et al. EAU guidelines on prostate cancer. Part 1: screening, diagnosis, and treatment of clinically localised disease. Eur Urol 2011;59(1):61–71.

162. Pucar D, Sella T, Schoder H. The role of imaging in the detection of prostate cancer local recurrence after radiation therapy and surgery. Curr Opin Urol 2008;18(1):87–97.

163. Rouviere O, Valette O, Grivolat S, et al. Recurrent prostate cancer after external beam radiotherapy: value of contrast-enhanced dynamic MRI in localizing intraprostatic tumor–correlation with biopsy findings. Urology 2004;63(5):922–7.

164. Tamada T, Sone T, Jo Y, et al. Locally recurrent prostate cancer after high-dose-rate brachytherapy: the value of diffusion-weighted imaging, dynamic contrast-enhanced MRI, and T2-weighted imaging in localizing tumors. AJR Am J Roentgenol 2011;197(2):408–14.

165. Haider MA, Chung P, Sweet J, et al. Dynamic contrast-enhanced magnetic resonance imaging for localization of recurrent prostate cancer after external beam radiotherapy. Int J Radiat Oncol Biol Phys 2008;70(2):425–30.

166. Kim CK, Park BK, Lee HM. Prediction of locally recurrent prostate cancer after radiation therapy: incremental value of 3T diffusion-weighted MRI. J Magn Reson Imaging 2009;29(2):391–7.

167. Pickett B, Kurhanewicz J, Coakley F, et al. Use of MRI and spectroscopy in evaluation of external beam radiotherapy for prostate cancer. Int J Radiat Oncol Biol Phys 2004;60(4):1047–55.

168. Nguyen PL, Chen MH, D'Amico AV, et al. Magnetic resonance image-guided salvage brachytherapy after radiation in select men who initially presented with favorable-risk prostate cancer: a prospective phase 2 study. Cancer 2007;110(7):1485–92.

169. Albrecht S, Buchegger F, Soloviev D, et al. (11)C-acetate PET in the early evaluation of prostate cancer recurrence. Eur J Nucl Med Mol Imaging 2007;34(2):185–96.

170. Perlmutter MA, Lepor H. Prostate-specific antigen doubling time is a reliable predictor of imageable metastases in men with biochemical recurrence after radical retropubic prostatectomy. Urology 2008;71(3):501–5.

171. Choueiri TK, Dreicer R, Paciorek A, et al. A model that predicts the probability of positive imaging in prostate cancer cases with biochemical failure after initial definitive local therapy. J Urol 2008; 179(3):906–10 [discussion: 910].

172. Langsteger W, Balogova S, Huchet V, et al. Fluorocholine (^{18}F) and sodium fluoride (^{18}F) PET/CT in the detection of prostate cancer: prospective comparison of diagnostic performance determined by masked reading. Q J Nucl Med Mol Imaging 2011;55(4):448–57.

173. Schmidt GP, Kramer H, Reiser MF, et al. Whole-body magnetic resonance imaging and positron emission tomography-computed tomography in oncology. Top Magn Reson Imaging 2007;18(3):193–202.

174. Giovacchini G, Picchio M, Coradeschi E, et al. Predictive factors of [(11)C]choline PET/CT in patients with biochemical failure after radical prostatectomy. Eur J Nucl Med Mol Imaging 2010;37(2):301–9.

175. Scattoni V, Picchio M, Suardi N, et al. Detection of lymph-node metastases with integrated [^{11}C] choline PET/CT in patients with PSA failure after radical retropubic prostatectomy: results confirmed by open pelvic-retroperitoneal lymphadenectomy. Eur Urol 2007;52(2):423–9.

Imaging Prostate Cancer

Adam J. Jung, MD, PhD, Antonio C. Westphalen, MD, MAS*

KEYWORDS

- Prostate cancer • Magnetic resonance imaging • Magnetic resonance spectroscopic imaging
- Diffusion-weighted imaging • Dynamic contrast enhancement

KEY POINTS

- The primary diagnostic challenge in caring for patients with prostate cancer is our limited ability to accurately characterize the disease as indolent or aggressive at the time of presentation, and stratify management from active surveillance through definitive surgery or radiation accordingly.
- Recent advances in multiparametric endorectal magnetic resonance (MR) imaging promise to improve the characterization of prostate cancer.
- With the need to prevent overdiagnosis and overtreatment of clinically insignificant prostate cancers, MR imaging is playing an increasing role in the clinical management of patients.
- Although acceptance has increased substantially in the last few years, MR imaging of the prostate is standard of care in only a few large medical centers.
- Ultimately, new, faster, and more reproducible MR imaging techniques will emerge and new MR-based paradigms will result in improved risk assessment and personalized treatment for men with prostate cancer.

INTRODUCTION

With more than 241,000 new cases and 28,000 deaths predicted for 2012 in the United States, prostate cancer remains the most common noncutaneous cancer and second most common cause of death from cancer in men.[1] However, the large majority of cancers that are diagnosed through prostate-specific antigen (PSA) screening remain clinically insignificant, and the clinical decision to undergo definitive treatment versus more conservative active surveillance remains challenging.

The debate around the necessity to screen men with PSA has recently intensified, especially in view of the results of 2 large clinical trials,[2,3] reinforcing the understanding that PSA screening has led to overdiagnosis and overtreatment of prostate cancer. The major challenge in caring for patients with prostate cancer is, therefore, our limited ability to accurately characterize the disease as indolent or aggressive at the time of presentation, and adequately stratify management

from active surveillance through focal treatment, to definitive surgery or radiation therapy.

Contemporary multiparametric magnetic resonance (MR) imaging techniques aid initial diagnosis in a subset of patients and, more broadly, improve local staging, assessment of cancer aggressiveness, and decision making on treatment. This article presents a detailed description of MR imaging–based prostate anatomy, relevant sequences, and imaging findings used to accurately detect and characterize prostate cancer.

ANATOMY

A clear understanding of the prostatic anatomy is very important for adequate interpretation of imaging studies but also to facilitate clinical interactions with referring urologists. Multiparametric MR imaging with an endorectal coil provides fine anatomic detail of the prostate. Numerous descriptions of prostate zonal anatomy have evolved over recent decades[4,5]; however, this article presents

Department of Radiology and Biomedical Imaging, University of California San Francisco, 350 Parnassus Avenue, Suite 307, San Francisco, CA 94143, USA
* Corresponding author.
E-mail address: antonio.westphalen@ucsf.edu

Radiol Clin N Am 50 (2012) 1043–1059
http://dx.doi.org/10.1016/j.rcl.2012.08.001

a contemporary radiologic description that is most relevant to MR imaging.

The prostate can be thought of as an inverted cone on coronal images. Similar to the human heart, the apex and base refer to the most caudal and cranial aspects of the prostate gland, respectively. The midgland is sandwiched in between these levels, resulting in the common cranial to caudal prostate levels: the base, midgland, and apex (**Figs. 1** and **2**). On sagittal imaging, the gland lies with its long axis parallel to the anterior rectal wall (**Fig. 3**). The prostate is bordered along its superior aspect by the bladder ventrally and the seminal vesicles more dorsally. Similarly, the urogenital diaphragm demarcates the gland's inferiormost border. The prostate is separated from the rectum posteriorly by a thin (2–3 mm) fascial layer know as the Denovillier fascia. The levator ani and obturator interni muscles border the lateral walls of the prostate along its caudal and cranial margins, respectively. The Santorini plexus of veins and the pubic symphysis border the prostate anteriorly.

The prostate gland can be divided into glandular and nonglandular components. The fibromuscular stroma and prostatic urethra make up the nonglandular components. The fibromuscular stroma is located directly anterior to the urethra and is a common site of central-gland cancers.

The proximal prostatic urethra begins at the central prostate base and extends to the level of the midgland, where the ejaculatory ducts enter the prostatic urethra at the verumontanum. These paired ejaculatory ducts begin at the inferomedial aspect of the seminal vesicles and extend within the midline of the peripheral zone before angulating anteriorly toward the verumontanum (see **Fig. 3**). The more distal urethra also angulates slightly anteriorly at the verumontanum (see **Fig. 3**), and can sometimes be seen as an inverted "Y" or "V" on axial T2-weighted MR imaging (see **Fig. 2**). The preprostatic and distal prostatic sphincters are largely responsible for urinary continence. The preprostatic sphincter encases the urethra and periurethral glandular tissue, extending from the bladder neck to the verumontanum. The distal prostatic sphincter starts at the prostatic apex and continues through the urogenital diaphragm to the penile corpus spongiosum.[6]

The peripheral zone, central zone, transition zone, and periurethral glandular tissue constitute the glandular components of the prostate. More practically, the prostate can be divided into 2 major compartments consisting of the peripheral zone and the central gland. On imaging, it is analogous to a baseball within a baseball mitt whereby the ball represents the central gland and the mitt represents the peripheral gland (see **Fig. 2**). The peripheral zone encompasses nearly 70% of the prostate in young males. It surrounds the entire posterolateral aspect of the gland and extends anterolaterally toward the anterior fibromuscular stroma, but does not extend beyond it. The peripheral zone is high in water content, giving it its typical high-signal appearance on T2-weighted MR imaging. The radiologic description of the peripheral zone can be further divided and labeled as the anterior horn, lateral, and paramedian regions (**Fig. 4**). Seventy percent to 75% of prostate cancers arise in the peripheral zone.

The central gland consists of the transition zone, central zone, and periurethral glandular tissue. The periurethral glandular tissue represents less than 1% of the volume of the prostate. In the young male the transition and central zones consist of approximately 5% and 25% of the gland, respectively (**Fig. 5**). This allocation changes with the development of benign prostatic hyperplasia (BPH), the transition zone becoming the predominant component of the central gland (see **Fig. 5**). The enlargement of the transition zone condenses the surrounding central zone into a thin rim, which serves as the pseudocapsule used as the plane for surgical treatment of BPH. The true fibromuscular capsule of the prostate surrounds its external surface and has low signal intensity on T2-weighted MR images, but is not always clearly seen. The central gland is typically randomly heterogeneous on T2-weighted MR images, with foci of high and low signal intensity that are often

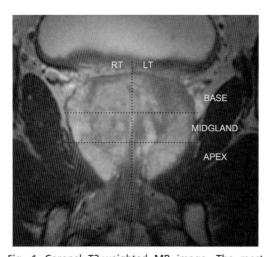

Fig. 1. Coronal T2-weighted MR image. The most superior aspect of the prostate is called the base, and the inferior portion is the apex. The midgland is situated between the apex and the base. Further subdivision of these levels into right and left derives the sextant nomenclature.

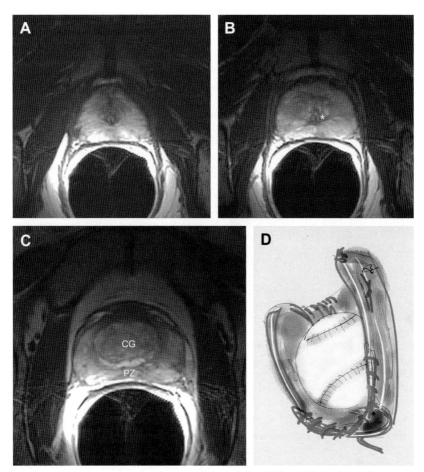

Fig. 2. Axial T2-weighted MR images depict the apex (*A*), midgland (*B*), and base (*C*) of the prostate. The apex is almost entirely made up of peripheral zone glandular tissue. The urethra is seen at the level of the verumontanum as an inverted "V" in the midgland (*asterisk* in *B*). The relationship between the peripheral zone and the central gland is similar to that of a baseball in a baseball mitt (*D*). The ball represents the central gland and the mitt, the peripheral zone. CG, central gland; PZ, peripheral zone.

nodular in appearance. BPH nodules very often demonstrate a thin, well-defined rim of low T2 signal intensity (**Fig. 6**). Lack of this capsule has been described as a sign associated with central-gland cancers. Signal characteristics of BPH on T2-weighted MR imaging are largely related to the composition of the BPH nodules, with predominantly stromal and collagen-filled nodules being hypointense and highly glandular BPH nodules being hyperintense.

The seminal vesicles are paired lobulated glands found immediately superior to the prostate base and posteroinferiorly to the bladder. These vesicles taper distally into a small duct that joins the vas deferens to form the ejaculatory duct. The seminal vesicles can be best visualized on coronal and axial T2-weighted MR images as elongated, multiseptated, fluid-filled structures. Seminal vesicles may be fully or partially expanded.

IMAGING FINDINGS

Transrectal Ultrasonography and Transrectal Ultrasound–Guided Biopsy

The diagnosis, management, and prognosis of prostate cancer are largely dependent on histopathological features obtained by transrectal ultrasonography and transrectal ultrasound (TRUS)-guided biopsy. TRUS-guided biopsy uses B-mode and color Doppler imaging to localize the prostate, target suspicious areas, and systematically obtain anywhere from 6 to more than 40 18-gauge biopsy cores. Typically the prostate gland is scanned in the axial plane, from the apex to the base. The seminal vesicles are identified bilaterally, using an oblique sagittal view that also demonstrates the ampulla of the vas deferens. The peripheral zone has high echogenicity and is routinely distinguished from the

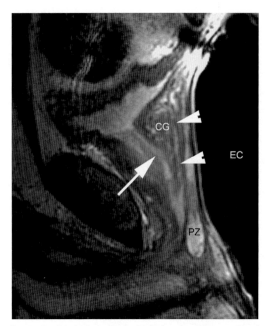

Fig. 3. Sagittal T2-weighted MR image. The urethra is identified centrally as an ill-defined line of high signal intensity (*arrow*), and an ejaculatory duct is seen entering the urethra at the level of the verumontanum (*arrowheads*). CG, central gland; EC, endorectal coil; PZ, peripheral zone.

central gland, which is typically hypoechoic and heterogeneous owing to BPH (**Fig. 7**). Prostate cancer is characteristically identified as a round or oval focus of low echogenicity in the peripheral zone (**Fig. 8**). Transrectal ultrasonography, however, does not visualize all malignant foci because 37% to 50% of cancers are isoechoic or only slightly hypoechoic when compared with the peripheral zone.[7] B-mode transrectal ultrasonography has very limited ability to identify tumors in the central gland. It has been shown that some prostate cancers demonstrate increased flow on color Doppler, a feature that is also used to guide biopsies.[8] Because of these sampling errors,

however, the reported false-negative rate of TRUS-guided biopsy reaches up to 30%.[9] In addition, Gleason scores established through TRUS-guided biopsy are often discordant with prostatectomy specimens. TRUS-guided biopsy underestimates the score of cancer in up to 38% of patients, therefore misrepresenting tumor aggressiveness.[10] The volume of disease can be estimated based on the number of positive biopsy cores and on the percentage of tumor seen in positive cores. These criteria, however, are also dependent on the accuracy of TRUS-guided biopsy. Multiple risk-stratification schemes are available to predict prognosis and aid in the decision to undergo active surveillance versus definitive forms of treatment.[11,12] These criteria rely heavily on the histopathologic findings of Gleason grade and extent of tumor seen in the TRUS-guided core biopsy specimens, which in turn are inextricably related to the region of the prostate that is sampled.

Computed Tomography

Computed tomography (CT) has no established role in the diagnosis of prostate cancer, but may be considered for the staging of men with high-risk prostate cancer. High risk is usually defined as total serum PSA greater than 20.0 ng/mL, locally advanced disease on clinical assessment, or Gleason score greater than or equal to 8. Identification of pelvic lymphadenopathy on CT depends on lymph node enlargement, and the correlation between nodal size and metastatic involvement is poor. Even in patients with high-risk cancer, the sensitivity of CT scanning for detecting positive nodes is only about 35%. Although osseous metastases can be identified on CT, the method is usually used to follow up patients with known metastatic disease rather than to diagnose it. Bone scintigraphy is significantly more sensitive than CT for the detection of bone metastasis, and many patients with positive radionuclide scans have normal CT. Metastatic prostate cancer is an osteoblastic process and treated disease is characterized by increased density of the lesion, therefore care must be taken not to overcall osseous metastasis, especially following systemic therapy (**Fig. 9**).

Radionuclide Scans

Whole-body bone scintigraphy is the method of choice for the detection of bone metastases in patients with prostate cancer. A bone scan will identify osseous metastases in fewer than 5% of men with a serum PSA equal to or less than 20 ng/mL, whereas approximately 15% of men with PSA levels greater than 20.0 ng/mL have a positive

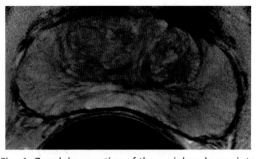

Fig. 4. Zonal demarcation of the peripheral zone into the anterior horn (*blue*), lateral (*red*), and paramedian (*green*) regions. Central gland is highlighted in yellow.

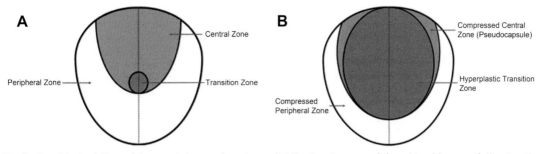

Fig. 5. Graphic depiction of the prostate zonal anatomy distribution in young (*A*) and in older men following the development of benign prostatic hyperplasia (BPH) (*B*).

scan. Accordingly, a bone scan is not recommended to all patients and is typically reserved for men with high-risk disease, symptomatic patients, or patients whose examination suggests the presence of metastases. Osseous metastases of prostate cancer usually present as focal areas of radiotracer uptake in the axial skeleton, in particular pelvic bones (**Fig. 10**). Bone scans are also used to monitor disease after systemic therapy, and good response to treatment is characterized by progressive decrease of radiotracer uptake. In some patients, however, a flare phenomenon may be seen in the first weeks after therapy. The flare phenomenon is characterized by increased uptake of radiotracer because of increased osteoclast turnover associated with healing. Single-photon emission CT (SPECT) is another method

used to detect bone metastases. SPECT is essentially the same examination as a planar scintigraphy, except that it is a tomographic technique, and therefore more accurately localizes disease. Other radionuclide examinations, including positron emission tomography/CT, are not routinely used to investigate patients with prostate cancer.

Magnetic Resonance Imaging

Endorectal multiparametric MR imaging uses anatomic T1-weighted and T2-weighted MR imaging, diffusion-weighted MR imaging (DWI), MR spectroscopic imaging (MRSI), and perfusion-based dynamic contrast-enhanced (DCE) MR imaging to localize, characterize, and stage prostate cancers. In addition, studies have shown that MR imaging may provide prognostic information that is incremental to that obtained with commonly used risk assessment/stratification tools.[13,14]

T1-weighted MR imaging
The prostate demonstrates homogeneous low signal intensity on T1-weighted MR images, making it difficult to discern the zonal anatomy and extremely difficult to identify cancer. T1-weighted MR images are obtained to evaluate for postbiopsy

Fig. 6. Axial T2-weighted MR image. BPH is characterized by hypertrophy of the transitional zone with associated compression of the central zone, creating the pseudocapsule (*arrowheads*). The peripheral zone can also be compressed with extensive BPH changes (PZ). Note the typical appearance of a BPH nodule with its thin rim of low signal intensity (*arrow*). CG, central gland.

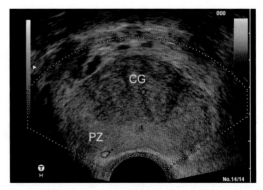

Fig. 7. Axial power Doppler transrectal ultrasound image depicts the typical echogenicities of the peripheral zone (PZ) and central gland (CG). No focal abnormalities are seen.

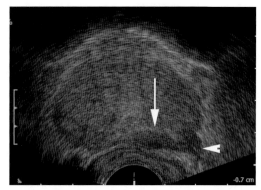

Fig. 8. Axial gray-scale transrectal ultrasound image. Prostate cancer typically has low echogenicity when compared with the peripheral zone (*arrow*). Note the presence of extracapsular extension (*arrowhead*).

hemorrhage and to assess lymph nodes and osseous structures.

Postbiopsy hemorrhage appears as areas of high T1 signal intensity within the otherwise homogeneous prostate. On T2-weighted images, however, postbiopsy hemorrhage has low signal intensity and can mimic the appearance of cancer and/or lead to an inaccurate estimate of its volume (**Fig. 11**). Postbiopsy hemorrhage has also been shown to affect the diagnostic accuracy of DCE, DWI, and MRSI.[15,16] Hence, an interval of 6 to 8 weeks between a prostate biopsy and MR imaging is recommended to allow for the resorption of all blood products (see **Fig. 11**). It is interesting, however, that in some patients postbiopsy hemorrhage can outline the tumor, allowing for its identification of T1-weighted MR images.

As with CT, lymph node evaluation is limited on MR imaging because size thresholds have limited sensitivity and specificity for detecting metastases. The availability of new lymphotropic paramagnetic iron oxide particle agents in the future may increase the overall accuracy for the detection of metastatic lymph nodes.

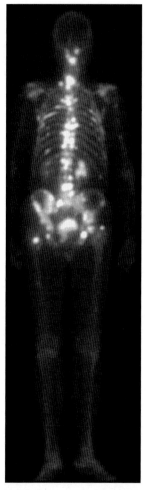

Fig. 10. Total body bone scan, anteroposterior projection. Multiple focal areas of uptake are seen, in particular in the axial skeleton, consistent with metastatic disease.

T2-weighted MR imaging

High-resolution T2-weighted MR imaging offers superior soft-tissue contrast and clear depiction of prostatic zonal anatomy in multiple planes,

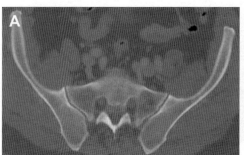
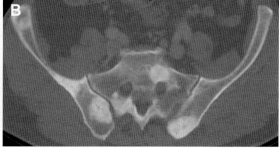

Fig. 9. Axial contrast-enhanced CT images of the pelvic bones. Pretreatment image did not identify any focal abnormalities (*A*). A follow-up 6 months after treatment (*B*) demonstrates multiple sclerotic foci, consistent with treatment response in this man with very low serum PSA.

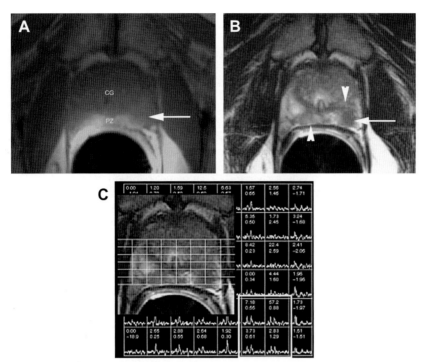

Fig. 11. Axial T1-weighted and T2-weighted MR images, and MR spectroscopic image. High signal intensity within the peripheral zone on the T1-weighted MR image is consistent with postbiopsy hemorrhage (*A*). Note a focal round area in the left peripheral zone that is spared of hemorrhage (*arrow* in *A*). This finding is consistent with the presence of prostate cancer (T1 halo sign). On the T2-weighted MR image this area has low signal intensity, consistent with prostate cancer (*arrow* in *B*); its boundaries, however, are indistinct because of the presence of adjacent low signal secondary to postbiopsy hemorrhage (*arrowheads* in *B*). Cancerous metabolism is seen on the MR spectroscopic image (highlighted with *thicker white border* in *C*). CG, central gland; PZ, peripheral zone.

and is the mainstay of MR imaging of the prostate. More than 95% of prostate cancers are adenocarcinoma, of which more than 70% occur within the peripheral zone. Most of these cancers demonstrate low signal intensity on the background of bright peripheral zone tissue (**Fig. 12**), because of the loss of the normal glandular (ductal) morphology that occurs in prostate cancer. Other benign abnormalities (eg, inflammation, stromal BPH, fibrosis/scarring) and therapeutic changes (eg, radiation, hormone ablation) may also demonstrate low T2 signal intensity on MR images.[17] Nevertheless, an infiltrating prostate cancer may cause minimal reduction in glandular morphology and be isointense on T2-weighted imaging.[17] Signal intensity is also likely related to the amount of mucin associated with the cancer, which is particularly evident during the assessment of mucinous adenocarcinomas.[18,19] Consequently, T2-weighted MR imaging alone has demonstrated limited ability to diagnose prostate cancer. Rosenkrantz and colleagues[20] recently reported an overall diagnostic accuracy of approximately 60% for two separate readers. Accuracy declines further in posttherapeutic glands because of

atrophy and homogeneous reduction in signal intensity as well as loss of zonal anatomy on T2-weighted MR imaging.[6,21,22] Overall detection and characterization of prostate cancer can be significantly improved through the addition of various functional sequences to anatomic imaging and by performing the multiparametric examination at higher magnetic-field strengths.[23]

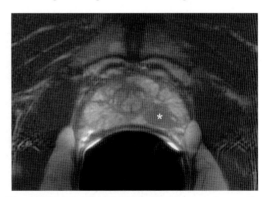

Fig. 12. Axial T2-weighted MR image shows the typical appearance of prostate cancer within the peripheral zone: a focal round area of low signal intensity (*asterisk*).

Central-gland tumors represent the remaining 20% to 30% of prostate cancers. These tumors also usually have low signal intensity of T2-weighted MR images and are difficult to distinguish from normal central-gland tissue, in particular in the presence of BPH. Central-gland tumors can be identified as an ill-defined flat area of low signal intensity that infiltrates or replaces the more random and heterogeneous appearance of BPH (**Fig. 13**).

T2-weighted MR imaging is also the primary sequence used to evaluate locoregional spread of cancer.[24–33] Prognosis, management, and treatment options of prostate cancer are greatly affected by cancer stage. Specifically, cancers with extracapsular extension (ECE) and/or seminal vesicle invasion (SVI), denoted as stage T3A and T3B, respectively, have worse prognosis and are more likely to recur following surgical or radiation therapy. T2-weighted axial MR imaging criteria for ECE include: (1) asymmetry of neurovascular bundles, (2) obliteration of the rectoprostatic angle, (3) bulging of the prostatic contour, and (4) capsular irregularity associated with tumor signal in the periprostatic fat (**Fig. 14**). The true prostatic capsule is incompletely identified as a thin 1-mm line of low T2-weighted signal that surrounds the gland, and care must be taken not to overcall ECE. The neurovascular bundle is best appreciated on T2-weighted axial images as small lines and dots of low signal clustered in the bilateral rectoprostatic angles (see **Fig. 14**). Prostate cancer frequently extends beyond the capsule following the course of the neurovascular bundles, as these are regions of capsular vulnerability. Cancers in the prostatic base can extend directly into the adjacent seminal vesicles. Seminal-vesicle invasion is usually the result of direct extension of a tumor located at the base of the prostate. It is best appreciated on axial and coronal T2-weighted images as foci of low signal intensity that partly or entirely obliterates the lumen on the seminal vesicle (**Fig. 15**).

Diffusion-weighted MR imaging/apparent diffusion coefficient maps

DWI has quickly evolved to become one of the most relevant sequences for imaging prostate cancer. DWI uses changes in the Brownian motion of water molecules in tissues at the microscopic scale. The rate of diffusion in soft tissues is lower than in free solution and is described by the apparent diffusion coefficient (ADC), which correlates inversely with tissue cellularity. In prostate cancer, the increased cellularity and associated loss of ductal morphology results in a smaller extracellular space, resulting in the restriction of water diffusion and a corresponding reduction in ADC values (**Fig. 16**).[34] A recent meta-analysis demonstrated the sensitivity and specificity of DWI when added to T2-weighted imaging to range from 65% to 84% and 77% to 87%, respectively.[35] Other studies have demonstrated an inverse relationship between Gleason grade and ADC values in peripheral-zone cancers and its ability to discriminate between low-, intermediate-, and high-grade tumors.[36–39] Diffusion restriction is especially useful in detecting anterior central-gland cancer (see **Fig. 13**). There is, however, significant overlap of ADC values of benign and malignant tissues, and ADC findings should be used in conjunction with T2-weighted MR imaging and other available imaging parameters. DWI is also an important technique for the identification of locally recurrent disease after treatment, in particular after radiation therapy (**Fig. 17**).[40]

Proton (¹H) MR spectroscopy imaging

Proton (¹H) MR spectroscopy imaging (MRSI) depicts the metabolic profile of the various tissues found in the prostate.

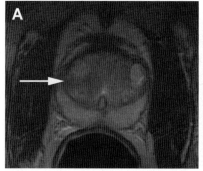
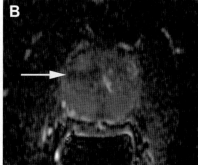

Fig. 13. Axial T2-weighted MR image and apparent diffusion coefficient (ADC) map shows a right central-gland tumor. On the T2-weighted MR image, the tumor has low signal intensity, ill-defined borders, and infiltrative pattern (*arrow in A*). The tumor is much more distinct on the ADC map, which demonstrates marked diffusion restriction (*arrow in B*).

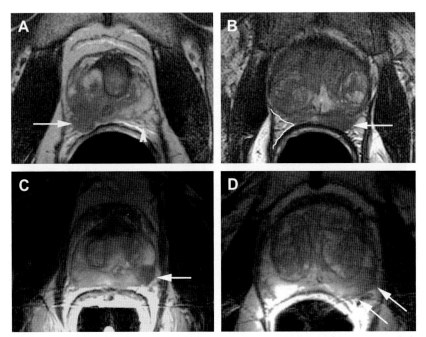

Fig. 14. Axial T2-weighted MR images depict 4 imaging patterns of extracapsular extension: asymmetry of the neurovascular bundles (*A*), obliteration of the rectoprostatic angle (*B*), bulging of the prostatic contour (*C*), and capsular irregularity associated with tumor signal in the periprostatic fat (*D*). The normal left neurovascular bundle (*arrowhead*) and right-sided extracapsular extension (*arrow*) are depicted in *A*. The normal right rectoprostatic angle (*white line*) and left-sided obliteration (*arrow*) are depicted in *B*. Bulging of a left peripheral zone tumor beyond the expected contour of the prostate is shown in *C* (*arrow*). A "spiculated" contour of the prostate, or capsular irregularity, caused by extracapsular extension of a left peripheral zone tumor is shown in *D* (*arrows*).

Metabolic spectra from volumes of interest (voxels) that encompass prostate cancer demonstrate increased levels of choline (Cho) and decreased levels of citrate (Cit) and polyamines (Fig. 18). The elevation in the concentration of Cho is mostly related to the increased cell membrane turnover associated with neoplastic proliferation. Cit and polyamines are abundantly found in normal prostatic tissue, which is replaced by abnormal cells. A creatine (Cr) peak is also visualized and serves as an internal reference. The areas under each metabolite peak represent the relative metabolite concentrations, and these are usually quantified using the (Cho + Cr)/Cit ratio. ^{1}H-MRSI findings can then be quantified and scored from 1 to 5, with higher scores representing higher likelihood of cancer. This quantitative approach to ^{1}H-MRSI has been standardized and is depicted in Fig. 19.[41] When the (Cho + Cr)/Cit ratio is 3 or more standard deviations above the normal value, there is minimal overlap between spectroscopic voxels from regions of cancer and healthy

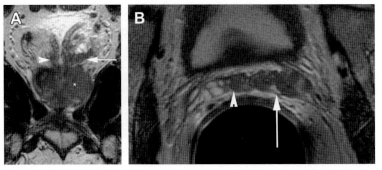

Fig. 15. Coronal and axial T2-weighted MR images show direct extension of a large central-gland tumor (*asterisk* in *A*) into the right and left seminal vesicles (*arrows* and *arrowheads* in *A* and *B*).

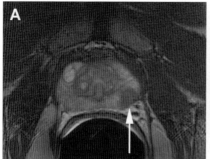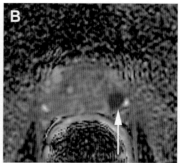

Fig. 16. Axial T2-weighted MR image (*A*) and ADC map (*B*) show a left peripheral zone cancer (*arrow*) at the level of the midgland. ADC map depicts avid diffusion restriction.

peripheral-zone tissues.[42] It has also been shown that the magnitude of elevation of the (Cho + Cr)/Cit ratio positively correlates with grade of prostate cancer.[43–45] Qualitatively, ^{1}H-MRSI data can be quickly interpreted by drawing a line from the top of the Cho peak to the top of the Cit peak. The more negative the slope, the more likely it is to represent a cancer-containing voxel. A positive slope indicates a noncancerous voxel (**Fig. 20**).

Previous studies have demonstrated that the addition of ^{1}H-MRSI to T2-weighted MR imaging improves tumor localization,[46] volume estimation,[47] staging,[31] tissue characterization,[44] and identification of recurrent disease after therapy (see **Fig. 17**).[48] A recent multicenter study supported by the American College of Radiology Imaging Network, however, showed that the combination of ^{1}H-MRSI and T2-weighted MR images does not improve tumor detection in patients with low-grade, low-volume disease selected to undergo radical prostatectomy.[49] These results suggest that positive ^{1}H-MRSI findings are more likely to reflect higher tumor grade and/or volume, as demonstrated by Shukla-Dave and Colleagues[50] in a study that

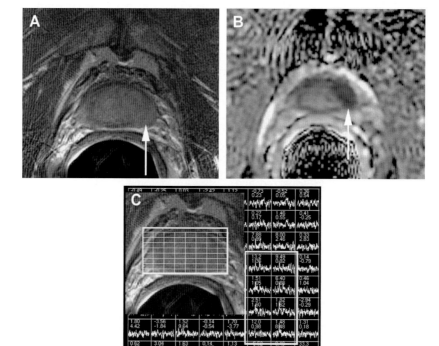

Fig. 17. Axial T2-weighted MR image (*A*), ADC map (*B*), and MR spectroscopic image obtained after radiation therapy in a man with rising PSA. Recurrent cancer is inconspicuous on T2-weighted MR imaging (*arrow* in *A*), but easily characterized on the ADC map (*arrow* in *B*) and MR spectroscopic image (neoplastic metabolism highlighted with *thicker white border* in *C*).

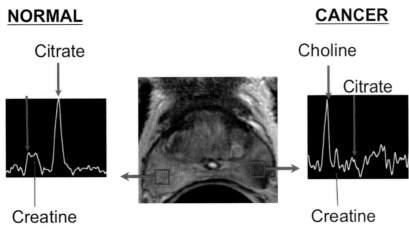

Fig. 18. Normal prostatic tissue is characterized by low choline and high citrate (*right*), whereas cancerous tissue demonstrates elevated choline (*left*) in the regions of corresponding T2-weighted image abnormality.

found ¹H-MRSI to improve the prediction of insignificant prostate cancer in low-risk patients.

Dynamic contrast-enhanced MR imaging

DCE MR imaging relies on tumor neoangiogenesis for detection and characterization of prostate cancer. In prostate cancer, the number of vessels (microvascular density) is increased in comparison with the surrounding normal tissue, leading to greater relative tumoral enhancement. Also, these new vessels demonstrate poor organization and wall integrity, which result in increased wall permeability and contrast leakage in the extravascular-extracellular space (EES).

DCE MR imaging can be evaluated both qualitatively and quantitatively. The former uses direct visualization of early and intense enhancement and rapid washout seen in prostate cancer. Intensity-versus-time curves can then be generated to evaluate time to peak, maximum uptake slope, peak enhancement, area under the enhancement curve, and washout rates. Newer software is able to generate these curves along with color maps for easier interpretation (**Fig. 21**). This qualitative approach to DCE MR imaging tends to be more accurate for large and high-grade cancers because of reader subjectivity, interscanner and interpatient variability, and significant overlap of enhancement characteristics with benign tissues, for example, prostatitis and hypervascular stromal BPH nodules.

The quantitative approach uses pharmacokinetic parameters to describe tissue vascularization

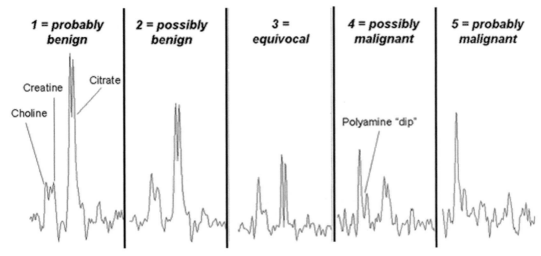

Fig. 19. Standardized evaluation and scoring of MRSI data on a scale of 1 to 5 based on changes in choline, citrate, polyamines, and signal-to-noise ratio. (*Data from* Jung JA, Coakley FV, Vigneron DB, et al. Prostate depiction at endorectal MR spectroscopic imaging: investigation of a standardized evaluation system. Radiology 2004;233:701–8.)

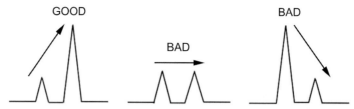

GOOD   BAD   BAD

Fig. 20. Pattern approach to interpretation of MR spectroscopic imaging. The slope of a line drawn from the choline to citrate peak can be used to qualitatively and quickly assess the likelihood of a cancer within a voxel. A positive slope indicates a benign voxel. Flat or negative slopes indicate an increasing likelihood of cancer.

and blood flow. These pharmacokinetic parameters are derived from mathematical pharmacokinetic models. The model most commonly used in prostate cancer was developed by Tofts.[51] This model assumes that gadolinium contrast transfers between 2 compartments, the intravascular space and the EES, and that this exchange is secondary to blood flow and vascular permeability. Three values are important for this particular model: the inflow kinetic constant K^{trans}, the outflow kinetic constant k_{ep}, and the volume v_e, or leakage space, which is the ratio of volume of EES per unit volume of tissue. Prostate cancer demonstrates increases in v_e, and K^{trans} and k_{ep} rate constants.[52] Newer software can generate v_e, K^{trans}, and k_{ep} maps, making interpretation less cumbersome.

The arterial input function (AIF) is another crucial value for DCE MR imaging. AIF is the concentration of gadolinium in the arterial blood plasma that is being supplied to a tissue. A direct measure of AIF is difficult, as the relationship between signal intensity and gadolinium concentration is not linear as with CT-based contrast agents. To overcome this problem, the Tofts model uses a population-averaged AIF; other models calculate individual values from T1 map datasets that must be generated to convert signal intensity seen on T1-weighted imaging into time-dependent gadolinium concentration curves.

Overall, DCE imaging has reported sensitivities and specificities ranging from 46% to 96% and 75% to 96%, respectively.[53] DCE imaging can

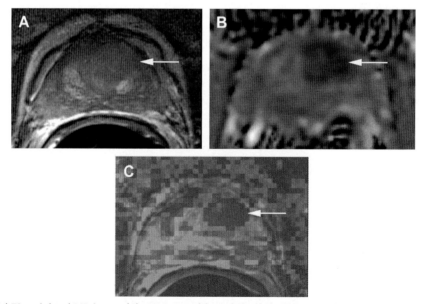

Fig. 21. Axial T2-weighted MR image (A), ADC map (B), and dynamic contrast-enhanced MR image (C). A large anterior central-gland tumor missed on transrectal ultrasound-guided biopsy is shown (arrows in A, B and C). On T2-weighted MR imaging, the tumor has a more flat appearance compared with the replaced heterogeneity of BPH. The ADC map demonstrates clear restriction of diffusion. A color map of peak enhancement depicts rapid contrast uptake by the tumor.

also potentially provide information on cancer aggressiveness based on histologic grade. Initial data also suggest that DCE imaging may be able to detect residual or recurrent cancer after therapy, based on a more dramatic contrast uptake and washout in comparison with surrounding regions of atrophy and benign tissues.

DIAGNOSTIC CRITERIA FOR PROSTATE CANCER

- T2-weighted imaging: Round/ellipsoid focus of low signal in the peripheral zone, ill-defined infiltrative pattern in the central gland
- DWI: Diffusion restriction (ie, low signal on ADC maps)
- ^{1}H-MRSI: Elevated Cho, decreased Cit and polyamine peaks, high (Cho + Cr)/Cit ratio, negative slope on qualitative interpretation
- DCE: Early and high peak enhancement, increased area under the enhancement curve, rapid washout; elevated v_e, K^{trans}, and k_{ep} using quantitative models

DIFFERENTIAL DIAGNOSIS

- Low signal on T2-weighted MR imaging can be seen with fibrosis/scarring, stromal BPH, inflammation, dysplasia/high-grade prostatic intraepithelial neoplasia (HGPIN), infection, treatment effects, and postbiopsy hemorrhage.
- Increased diffusion restriction can be seen in fibrosis/scarring, dysplasia/HGPIN, and stromal BPH.
- Elevated (Cho + Cr)/Cit ratios can be seen in prostatitis.
- Increased rate and total enhancement can be seen in prostatitis and hypervascular or stromal BPH.

PEARLS, PITFALLS, AND VARIANTS

- Take advantage of all MR imaging parameters available, with an emphasis on T2-weighted imaging for anatomic descriptions.
- Rely on DWI (ADC maps) for assessment of central-gland tumors.
- Tumors with high Gleason score (ie, more aggressive lesions) tend to demonstrate more apparent imaging findings on all parameters.
- Metastases to bones and lymph nodes are not common, in particular in the population undergoing MR imaging.
- Evaluate for postbiopsy hemorrhage on T1-weighted imaging.

- Ignore nonspecific, streaky regions of decreased signal on T2-weighted MR imaging, in particular when not associated with abnormalities in other sequences.

MR IMAGING PROTOCOL

Multicoil MR imaging using the body coil for excitation and combined endorectal and phased-array coils for signal reception has been established as an adequate technique for both 1.5-T and 3-T systems.[32,54,55] The theoretical 2-fold increase in the signal-to-noise ratio achieved on 3-T relative to 1.5-T systems can be used to increase spatial resolution, to increase temporal resolution of DCE studies, or to diminish overall scan time. **Table 1** describes in detail the acquisition parameters used in the authors' institution.

T1-Weighted Images

Axial plane, non–fat-saturated gradient-echo T1-weighted images are obtained from the pubic symphysis to the aortic bifurcation. This sequence is the only large field-of-view sequence of the pelvis that is obtained, and is used primarily to evaluate for the presence of postbiopsy hemorrhage in the prostate, pelvic lymphadenopathy, and, albeit partly, pelvic osseous metastases.

T2-Weighted MR Imaging

Small field-of-view multiplanar, fat-saturated, high-resolution turbo-spin-echo T2-weighted image of the prostate is the primary sequence used for assessment of prostate cancer. Images are acquired in the axial, sagittal, and coronal planes.

DWI/ADC Maps

Axial-plane, single-shot echo-planar DWI and ADC maps are used in adjunct to T2-weighted MR imaging to increase overall accuracy of detection of prostate cancer in regions of concurrent low or normal T2 signal intensity. The degree of ADC signal loss is also useful for approximating cancer aggressiveness. It is particularly useful for tumors located in the central gland.

^{1}H-MRSI

^{1}H-MRSI of the prostate is acquired using a combination of point-resolved spectroscopy volume localization and 3-dimensional chemical shift imaging to acquire arrays of ^{1}H spectra from the entire prostate gland.[56] Acquisition of prostate ^{1}H-MRSI data requires very accurate volume selection and efficient outer volume suppression techniques. MRSI data provide a metabolic profile of the gland and are helpful in characterizing

Table 1
Prostate imaging prescriptions for pelvic-phased array and medrad endorectal coils

	T1-Weighted	T2-Weighted	T2-Weighted	T2-Weighted	MRSI (GE)	DCE (Pre/Post)	EPI Diffusion
Plane	Axial	Sagittal	Axial	Coronal	Axial	Axial	Axial
Pulse sequence	3D FSPGR (24° flip)	T2 FSE	T2 FSE	T2 FSE	PROSE 3D MRSI	3D FSPGR (12° flip)	2D EPI
TE	In phase	102	96	102	130 (85)	2.1	Minimum
TR	5650	5650	6000	4825 (6000)	1000 (1300)	5	5000
FOV	24	14	14	16 (14)	11	460	24
Thickness	4	3	3	3	50	2.7	4
Spacing	0	0	0	0	6.9	0	0
Frequency	192	256	256	256	16 (12)	192	256 (128)
Phase	128	192	192	192	8	128	128
NEX	3	3	3	3	1	1	4
Frequency direction	A/P	R/L	A/P	A/P	R/L	A/P	R/L
Other						Temporal resolution: 6.5 s, 50 time points / Injection rate: 2 mL/s; delay 0.25 s	Minimum b = 800

Parameters are for 1.5 T and 3 T; however, values in parentheses are prescribed differently for 3-T examinations.

Abbreviations: 2D, 2-dimensional; 3D, 3-dimensional; A/P, anterior/posterior; DCE, dynamic contrast enhanced; EPI, echo planar imaging; FOV, field of view; FSE, fast spin echo; FSPGR, fast spoiled gradient echo; GE, gradient echo; MRSI, magnetic resonance spectroscopy imaging; NEX, number of excitations; PROSE, prostate spectroscopy and imaging exam; R/L, right/left; TE, echo time; TR, repetition time.

suspicious foci on T2-weighted MR imaging and DWI. Spectroscopic abnormalities have also been shown to correlate with Gleason score.

DCE MR Imaging

Axial pregadolinium- and postgadolinium-enhanced contrast images are obtained using a 3-dimensional T1-weighted gradient-echo sequence over a 4-minute period using high temporal (5–10 seconds) and spatial resolutions to evaluate the perfusional characteristics of prostate cancer. This sequence is used in conjunction with T2-weighted MR imaging, DWI, and ¹H-MRSI to improve cancer detection. It is particularly useful for tumors located in the peripheral zone.

INFORMATION FOR REFERRING PHYSICIANS

- MR imaging with an endorectal coil is the optimal technique for staging prostate cancer. MR imaging is recommended, but not required, for the detection and localization of prostate cancer.
- Patients tolerate the endorectal coil very well, and complications are extremely rare.
- If an endorectal coil is not going to be used, it is recommended that imaging is performed using a 3.0-T MR scanner.

SUMMARY

The primary diagnostic challenge in caring for patients with prostate cancer is our limited ability to accurately characterize the disease as indolent or aggressive at the time of presentation, and to stratify management from active surveillance through definitive surgery or radiation accordingly. A major contributing factor to this problem is the known inaccuracies in disease detection and characterization of current clinical and imaging methods. Recent advances in multiparametric endorectal MR imaging promise to improve the characterization of prostate cancer. With the need to prevent overdiagnosis and overtreatment of clinically insignificant prostate cancers, MR imaging is playing an increasing role in the clinical management of patients. Although acceptance has increased substantially in the last few years, MR imaging of the prostate is standard of care in only a few large medical centers. Ultimately, new, faster, and more reproducible MR imaging techniques will emerge and new MR-based paradigms will result in improved risk assessment and personalized treatment for men with prostate cancer, and more accurately answer the fundamental question: "Do I need to undergo treatment for my prostate cancer?"

ACKNOWLEDGMENTS

The authors would like to thank Dr Fergus V. Coakley for his suggestions and help in preparing this article.

REFERENCES

1. American Cancer Society. Cancer facts and figures 2012. Atlanta: American Cancer Society; 2012.
2. Chustecka Z. Recommendation against routine PSA screening in US. Medscape Urology News 2011. Available at: www.medscape.com/viewarticle/751159. Accessed August 27, 2012.
3. Djavan B. Screening for prostate cancer: practical analysis of the ERSPC [corrected] and PLCO trials [editorial]. Eur Urol 2011;59(3):365–9.
4. Myers RP, Cheville JC, Pawlina W. Making anatomic terminology of the prostate and contiguous structures clinically useful: historical review and suggestions for revision in the 21st century. Clin Anat 2010;23(1):18–29.
5. McNeal JE. Anatomy of the prostate: an historical survey of divergent views. Prostate 1980;1(1):3–13.
6. Coakley FV, Hricak H. Radiologic anatomy of the prostate gland: a clinical approach. Radiol Clin North Am 2000;38(1):15–30.
7. Vo T, Rifkin MD, Peters TL. Should ultrasound criteria of the prostate be redefined to better evaluate when and where to biopsy. Ultrasound Q 2001;17(3):171–6.
8. Ismail M, Gomella LG. Ultrasound for prostate imaging and biopsy [review]. Curr Opin Urol 2001;11(5):471–7.
9. Rabbani F, Stroumbakis N, Kava BR, et al. Incidence and clinical significance of false-negative sextant prostate biopsies. J Urol 1998;159(4):1247–50.
10. Kvale R, Moller B, Wahlqvist R, et al. Concordance between Gleason scores of needle biopsies and radical prostatectomy specimens: a population-based study. BJU Int 2009;103(12):1647–54.
11. D'Amico AV, Tempany CM, Cormack R, et al. Transperineal magnetic resonance image guided prostate biopsy. J Urol 2000;164(2):385–7.
12. Epstein JI, Walsh PC, Carmichael M, et al. Pathologic and clinical findings to predict tumor extent of nonpalpable (stage T1c) prostate cancer [see comments]. JAMA 1994;271(5):368–74.
13. Westphalen AC, Koff WJ, Coakley FV, et al. Prostate cancer: prediction of biochemical failure after external-beam radiation therapy—Kattan nomogram and endorectal MR imaging estimation of tumor volume. Radiology 2011;261(2):477–86.
14. Wang L. Prostate cancer: incremental value of endorectal MR imaging findings for prediction of

extracapsular extension. Radiology 2004;232(1): 133–9.

15. Qayyum A, Coakley FV, Lu Y, et al. Organ-confined prostate cancer: effect of prior transrectal biopsy on endorectal MRI and MR spectroscopic imaging. AJR Am J Roentgenol 2004;183(4): 1079–83.

16. Tamada T, Sone T, Jo Y, et al. Prostate cancer: relationships between postbiopsy hemorrhage and tumor detectability at MR diagnosis. Radiology 2008;248(2):531–9.

17. Hom JJ, Coakley FV, Simko JP, et al. Endorectal MR and MR spectroscopic imaging of prostate cancer: histopathological determinants of tumor visibility. AJR Am J Roentgenol 2005;184(Suppl 4):S62.

18. Schiebler ML, Schnall MD, Outwater E. MR imaging of mucinous adenocarcinoma of the prostate. J Comput Assist Tomogr 1992;16(3):493–4.

19. Westphalen AC, Coakley FV, Kurhanewicz J, et al. Mucinous adenocarcinoma of the prostate: MR imaging and MR spectroscopic imaging features. AJR 2009;193(3):W238–43.

20. Rosenkrantz AB, Mannelli L, Kong X, et al. Prostate cancer: utility of fusion of T2-weighted and high b-value diffusion-weighted images for peripheral zone tumor detection and localization. JMRI 2011; 34(1):95–100.

21. Chen M, Hricak H, Kalbhen CL, et al. Hormonal ablation of prostatic cancer: effects on prostate morphology, tumor detection, and staging by endorectal coil MR imaging. AJR Am J Roentgenol 1996; 166(5):1157–63.

22. Westphalen AC, Kurhanewicz J, Cunha RM, et al. T2-Weighted endorectal magnetic resonance imaging of prostate cancer after external beam radiation therapy. Int Braz J Urol 2009;35(2):171–80 [discussion: 81–2].

23. Kurhanewicz J, Vigneron D, Carroll P, et al. Multi-parametric magnetic resonance imaging in prostate cancer: present and future. Curr Opin Urol 2008; 18(1):71–7.

24. Wang L, Akin O, Mazaheri Y, et al. Are histopathological features of prostate cancer lesions associated with identification of extracapsular extension on magnetic resonance imaging? BJU Int 2010; 106(9):1303–8.

25. Nogueira L, Wang L, Fine SW, et al. Focal treatment or observation of prostate cancer: pretreatment accuracy of transrectal ultrasound biopsy and T2-weighted MRI. Urology 2010;75(2):472–7.

26. Westphalen AC, McKenna DA, Kurhanewicz J, et al. Role of magnetic resonance imaging and magnetic resonance spectroscopic imaging before and after radiotherapy for prostate cancer. J Endourol 2008; 22(4):789–94.

27. McKenna DA, Coakley FV, Westphalen AC, et al. Prostate cancer: role of pretreatment MR in predicting outcome after external-beam radiation therapy—initial experience. Radiology 2008;247(1):141–6.

28. Wang L, Hricak H, Kattan MW, et al. Prediction of organ-confined prostate cancer: incremental value of MR imaging and MR spectroscopic imaging to staging nomograms. Radiology 2006;238(2):597–603.

29. Sala E, Eberhardt SC, Akin O, et al. Endorectal MR imaging before salvage prostatectomy: tumor localization and staging. Radiology 2006;238(1): 176–83.

30. Hricak H, Wang L, Wei DC, et al. The role of preoperative endorectal magnetic resonance imaging in the decision regarding whether to preserve or resect neurovascular bundles during radical retropubic prostatectomy. Cancer 2004;100(12):2655–63.

31. Yu KK, Scheidler J, Hricak H, et al. Prostate cancer: prediction of extracapsular extension with endorectal MR imaging and three-dimensional proton MR spectroscopic imaging. Radiology 1999;213(2):481–8.

32. Hricak H, White S, Vigneron D, et al. Carcinoma of the prostate gland: MR imaging with pelvic phased-array coils versus integrated endorectal-pelvic phased-array coils. Radiology 1994;193(3):703–9.

33. Rosen MA, Goldstone L, Lapin S, et al. Frequency and location of extracapsular extension and positive surgical margins in radical prostatectomy specimens. J Urol 1992;148(2 Pt 1):331–7.

34. Zelhof B, Lowry M, Rodrigues G, et al. Description of magnetic resonance imaging-derived enhancement variables in pathologically confirmed prostate cancer and normal peripheral zone regions. BJU Int 2009;104(5):621–7.

35. Wu LM, Xu JR, Ye YQ, et al. The clinical value of diffusion-weighted imaging in combination with t2-weighted imaging in diagnosing prostate carcinoma: a systematic review and meta-analysis. AJR Am J Roentgenol 2012;199(1):103–10.

36. Woodfield CA, Tung GA, Grand DJ, et al. Diffusion-weighted MRI of peripheral zone prostate cancer: comparison of tumor apparent diffusion coefficient with Gleason score and percentage of tumor on core biopsy. Am J Roentgenol 2010;194(4):W316–22.

37. Hambrock T, Somford DM, Huisman HJ, et al. Relationship between apparent diffusion coefficients at 3.0-T MR imaging and Gleason grade in peripheral zone prostate cancer. Radiology 2011;259(2):453–61.

38. Verma S, Rajesh A, Morales H, et al. Assessment of aggressiveness of prostate cancer: correlation of apparent diffusion coefficient with histologic grade after radical prostatectomy. AJR Am J Roentgenol 2011;196(2):374–81.

39. Bittencourt LK, Barentsz JO, de Miranda LC, et al. Prostate MRI: diffusion-weighted imaging at 1.5T correlates better with prostatectomy Gleason grades than TRUS-guided biopsies in peripheral zone tumours. Eur Radiol 2012;22(2):468–75.

40. Westphalen AC, Reed GD, Vinh PP, et al. Multiparametric 3T endorectal MRI after external beam radiation therapy for prostate cancer. J Magn Reson Imaging 2012;36(2):430–7.

41. Jung JA, Coakley FV, Vigneron DB, et al. Prostate depiction at endorectal MR spectroscopic imaging: investigation of a standardized evaluation system. Radiology 2004;233(3):701–8.

42. Kurhanewicz J, Vigneron DB, Hricak H, et al. Three-dimensional H-1 MR spectroscopic imaging of the in situ human prostate with high (0.24-0.7-cm^3) spatial resolution. Radiology 1996;198(3):795–805.

43. Kurhanewicz J, Swanson MG, Nelson SJ, et al. Combined magnetic resonance imaging and spectroscopic imaging approach to molecular imaging of prostate cancer. J Magn Reson Imaging 2002; 16(4):451–63.

44. Westphalen AC, Coakley FV, Qayyum A, et al. Peripheral zone prostate cancer: accuracy of different interpretative approaches with MR and MR spectroscopic imaging. Radiology 2008;246(1):177–84.

45. Zakian KL, Sircar K, Hricak H, et al. Correlation of proton MR spectroscopic imaging with Gleason score based on step-section pathologic analysis after radical prostatectomy. Radiology 2005;234(3): 804–14.

46. Futterer JJ, Heijmink SW, Scheenen TW, et al. Prostate cancer localization with dynamic contrast-enhanced MR imaging and proton MR spectroscopic imaging. Radiology 2006;241(2):449–58.

47. Coakley FV, Kurhanewicz J, Lu Y, et al. Prostate cancer tumor volume: measurement with endorectal MR and MR spectroscopic imaging. Radiology 2002;223(1):91–7.

48. Westphalen AC, Coakley FV, Roach M 3rd, et al. Locally recurrent prostate cancer after external beam radiation therapy: diagnostic performance of 1.5-T endorectal MR imaging and MR spectroscopic imaging for detection. Radiology 2010;256(2):485–92.

49. Weinreb JC, Blume JD, Coakley FV, et al. Prostate cancer: sextant localization at MR imaging and MR spectroscopic imaging before prostatectomy—results of ACRIN prospective multi-institutional clinicopathologic study. Radiology 2009;251(1):122–33.

50. Shukla-Dave A, Hricak H, Akin O, et al. Preoperative nomograms incorporating magnetic resonance imaging and spectroscopy for prediction of insignificant prostate cancer. BJU Int 2012;109(9):1315–22.

51. Tofts PS. Modeling tracer kinetics in dynamic Gd-DTPA MR imaging. J Magn Reson Imaging 1997; 7(1):91–101.

52. van Dorsten FA, van der Graaf M, Engelbrecht MR, et al. Combined quantitative dynamic contrast-enhanced MR imaging and 1H MR spectroscopic imaging of human prostate cancer. J Magn Reson Imaging 2004;20(2):279–87.

53. Verma S, Turkbey B, Muradyan N, et al. Overview of dynamic contrast-enhanced MRI in prostate cancer diagnosis and management. AJR Am J Roentgenol 2012;198(6):1277–88.

54. Heijmink SW, Fütterer JJ, Hambrock T, et al. Prostate cancer: body-array versus endorectal coil MR imaging at 3 T—comparison of Image quality, localization, and staging performance. Radiology 2007; 244(1).184–95.

55. Fütterer JJ, Engelbrecht MR, Jager GJ, et al. Prostate cancer: comparison of local staging accuracy of pelvic phased-array coil alone versus integrated endorectal–pelvic phased-array coils. Eur Radiol 2007;17(4):1055–65.

56. Kurhanewicz J, Vigneron DB, Nelson SJ. Three-dimensional magnetic resonance spectroscopic imaging of brain and prostate cancer. Neoplasia 2000;2(1–2):166–89.

Role of Transrectal Ultrasonography in Prostate Cancer

Sangeet Ghai, MD, FRCR[a,b,*], Ants Toi, MD, FRCPC[a,b,c,d]

KEYWORDS

- Transrectal ultrasound • Prostate cancer • Screening • Targeted biopsy

KEY POINTS

- Prostate cancer is the most frequently diagnosed cancer in men, about 2 or 3 times more than lung and colorectal cancer.
- Transrectal ultrasound-guided systematic biopsy of the prostate is the gold standard for detecting prostate cancer.
- Prostate cancer may be visible on TRUS and is usually seen as hypoechoic nodules, if visible.
- With increased PSA screening, the stage at diagnosis of prostate cancer has been decreasing, and most patients presenting today have low-grade and organ-confined disease.
- With recent advances in multiparametric MRI, and in newer ultrasound techniques, such as contrast-enhanced ultrasound and elastography, its role may evolve toward targeted biopsies rather than systematic biopsy, as we question which kinds of lesions do we want to discover.

INTRODUCTION

Transrectal ultrasound (TRUS) was first developed in the 1960s and 1970s by Japanese investigators who published their experience with a radial scanner placed on a chair.[1,2] Since then, the technique has evolved, with the development of smaller probes, gray-scale real-time imaging, improved transducer design, and introduction of biopsy guidance devices. An additional breakthrough was the development of the "biopsy gun" by Lindgren in Sweden. TRUS-guided systematic biopsy of the prostate is now the gold standard diagnostic modality of prostate cancer and has replaced the "blind" finger-guided transrectal and the earlier transperineal approaches.

PROSTATE CANCER AND SCREENING

Prostate cancer is the most frequently diagnosed cancer in men, about 2 or 3 times more than lung and colorectal cancer. It is also the second leading cause of deaths in men, after lung cancer, in North America and kills about 45,000 men each year. It primarily affects men older than 50 years. About 1 in 7 men is affected by the disease during his lifetime[3] and 1 in 28 will die from prostate cancer The risk is higher in African American men and those with a family history of prostate cancer.[4–7] The risk doubles with a single affected relative and is even higher with multiple affected relatives. More than 95% of primary malignant tumors of the prostate are adenocarcinomas that develop in the acini of

[a] University of Toronto, Toronto, Ontario, Canada; [b] Joint Department of Medical Imaging, University Health Network, Mount Sinai Hospital, Women's College Hospital, Toronto, Ontario, Canada; [c] Radiology, University of Toronto, Toronto, Ontario, Canada; [d] Obstetrics and Gynecology, University of Toronto, Toronto, Ontario, Canada
* Corresponding author. Department of Medical Imaging, Toronto General Hospital, NCSB - 1C544, 585 University Avenue, Toronto M5G 2N2, Ontario, Canada.
E-mail address: sangeet.ghai@uhn.ca

Radiol Clin N Am 50 (2012) 1061–1073
http://dx.doi.org/10.1016/j.rcl.2012.08.007
0033-8389/12/$ – see front matter © 2012 Elsevier Inc. All rights reserved.

the prostatic ducts. About 80% of cancers occur in the peripheral zone of the prostate, 15% in the transition zone, and the remaining 5% in the central zone (**Fig. 1** showing normal zonal anatomy of the prostate on TRUS).[8] Prostate cancer is described by stage (clinical extent) and histologic dedifferentiation (grade). For staging, the TNM staging system is used. Histologic grading uses the Gleason grade (range 1–5, grade 1 being well differentiated and grade 5, poorly differentiated) and score (the sum of the 2 most prevalent histologic patterns) are used to quantify the histologic characteristics of prostate tumors.[9–11] Ten-year mortality with intermediate-grade tumors (Gleason 5–7) is 13% to 24% and with high-grade tumors (Gleason 8–10) is 44% to 66%.[12] Rarely, other tumors may affect the prostate, including transitional-cell carcinoma, sarcomas, and lymphoma.[13]

Prostate cancer screening attempts to detect clinically significant prostate cancer in asymptomatic men at an early stage, when curative therapy is possible and outcomes can be improved. The stage at diagnosis of prostate cancer has been decreasing since the 1990s, partly because of the introduction of screening, and most patients presenting today have organ-confined disease.[14] Screening for prostate cancer has come under discussion recently. Two major studies of population screening have been carried out: the European Randomized Screening for Prostate Cancer (ERSPC) trial and the American Prostate, Lung, Colorectal, Ovary (PLCO) study.[15,16] Both trials

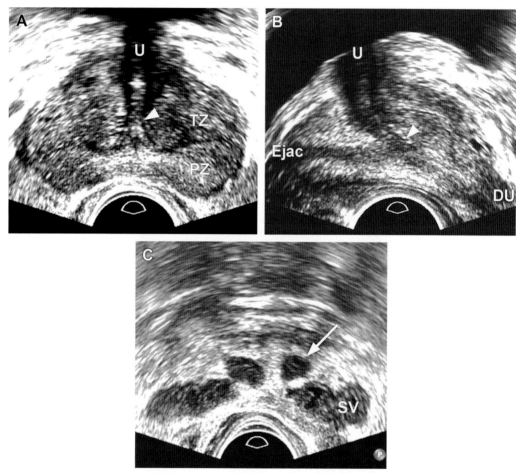

Fig. 1. Normal appearances of prostate at transrectal ultrasound. (*A*) Axial view shows peripheral zone (PZ) and transition zone (TZ) separated by a hypoechoic line representing the surgical capsule. Internal urethra and muscular internal urethral sphincter form a hypoechoic band (U). The arrowhead shows the veru montanum. (*B*) Sagittal view with patient's head to left side. Note hypoechoic internal urethral sphincter (U) coursing toward veru montanum (*arrowhead*). At this point, the urethra angles slightly and ultimately leaves the prostate at its apex at the distal urethra (DU). The ejaculatory ducts (Ejac) course horizontally from prostate base to join the urethra at the veru (*arrowhead*). (*C*) Axial view of right and left seminal vesicle (SV) and vas with only left side labeled. The arrow is pointing to the vas.

Prostate cancer facts:

- The most common cancer in men
- Second leading cause of cancer death in men (after lung)
- Best screen is PSA and DRE but screening only done after discussion
- New screening tests are being developed
- The diagnostic test is TRUS with biopsy
- Many men have microscopic cancers that do not affect longevity
- Multiple therapeutic options exist depending on circumstances
- Curative treatments commonly affect quality of life

examined mortality as the end point, and both found little effect on mortality from screening. The rising gap between incidence and mortality rates in the prostate-specific antigen (PSA) screening era may be indicative of increased rates of overdiagnosis.[17] The ERSPC trial, however, did find a small benefit in favor of screening and that survival advantage of screened men increases with time. The study also suggested that the population that benefited from screening was men between the ages of 55 and 69 years. The American PLCO study did not show benefit of screening for prostate cancer but it had a major flaw because many men in the nonscreened group in fact were screened with PSA. Heavy pre-screening before randomization is likely to have reduced the number of aggressive cancers in both arms and thereby outcomes.[18] Most professional organizations recommend for screening but only after discussion and patient consent. Recently however, the US Preventative Services Task Force has recommended against screening with concerns regarding potential risks involved with diagnosis and potential for overtreatment. This opinion is strongly contested by other organizations.

Screening is done with digital rectal examination (DRE) and PSA. PSA is a normally occurring enzyme secreted by the epithelial cells of prostate ducts and functions to liquefy the ejaculate. The prostate is the main source of PSA, and only trace amounts are found in other tissues in men and women. Small amounts leak into the serum and can therefore be measured.[19] Cancer is believed to produce 10 times as much PSA as benign tissue.[20,21] In the serum, PSA is partly free and partly bound to proteins. The ratio of free to total PSA in the serum tends to be low in cancer and chronic prostatitis.[22,23] A free/total ratio of less than 20% in 4 to 10 ng/mL PSA range will detect 95% of cancers on biopsy;

however, 5% of clinically significant cancers may be missed and therefore an exact cutoff value is not universally accepted.[24]

PSA is a nonspecific test of prostate abnormality and irritation. Elevated levels are seen in cancer, but also in benign conditions, including benign prostatic hyperplasia (BPH), inflammation, after ejaculation, following DRE, biopsy, and cystoscopy. On the other hand, PSA levels can be artificially reduced with antiandrogenic medications, such as dutasteride (Avodart) and finasteride (Proscar), which decrease PSA levels by about 50%. The recommendations for using PSA levels to direct biopsy are changing, and currently there is no longer a general consensus for a lower limit. Generally, PSA level of 4 mg/mL (and more recently, 2.5 mg/mL) is considered as an indication for biopsy. Men with a PSA level greater than 2.5 ng/mL have a 20% chance of finding prostate cancer at biopsy, and this increases to 50% if the PSA level is greater than 10 ng/mL.[25] The rate of PSA rise (PSA velocity) of more than 0.75 ng/mL per year, irrespective of PSA level, is also considered as an indication for prostate biopsy.[20,21,23,26] On the other hand, not all cancers produce PSA, and 20% to 40% of men with clinically significant cancer have normal PSA. Therefore, biopsy is indicated if there is a nodule felt at palpation on DRE, irrespective of the PSA level.[25,27]

SONOGRAPHIC APPEARANCE OF PROSTATE CANCER

Typically, cancer is a hypoechoic area, especially in the peripheral zone, that cannot be attributed to benign causes (**Fig. 2**).[28,29] About 40% to 60% of prostate cancers are not visible at TRUS, in particular the low-grade cancers. Normal appearance on TRUS does not imply absence of cancer and so patients clinically suspected to have cancer, based on PSA levels or velocity and findings on DRE, should be referred for TRUS with biopsy and not just TRUS alone. Search for suspicious areas remains important, however, as biopsies from such areas are twice as likely to demonstrate high-grade and high-volume cancer as systematic biopsy.[25]

Lee and colleagues[28] first demonstrated the hypoechoic appearance of prostate cancer in 1985. Subsequently, other studies also showed similar findings of hypoechoic appearance of prostate cancers in the peripheral zone.[30,31] The proposed cause of the hypoechoic appearance on TRUS is the replacement of normal loose glandular tissue by a packed mass of tumor cells with fewer reflecting interfaces. The more infiltrative tumors or those with glandular structure will preserve interfaces and

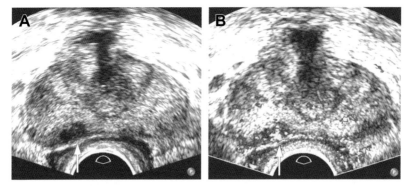

Fig. 2. Typical cancer visible as hypoechoic vascular nodule. (*A*) Hypoechoic nodule in peripheral zone (*arrow*). (*B*) Increased vascularity shown in the nodule (*arrow*).

echogenicity and therefore not be visible on ultrasound.[30] Because most prostate cancers are infiltrative rather than with well-defined margins, many are not visible on ultrasound. In an attempt to correlate the echogenicity of neoplasms on TRUS with pathology, Shinohara and colleagues[31] found that hypoechoic lesions tend to be more aggressive than the isoechoic or the "not visible" cancers on ultrasound. Conversely, only about 50% of hypoechoic areas are cancer.[32] Other lesions that may be hypoechoic include hyperplasia, prostatitis, benign glandular ectasia, fibrosis, and cysts.[30]

Infrequently, prostate cancer may have a hyperechoic appearance on ultrasound. This is thought to be secondary to a desmoplastic response of the surrounding glandular tissue to the tumor. Tumor infiltration in areas of BPH and preexisting degenerative calcification can also have a hyperechoic appearance.[33,34] Uncommon histologic types of cancer, including the cribriform pattern and comedonecrosis with focal calcification, may also have an echogenic or "starry sky" appearance on ultrasound (**Fig. 3**).[35]

More than 30% of prostate cancers are isoechoic and not visible on TRUS and therefore impossible to detect, without systematic biopsies.

Prostate cancer and screening

- There is much debate on type, grade, and volume of prostate cancer detected on systematic TRUS-guided prostate biopsies

- Two major prospective studies, ERSPC trial and the American PLCO study, found little benefit on mortality from prostate screening.

- With advances in multiparametric MRI, contrast-enhanced ultrasound, and elastography, the role of TRUS-guided biopsy in detection of prostate cancer may evolve to targeted biopsies rather than systematic biopsies.

Secondary signs, such as gland asymmetry, capsular bulge, and posterior attenuation, may sometimes help direct biopsies to these isoechoic tumors.[35] Another group of difficult cancers to detect on TRUS are those in the very heterogeneous transition zone and the far anterior tumors. These tumors are far from the probe in the rectum, and may also be obstructed by shadowing from the urethra. Also, many operators are simply not aware of the presence and appearance of anterior cancer at ultrasound (**Fig. 4**). Systematic transition zone biopsy may also miss them because of their anterior location and deliberate avoidance of the urethra at time of biopsy.[36]

Color and Power Doppler Ultrasound

Doppler imaging has been evaluated to detect increased vascularity that can be associated with cancer, especially in attempts to recognize cancers

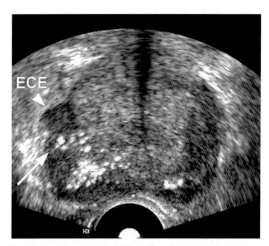

Fig. 3. Focal spotty calcifications (starry sky) that can be associated with cancer (*arrow*). The cancer is hypoechoic and can be seen to have extracapsular extension (ECE) where it breaks the prostate contour (*arrowhead*).

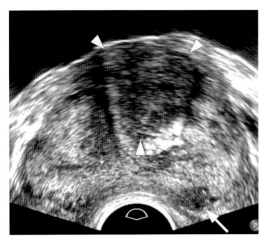

Fig. 4. Small posterior cancer (*arrow*) and much larger anterior cancer (*arrowheads*). It is important to search for and biopsy anterior hypoechoic areas.

that are isoechoic, because cancers may have increased microvessel density.[37] Studies have, however, shown only a 5% to 17% increase in cancer detection using color Doppler over gray-scale imaging.[37] Hypoechoic nodules that are vascular tend to have a larger tumor volume and also a higher Gleason score.[38] Vascularity, however, may be increased in benign conditions, such as infection and inflammation (**Fig. 5**).

RECENT ADVANCES IN TRUS

Because not all cancer is visible at TRUS and not detected by systematic prostate biopsy (the current gold standards for detecting prostate cancer), there is continuing search for imaging techniques to detect prostate cancer and allow directed biopsy. When evaluating new techniques,

it is important to evaluate the added value of the published technique to conventional TRUS and not just the reported sensitivity and specificity of the new technique.

Contrast-Enhanced Ultrasound

Cancer in general is associated with an increased microvessel density owing to proliferation of neo-vessels. Conventional color/power Doppler US imaging cannot detect micro-neovascularity, but microbubble contrast-enhanced US may demonstrate neovascularity in some instances.[39] US contrast agents increase signal-to-noise ratio and thereby enable improved detection of low-volume blood flow. Modern contrast-specific imaging techniques, such as gray-scale harmonic US, use the nonlinear behavior of the microbubbles to detect signals reflected by the microbubbles and allow for improved visibility at US. Harmonic gray-scale US can also be performed with an intermittent imaging mode, which improves the survival time of microbubbles by lowering the energy deposition into tissue.[40] Other more sensitive contrast-enhanced US techniques, such as cadence contrast-pulse sequence have recently been made available. At present, contrast-enhanced US of the prostate remains investigational.[41]

In different studies,[42–44] the authors noted that following contrast-enhanced US, targeted biopsy allowed for the detection of some cancers not found on systematic biopsy, but adding systematic biopsy samples allows for maximal cancer detection, as not all cancers were identified by the contrast agents. They concluded that contrast-enhanced US had higher sensitivity of detecting cancer than unenhanced US, but the difference in specificity was not significant. In another study, Mitterberger and colleagues[45] found significantly higher Gleason

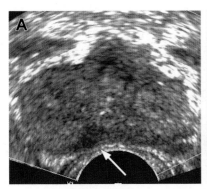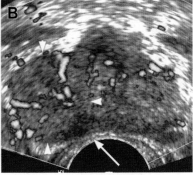

Fig. 5. Isoechoic cancer detected with power Doppler. (*A*) There is a small obvious posterior hypoechoic cancer nodule (*arrow*). (*B*) Power Doppler shows that the small nodule is not vascular (*arrow*) even though it is cancer; however, there is abnormal vascularity throughout the right lobe (*arrowheads*) that indicates a much larger area of isoechoic cancer. In retrospect in Fig. 5A, there are subtle changes suggesting cancer throughout: the entire right lobe is enlarged and deformed, and the surgical capsule is effaced.

score in cancers detected by contrast-enhanced targeted biopsy as compared with systematic biopsy. They also found that premedication with dutasteride (a dual 5 alpha reductase inhibitor) for 7 to 14 days before biopsy, improved cancer detection with contrast-enhanced US, by reducing prostatic blood flow in benign prostatic tissue.[46]

Using gray-scale and wide-band harmonic US, Halpern and colleagues[47] compared areas of contrast material enhancement in the prostate with whole-mount radical prostatectomy and noticed that it improved sensitivity for the detection of cancers in the outer gland, but focal enhancement also occurred in areas of benign hyperplasia. In another study with gray scale and harmonic ultrasound, Halpern and colleagues[48] suggested that a suspicious site on contrast-enhanced US was 5 times more likely to have a positive finding on prostate biopsy than a standard sextant site.

Elastography

Elastography is an imaging technique that evaluates the change in elasticity or stiffness of the tissue. Cancerous tissue typically has an increase in cellular tissue density and vessel density. Although various contrast-enhanced US techniques described previously attempt to differentiate cancer from benign tissue based on increased vascularity in cancer, elastography techniques attempt to detect cancer based on increased tissue stiffness with cancer and concommitant change in tissue elasticity (**Fig. 6**).

In a recent prospective study,[49] areas suspicious for prostate cancer on elastography were compared with histologic specimens after surgery. Real-time elastography detected 28 of 32 foci of prostate cancer (88% sensitivity). Konig and colleagues[50] detected 127 of 151 cancers using real-time elastography as an additional diagnostic feature and concluded that it is possible to detect prostate cancer with a high degree of sensitivity using real-time elastography in conjunction with conventional diagnostic methods for guided prostate biopsies. Pallwein and colleagues[51] compared cancer detection rates between real-time elastography targeting 5 peripheral zone sites versus 10 core systematic biopsies. The overall cancer detection rate by patient was not significantly different in the 2 groups, although the detection rate for biopsy cores was significantly better in the elastography-targeted cores (12.7%) than in the systematic biopsies (5.6%).

ROLE OF TRANSRECTAL ULTRASOUND

Currently, the main roles of TRUS in prostate cancer include guiding both biopsy and therapy. Therapy guidance includes placement of fiducial markers for external beam radiotherapy, and guidance for brachytherapy, cryoablation, and high-intensity focused ultrasound (HIFU). Prostate volume measurement helps determine suitability for brachytherapy. TRUS is moderately accurate for local staging including evaluation for extracapsular extension and seminal vesicle involvement. MRI has proved more accurate in demonstrating

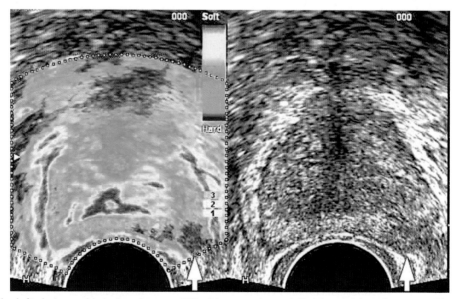

Fig. 6. The left elastographic image shows a stiffer blue area (*arrow*) that is suspicious for cancer. The cancer is much less conspicuous on the matching right gray-scale image (*arrow*).

> *Transrectal ultrasound and prostate cancer:*
>
> - TRUS alone is not the primary technique to find cancer, biopsy is needed
> - Classic appearance of cancer is hypoechoic nodule in peripheral zone
> - Only about 50% to 70% of cancers are visible at TRUS
> - Only about 50% of hypoechoic nodules are cancer
> - TRUS has 3 main roles
>   - Guide biopsy
>   - Guide therapy
>   - Measure volume of prostate

extracapsular extension and seminal vesicle involvement and can also evaluate lymphadenopathy (**Fig. 7**).

Prostate Biopsy

TRUS-guided prostate biopsy is performed in an ambulatory setting. Preparation includes antibiotic prophylaxis and anticoagulant avoidance. Rectal cleansing with enema or laxative can improve visibility and some claim infection-reducing effects.[52]

Unlike percutaneous biopsies at other sites, an aseptic environment cannot be maintained at the time of transrectal biopsies. Therefore, all patients have to be administered antibiotics in the periprocedure period. The usual recommendation is use of broad-based gram-negative fluoroquinolones (such as ciprofloxacin). However, fluoroquinolone resistance is rising and prophylactic antibiotic

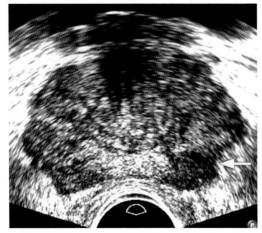

Fig. 7. Extracapsular extension of cancer visible as a hypoechoic nodule that clearly bulges through the capsule (*arrow*).

selection is best done with infectious disease specialist consultation. Adding intravenous aminoglycoside to fluoroquinolones may minimize the risk of urinary tract infection following prostate biopsy.[52–54] Biopsy should always be avoided during urinary infection and for 4 to 6 weeks thereafter. Endocarditis prophylaxis is no longer recommended for prostate biopsy.

Some recent prospective studies on TRUS biopsy with continued use of low-dose aspirin (ASA) showed no increased risk of clinically significant bleeding or hematuria.[55–57] Most practitioners recommend discontinuation of antiplatelet agents to minimize the risk of bleeding complications in an elective procedure, however. ASA and NSAIDs should be stopped for 5 days before the biopsy. Other antiplatelet agents, such as clopidogrel (Plavix) should be stopped for 7 to 10 days, and ticlopidine for 14 days before the biopsy. Antiplatelet medicines should be interrupted only after consultation with the treating physician to determine safety of stopping during biopsy.[52] Coumadin (Warfarin) should be stopped for 5 days and patients coagulation tested before biopsy.[52] Dibigatran (Pradaxa) should be discontinued for 3 days before biopsy. The agents may be restarted within 24 hours of biopsy if there is no major bleeding. Hematology consult is advised for discussion of bridging anticoagulation in patients with mechanical heart valves, atrial fibrillation with prior neurologic event, and recurrent or recent (<1 year ago) venous thromboembolism.[58]

Although TRUS biopsy is well tolerated, it is associated with pain if performed without local anesthesia, more so if increased numbers of cores are obtained. The most commonly used anesthetic agent is 5 to 10 mL of 1% or 2% injectable lidocaine without epinephrine, injected bilaterally at the site of the neurovascular bundle at the base of the gland just lateral to the junction between the prostate and seminal vesicle.[59] In a randomized prospective study in our practice, we found no extra benefit of apical periprostatic lidocaine infiltration. Direct injections into the gland may also be given for instant effect, but we have noticed increased vasovagal reactions with intragland lidocaine injections in our practice.

During the procedure, patients are positioned in the left lateral decubitus position. DRE is performed before placement of the probe. A variety of probes and guides are available. Ching and colleagues[60] suggested that end-fire probes/guides provide better sampling than side-fire devices. Electronic guidelines direct the needle path. The automated biopsy gun with 18-guage needles has been shown to obtain good samples with remarkable patient acceptance and safety.[56]

If the TRUS queries suspicious areas, these sites should be sampled first, in case the patient is unable to tolerate the entire procedure.[29] Biopsy through the urethra, internal urethral sphincter, and ejaculatory ducts is avoided because it can result in considerable bleeding and potential injury to these structures. Once the procedure is completed, pressure with probe or the finger may be applied for a minute to help stop bleeding. It is advisable to observe patients for about an hour after the biopsy before discharging them from the unit, as some patients may have delayed hypotensive or vasovagal reactions.

It is common to see minor blood in the urine, stool, and in ejaculate following prostate biopsy. It generally lasts only a few days, although the semen may remain discolored for 6 to 8 weeks. Complications requiring physician intervention occur infrequently following prostate biopsy, generally in 1% to 2% of patients, with infection and sepsis being the foremost, followed by rectal or urethral bleeding and retention. With increasing resistance to fluoroquinolones, the incidence of septic complications requiring therapy can be up to 5% despite prophylactic antibiotics. Patients should be advised to seek help promptly if they start feeling feverish or unwell. One has to carefully select the appropriate prophylactic antibiotic if the patient gives history of infection or sepsis following a previous prostate biopsy and infectious disease consult can be helpful. A hypotensive vasovagal reaction may occur in 1% to 6% of patients following prostate biopsy, usually within 30 to 60 minutes of a biopsy. Most of these patients recover spontaneously.[29]

PROSTATE BIOPSY SAMPLING PROTOCOLS

At initial biopsy, 10 to 12 samples are typically obtained in a systematic fashion and additional samples are taken if any suspicious areas are seen at time of TRUS (**Fig. 8**).

TRUS-guided prostate biopsy sampling protocols

- 10 to 12 samples in systematic fashion plus additional samples if suspicious areas on TRUS
- Follow-up biopsy protocols (if persistent suspicion despite negative biopsy, HGPIN, or ASAP on initial biopsy)
  - 12 to 17 systematic samples
  - 12-core systematic biopsy and additional targeted areas questioned on multiparametric MRI, contrast-enhanced US, or elastography, although many of these newer tests are investigational at this time

---

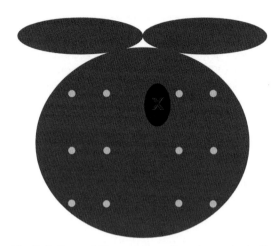

Fig. 8. Pattern of 12-core biopsy. Samples are typically taken from the medial and lateral aspects of the peripheral zone (*yellow dots*). Additional samples are taken from suspicious areas falling outside the systematic pattern (X).

Follow-up Extended Biopsy Protocols

These are typically used for follow-up when initial biopsy is negative but high clinical suspicion remains, or the initial biopsy shows atypical cells (atypical small acinar proliferation [ASAP]), high-grade prostate intraepithelial neoplasia (HGPIN), or micro-foci of cancer. Follow-up biopsy generally uses extended biopsy protocols, which recommend obtaining 12 to 17 biopsy samples under TRUS guidance. Cancer detection rates increase by 5% to 35% as opposed to sextant biopsies.[61–63] Even with the extended biopsy protocols, however, 17% to 35% of men with negative results on the first biopsy but with persistent clinical suspicion, will be diagnosed to have prostate cancer on subsequent biopsies.[61,62,64] Also, only 26% to 35% of patients with unilateral cancer on 10 to 12 core biopsies, have true unilateral disease at radical prostatectomy.[65–67] Similarly, systematic biopsies tend to substantially underestimate the true Gleason score found on prostatectomy specimens.[65]

Saturation Biopsy

Saturation biopsy refers to procedures in which more than 20 cores are obtained in a systematic manner. These protocols are used to evaluate extent of disease if focal therapy is planned or in men with high suspicion when repeated biopsy shows only low-volume disease. They are generally done with a template transperineal approach. Cancer detection rates are usually in the 30% to 40% range with saturation biopsy in men with prior negative biopsy,[62,68–70] and the risk of complications is about twice that of 12 to 18 core techniques[70,71]; however, saturation biopsy techniques may also miss significant cancers.[72]

MRI-ASSISTED BIOPSIES

As discussed previously, the negative predictive value of a systematic TRUS-guided biopsy is 36% to 89%.[73] Also, the positive predictive value of PSA is low, because numerous benign prostate conditions can increase PSA.[74] After an initial negative prostate biopsy, some men present with persistently elevated PSA levels.[75] Because a high proportion of tumors found at repeat biopsies are of clinical significance, patients with an initial negative biopsy, remain a great diagnostic problem for the urologists.[76]

MRI, especially multiparametric MRI (MP-MRI) has been shown to improve prostate cancer detection. MP-MRI of the prostate combines T2-weighted imaging with diffusion-weighted imaging (DWI) and perfusion imaging and has been extensively investigated in recent years.[77] It has a high sensitivity, particularly in detecting high-grade clinically significant carcinomas.[78] Using its localizing strength, MP-MRI of the prostate has increased opportunities for image-guided techniques.

In recent years, several groups have reported first results of in-bore MRI-guided biopsies (MRI-GB). Two studies have reported cancer detection rates of 41%[79] and 38%[80] respectively, whereas there have been other reports with biopsy yield of 59.0%[81] and 55.5%[82] in subjects with elevated PSA levels and prior negative biopsy, when biopsying MRI-identified targets in the magnet (MRI-GB). One of these recent studies[81] showed a fourfold increase in biopsy yield (59%) compared with TRUS biopsy in subjects with increased PSA levels and prior negative biopsy when biopsying MRI-identified targets (MRI-GB). But MRI-GB is not commonly available and is associated with other disadvantages. The biopsy device is expensive and has to be MR compatible. Magnetic environment increases the complexity of interventional procedures. The procedure is usually performed in the prone position and probably associated with higher patient discomfort. Also, the duration for 1 biopsy session is in the range of 34 to 80 minutes.[80,81] Another drawback of MRI-GB may be undersampling of sites other than the MRI targets.

MRI-directed/assisted TRUS biopsy (TRUS-GB), that is, using TRUS to sample the suspicious lesions questioned on MRI, currently uses anatomic landmarks (eg, shape of prostate, position of the veru montanum, distance from the apex or the base of the gland, presence of a cyst or a calcification) to assist in creating a mental image of where the suspicious lesion on MRI is likely to be on the TRUS-generated image.[83] This "mental fusion" of the images is operator dependent[84] and relies on the ability of the operator to mentally segment and register the site questioned on MRI at the time of TRUS biopsy. In a recent study,[85] prostate cancer was diagnosed in 11 of 16 patients (69% cancer detection rate) at the MRI sites using "mental fusion" TRUS-GB in patients with previous negative biopsy and increased PSA. The investigators attributed the very high success of the mental registration technique to a low rate of patients with suspicious lesions on MRI, and therefore concluded their biopsy yield rate could not be compared with the MRI-GB studies. Also, this study had a small cohort of 16 patients. In another recent study with a similar cohort of patients,[83] cancer detection rate was 28.8% in MRI-targeted cores (TRUS-GB) and 3.6% in standard cores, with overall cancer detection rate of 56% (in 46 of 82 patients). The transition zone remains a problem for MRI, as BPH nodules are heterogeneous at MRI and benign nodules may appear suspicious.

An ideal biopsy system would allow for sampling of MRI-identified target lesions with high accuracy, mapping of location of all tissue core samples on a 3-dimensional image of the prostate, while keeping the procedure's cost relatively stable. One solution to this problem may be to fuse previously acquired MRI data to the real-time TRUS, thus exploiting the advantages of both modalities.[86,87] Using these complementary methods, the needle can be directed into suspicious regions identified on the MRI using US guidance. MRI-TRUS fusion affords lower cost and can map the locations of all cores. This platform fuses pre-biopsy MRI with real-time TRUS imaging to identify and biopsy lesions suspicious for prostate cancer on the MP-MRI (MRI-TRUS fusion biopsy) (**Fig. 9**). A recent study using one such fusion platform[88] reported higher cancer per core for all lesions suspicious on MRI versus the standard 12-core TRUS biopsy alone in a heterogeneous cohort of patients and included patients with no prior, prior negative, and prior positive biopsy histories. The overall cancer detection rate in this study was 54.4%, although the cancer detection rate when biopsying MRI-identified targets alone was 45%. In 10 of the 55 subjects, prostate cancer was detected on 12-core TRUS biopsy alone. At present, however, there seem to be some limitations to accurate fusion biopsies, namely, patient movement and time-consuming motion compensation, and gland swelling following the initial biopsies leading to misregistration.

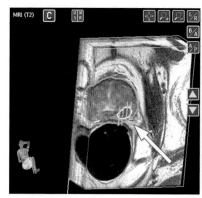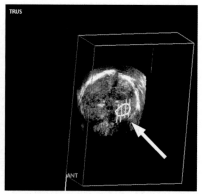

Fig. 9. MRI-ultrasound fusion. Left MRI (*arrow*) is fused with right 3-dimensional ultrasound image. The corresponding suspicious target is indicated on both images (*arrows*). Subsequently, this lesion is targeted for biopsy with TRUS guidance.

Future research in this area with randomized prospective trials comparing cancer detection rates following in-bore MRI biopsy, MRI-assisted mental registration biopsy, and MRI-TRUS fusion biopsy, will help to determine the more accurate and cost-effective means of prostate sampling in men with persistently elevated PSA levels and high clinical suspicion despite previous negative prostate biopsy.

SUMMARY

TRUS-guided prostate biopsy remains the gold standard for detecting prostate cancer. With recent advances in MP-MRI, and in newer US techniques, such as contrast-enhanced US and elastography, its role may evolve toward targeted biopsies rather than systematic biopsy, as we question which kind of lesions are we willing to discover.

REFERENCES

1. Watanabe H, Igari D, Tanahasi Y, et al. Development and application of new equipment for transrectal ultrasonography. J Clin Ultrasound 1974;2:91–8.
2. Watanabe H. History and applications of transrectal sonography of the prostate. Urol Clin North Am 1989;16:617–22.
3. Canadian cancer society. Statistics for 2011. Available at: http://www.cancer.ca. Accessed August 29, 2012.
4. Levy IG, Iscoe NA, Klotz LH. Prostate cancer. 1. The descriptive epidemiology in Canada. CMAJ 1998; 159:509–13.
5. Neal DE, Leung HY, Powell PH, et al. Unanswered questions in screening for prostate cancer. Eur J Cancer 2000;36:1316–21.
6. Rietbergen JB, Schroder FH. Screening for prostate cancer: more questions than answers. Acta Oncol 1998;37:515–32.
7. Bratt O. Hereditary prostate cancer: clinical aspects. J Urol 2002;168:906–13.
8. Sexton WJ, Spiess PE, Pisters LL, et al. Are there differences in zonal distribution and tumor volume of prostate cancer in patients with a positive family history? Int Braz J Urol 2010;36(5):571–82.
9. Che M, Sakr W, Grignon D. Pathologic features the urologist should expect on a prostate biopsy. Urol Oncol 2003;21:153–61.
10. Gleason DF, Mellinger GT. Prediction of prognosis for prostatic adenocarcinoma by combined histological grading and clinical staging. J Urol 1974;111:58–64.
11. Epstein JI, Allsbrook WC Jr, Amin MB, et al. Update on the Gleason grading system for prostate cancer: results of an international consensus conference of urologic pathologists. Adv Anat Pathol 2006;13:57–9.
12. Nam RK, Jewett MA, Krahn MD. Prostate cancer. 2. Natural history. CMAJ 1998;159:685–91.
13. Campbell MF, Wein AJ, Kavoussi LR, et al, editors. Campbell-Walsh urology. 9th edition. Philadelphia: Saunders; 2007.
14. Shao YH, Demissie K, Shih W, et al. Contemporary risk profile of prostate cancer in the US. J Natl Cancer Inst 2009;101:1280–3.
15. Schröder FH, Hugosson J, Roobol MJ, et al. Screening and prostate-cancer mortality in a randomized European study. N Engl J Med 2009;360: 1320–8.
16. Andriole GL, Crawford ED, Grubb RL 3rd, et al. Mortality results from a randomized prostate-cancer screening trial. N Engl J Med 2009;360: 1310–9.
17. Eckersberger E, Finkelstein J, Sadri H, et al. Screening for prostate cancer: a review of the ERSPC and PLCO trials. Rev Urol 2009;11(3): 127–33.
18. Schröder FH, Roobol MJ. ERSPC and PLCO prostate cancer screening studies: what are the differences? Eur Urol 2010;58(1):46–52.

19. Bunting PS, DeBoer G, Choo R, et al. Intraindividual variation of PSA, free PSA and complexed PSA in a cohort of patients with prostate cancer managed with watchful observation. Clin Biochem 2002;35: 471–5.

20. Polascik TJ, Oesterling JE, Partin AW. Prostate-specific antigen: a decade of discovery—what we have learned and where we are going. J Urol 1999;162:293–306.

21. Alapont Alacreu JM, Navarro Rosales S, Budia Alba A, et al. PSA and hK2 in the diagnosis of prostate cancer. Actas Urol Esp 2008;32:575–88 [in Spanish].

22. Jung K, Meyer A, Lein M, et al. Ratio of free-to-total prostate specific antigen in serum cannot distinguish patients with prostate cancer from those with chronic inflammation of the prostate. J Urol 1998; 159:1595–8.

23. Gonzalgo ML, Carter HB. Update on PSA testing. J Natl Compr Canc Netw 2007;5:737–42.

24. Thompson IM, Ankerst DP. Prostate-specific antigen in the early detection of prostate cancer. CMAJ 2007;176:1853–8.

25. Toi A, Neill MG, Lockwood GA, et al. The continuing importance of transrectal ultrasound identification of prostatic lesions. J Urol 2007;177:516–20.

26. Loeb S, Catalona WJ. What to do with an abnormal PSA test. Oncologist 2008;13:299–305.

27. Littrup PJ, Bailey SE. Prostate cancer: the role of transrectal ultrasound and its impact on cancer detection and management. Radiol Clin North Am 2000;38:87–113.

28. Lee F, Gray JM, McLeary RD, et al. Transrectal ultrasound in the diagnosis of prostate cancer: location, echogenicity, histopathology, and staging. Prostate 1985;7:117–29.

29. Toi A. The prostate. In: Rumack CM, Wilson SR, Carboneau WJ, et al, editors. Diagnostic ultrasound. Philadelphia: Elsevier; 2011. p. 392–428.

30. Shinohara K, Scardino PT, Carter SS, et al. Pathologic basis of the sonographic appearance of the normal and malignant prostate. Urol Clin North Am 1989;16:675–91.

31. Shinohara K, Wheeler TM, Scardino PT. The appearance of prostate cancer on transrectal ultrasonography: correlation of imaging and pathological examinations. J Urol 1989;142:76–82.

32. Dyke CH, Toi A, Sweet JM. Value of random ultrasound-guided transrectal prostate biopsy. Radiology 1990;176:345–9.

33. Dahnert WF, Hamper UM, Walsh PC, et al. The echogenic focus in prostatic sonograms, with xeroradiographic and histopathologic correlation. Radiology 1986;159:95–100.

34. Rifkin MD, Dahnert W, Kurtz AB. State of the art: endorectal sonography of the prostate gland. AJR Am J Roentgenol 1990;154:691–700.

35. Hamper UM, Sheth S, Walsh PC, et al. Bright echogenic foci in early prostatic carcinoma: sonographic and pathologic correlation. Radiology 1990;176: 339–43.

36. Lawrentschuk N, Haider MA, Daljeet N, et al. 'Prostatic evasive anterior tumours': the role of magnetic resonance imaging. BJU Int 2010;105:1231–6.

37. Amiel GE, Slawin KM. Newer modalities of ultrasound imaging and treatment of the prostate. Urol Clin North Am 2006;33:329–37.

38. Wijkstra H, Wink MH, de la Rosette JJ. Contrast-specific imaging in the detection and localization of prostate cancer. World J Urol 2004;22:346–50.

39. Pallwein L, Mitterberger M, Pelzer A, et al. Ultrasound of prostate cancer: recent advances. Eur Radiol 2008;18:707–15.

40. Halpern EJ, Ramey JR, Strup SE, et al. Detection of prostate carcinoma with contrast-enhanced sonography using intermittent harmonic imaging. Cancer 2005;104(11):2373–83.

41. Taverna G, Morandi G, Seveso M, et al. Colour Doppler and microbubble contrast agent ultrasonography do not improve cancer detection rate in transrectal systematic prostate biopsy sampling. BJU Int 2011;108:1723–7.

42. Bree RL. The role of color Doppler and staging biopsies in prostate cancer detection. Urology 1997; 49(Suppl 3A):31–4.

43. Pelzer A, Bektic J, Berger AP, et al. Prostate cancer detection in men with prostate specific antigen 4 to 10 ng/ml using a combined approach of contrast enhanced color Doppler targeted and systematic biopsy. J Urol 2005;173(6):1926–9.

44. Roy C, Buy X, Lang H, et al. Contrast enhanced color Doppler endorectal sonography of prostate: efficiency for detecting peripheral zone tumors and role for biopsy procedure. J Urol 2003;170(1):69–72.

45. Mitterberger M, Pinggera G, Horninger W, et al. Comparison of contrast enhanced colour Doppler targeted biopsy to conventional systematic biopsy: impact on Gleason score. J Urol 2007; 178(2):464–8.

46. Mitterberger M, Pinggera G, Horninger W, et al. Dutasteride prior to contrast-enhanced colour Doppler ultrasound prostate biopsy increases prostate cancer detection. Eur Urol 2008;53(1):112–7.

47. Halpern EJ, McCue PA, Aksnes AK, et al. Contrast-enhanced US of the prostate with Sonazoid: comparison with whole-mount prostatectomy specimens in 12 patients. Radiology 2002;222:361–6.

48. Halpern EJ, Frauscher F, Rosenberg M, et al. Directed biopsy during contrast-enhanced sonography of the prostate. AJR Am J Roentgenol 2002; 178(4):915–9.

49. Pallwein L, Mitterberger M, Struve P, et al. Real-time elastography for detecting prostate cancer: preliminary experience. BJU Int 2007;100(1):42–6.

50. Konig K, Scheipers U, Pesavento A, et al. Initial experiences with real-time elastography guided biopsies of the prostate. J Urol 2005;174(1):115–57.

51. Pallwein L, Mitterberger M, Struve P, et al. Comparison of sonoelastography guided biopsy with systematic biopsy: impact on prostate cancer detection. Eur Radiol 2007;17(9):2278–85.

52. El-Hakim A, Moussa S. CUA guidelines on prostate biopsy methodology. Can Urol Assoc J 2010;4(2): 89–94.

53. Tal R, Livne PM, Lask DM, et al. Empirical management of urinary tract infections complicating transrectal ultrasound guided prostate biopsy. J Urol 2003;169:1762–5.

54. Shigehara K, Miyagi T, Nakashima T, et al. Acute bacterial prostatitis after transrectal prostate needle biopsy: clinical analysis. J Infect Chemother 2008; 14:40–3.

55. Maan Z, Cutting CW, Patel U, et al. Morbidity of transrectal ultrasonography-guided prostate biopsies in patients after the continued use of low-dose aspirin. BJU Int 2003;91:798–800.

56. Rodriguez LV, Terris MK. Risks and complications of transrectal ultrasound-guided prostate needle biopsy: a prospective study and review of the literature. J Urol 1998;160:2115–20.

57. Herget EJ, Saliken JC, Donnelly BJ, et al. Transrectal ultrasound-guided biopsy of the prostate: relation between ASA use and bleeding complications. Can Assoc Radiol J 1999;50:173–6.

58. Kearon C, Hirsh J. Management of anticoagulation before and after elective surgery. N Engl J Med 1997;336:1506–11.

59. Nash PA, Bruce JE, Indudhara R, et al. Transrectal ultrasound guided prostatic nerve blockade eases systematic needle biopsy of the prostate. J Urol 1996;155:607–9.

60. Ching CB, Moussa AS, Li J, et al. Does transrectal ultrasound probe configuration really matter? End fire versus side fire probe prostate cancer detection rates. J Urol 2009;181:2077–82.

61. Dominguez-Escrig JL, McCracken SR, Greene D. Beyond diagnosis: evolving prostate biopsy in the era of focal therapy. Prostate Cancer 2011;2011: 386207.

62. Shariat SF, Roehrborn CG. Using biopsy to detect prostate cancer. Rev Urol 2008;10:262–80.

63. Eskew LA, Bare RL, McCullough DL. Systematic 5 region prostate biopsy is superior to sextant method for diagnosing carcinoma of the prostate. J Urol 1997;157:199–202.

64. Singh H, Canto EI, Shariat SF, et al. Predictors of prostate cancer after initial negative systematic 12 core biopsy. J Urol 2004;171:1850–4.

65. Taneja SS, Mason M. Candidate selection for prostate cancer focal therapy. J Endourol 2010;24:835–41.

66. Scales CD Jr, Presti JC Jr, Kane CJ, et al. Predicting unilateral prostate cancer based on biopsy features: implications for focal ablative therapy—results from the SEARCH database. J Urol 2007;178:1249–52.

67. Tsivian M, Kimura M, Sun L, et al. Predicting unilateral prostate cancer on routine diagnostic biopsy: sextant vs extended. BJU Int 2010;105:1089–92.

68. Walz J, Graefen M, Chun FK, et al. High incidence of prostate cancer detected by saturation biopsy after previous negative biopsy series. Eur Urol 2006;50: 498–505.

69. Stewart CS, Leibovich BC, Weaver AL, et al. Prostate cancer diagnosis using a saturation needle biopsy technique after previous negative sextant biopsies. J Urol 2001;166:86–91.

70. Ashley RA, Inman BA, Routh JC, et al. Reassessing the diagnostic yield of saturation biopsy of the prostate. Eur Urol 2008;53:976–81.

71. Pepe P, Aragona F. Saturation prostate needle biopsy and prostate cancer detection at initial and repeat evaluation. Urology 2007;70:1131–5.

72. Falzarano SM, Zhou M, Hernandez AV, et al. Can saturation biopsy predict prostate cancer localization in radical prostatectomy specimens: a correlative study and implications for focal therapy. Urology 2010;76:682–7.

73. Heijmink SW, van Moerkerk H, Kiemeney LA, et al. A comparison of the diagnostic performance of systematic versus ultrasound-guided biopsies of prostate cancer. Eur Radiol 2006;16:927–38.

74. Catalona WJ, Smith DS, Ratliff TL, et al. Measurement of prostate-specific antigen in serum as a screening test for prostate cancer. N Engl J Med 1991;324:1156–61.

75. Keetch DW, Catalona WJ, Smith DS. Serial prostate biopsies in men with persistently elevated serum prostate specific antigen values. J Urol 1994;151: 1571–4.

76. Djavan B, Ravery V, Zlotta A, et al. Prospective evaluation of prostate cancer detection on biopsies 1, 2, 3, 4: when should we stop? J Urol 2001;166: 1679–83.

77. Tanimoto A, Nakashima J, Kohno H, et al. Prostate cancer screening: the clinical value of diffusion-weighted imaging and dynamic MR imaging in combination with T2-weighted imaging. J Magn Reson Imaging 2007;25:146–52.

78. Sciarra A, Barentsz J, Bjartell A, et al. Advances in magnetic resonance imaging: how they are changing the management of prostate cancer. Eur Urol 2011;59:962–77.

79. Hoeks CM, Schouten MG, Bomers JG, et al. Three-tesla magnetic resonance-guided prostate biopsy in men with increased prostate-specific antigen and repeated, negative, random, systematic, transrectal ultrasound biopsies: detection of clinically

significant prostate cancers. Eur Urol 2012. [Epub ahead of print].

80. Engelhard K, Hollenbach HP, Kiefer B, et al. Prostate biopsy in the supine position in a standard 1.5T scanner under real time MR-imaging control using a MR-compatible endorectal biopsy device. Eur Radiol 2006;16:1237–43.

81. Hambrock T, Diederik SM, Hoeks C, et al. Magnetic resonance imaging guided prostate biopsy in men with repeat negative biopsies and increased prostate specific antigen. J Urol 2010;183:520–7.

82. Anastasiadis AG, Lichy MP, Nagele U, et al. MRI-guided biopsy of the prostate increases diagnostic performance in men with elevated or increasing PSA levels after previous negative TRUS biopsies. Eur Urol 2006;50:738–48.

83. Lee SH, Chung MS, Chung BH. Magnetic resonance imaging targeted biopsy in men with previously negative prostate biopsies. J Endourol 2012;26(7): 787–91.

84. Littrup PJ. Imaging and prostate cancer chemoprevention: current diagnosis and future directions. Urology 2001;57:121–3.

85. Arsov C, Quentin M, Rabenalt R, et al. Repeat transrectal ultrasound guided biopsies with additional targeted cores according to results of functional prostate MRI detects high-risk prostate cancer in patients with previous negative biopsy and increased PSA—a pilot study. Anticancer Res 2012;32:1087–92.

86. Kaplan I, Oldenburg NE, Meskell P, et al. Real time MRI-ultrasound image guided stereotactic prostate biopsy. Magn Reson Imaging 2002;20:295–9.

87. Xu S, Kruecker J, Turkbey B, et al. Real-time MRI-TRUS fusion for guidance of targeted prostate biopsies. Comput Aided Surg 2008;13:255–64.

88. Pinto PA, Chung PH, Rastinehad AR, et al. Magnetic resonance imaging/ultrasound fusion guided biopsy improves cancer detection following transrectal ultrasound biopsy and correlates with multiparametric magnetic resonance imaging. J Urol 2011;186:1281–5.

Imaging of Recurrent Prostate Cancer

Jurgen J. Fütterer, MD, PhD[a,b,*]

KEYWORDS

- Prostate cancer • Recurrence • MRI • Multi-parametric MRI • Imaging

KEY POINTS

- At least one functional magnetic resonance (MR) imaging technique next to anatomic T2-weighted images is needed to detect local recurrent prostate cancer.
- Whole-body MR imaging is superior to bone scintigraphy in the detection of bone metastases.
- Lymph node metastases detection with MR imaging has a poor sensitivity and good specificity.
- MR imaging plays an important role in the detection of local recurrent prostate cancer.

INTRODUCTION

The increasing incidence of prostate cancer, which is the most frequently diagnosed malignancy in the Western male population,[1] poses an increasing burden on health care. Prostate-specific antigen (PSA) screening and transrectal ultrasound-guided biopsy are revealing more and more patients with this disease. As long as prostate cancer is confined to the prostate (ie, no extracapsular extension, no seminal vesicle invasion, or no metastatic spread to lymph nodes or bones), treatment of the disease has a curative intent. Clinically localized prostate cancer is typically managed by well-established whole-gland therapies like radical prostatectomy or radiotherapy (brachytherapy or external beam radiotherapy).

Approximately 30% of patients who underwent radical prostatectomy will develop biochemical recurrent disease.[2,3] Biochemical failure (ie, a rising serum PSA in the absence of demonstrable metastases) is widely accepted as an appropriate end point for defining treatment failure in men with localized prostate cancer. The serum PSA is routinely used to monitor disease recurrence after definitive therapy because biochemical recurrence antedates metastatic disease progression and prostate cancer–specific mortality by an average of 7 and 15 years, respectively.[4–6] Patients with biochemical recurrence after radical prostatectomy have an 88% 10-year overall survival rate compared with a 93% in men without signs of biochemical recurrence.[7]

Approximately 25% to 30% of patients with newly diagnosed prostate cancer undergo external beam radiation therapy (EBRT) as their definitive treatment.[8–10] Unfortunately, up to 50% of patients develop biochemical failure, presumably caused by local recurrence after 5 years.[11–15] Currently, a serum PSA increase after radiotherapy is the best indicator of biologically active tumor.[16,17] Whenever such an elevation of serum PSA after nadir has taken place, imaging is required to investigate whether this increase is caused by local or systemic recurrent disease. Local recurrence (30%) may be amenable to salvage therapy, whereas systemic recurrence may be an indication for systemic treatment.[18–21]

The work-up of recurrent prostate cancer includes transrectal ultrasound-guided prostate biopsy and a bone scintigraphy. Transrectal ultrasound-guided biopsy is invasive and has limited

[a] Department of Radiology, Radboud University Nijmegen Medical Centre, P.O. Box 9101, Internal Postal Code 766, 6500 HB Nijmegen, The Netherlands; [b] MIRA Institute for Biomedical Technology and Technical Medicine, University of Twente, P.O. Box 217, 7500 AE Enschede, The Netherlands
* Department of Radiology, Radboud University Nijmegen Medical Centre, P.O. Box 9101, Internal Postal Code 766, 6500 HB Nijmegen, The Netherlands.
E-mail address: j.futterer@rad.umcn.nl

accuracy after radiation.[22,23] The latter work-up is performed because there is no absolute PSA cutoff value to accurately predict on an individual basis, if one is dealing with local recurrence and/or systemic disease.[17,24]

The emergence of novel local salvage therapeutic options, such as high-intensity focused ultrasound, laser ablation, or cryosurgery, is an additional factor driving the increased interest in a more detailed evaluation of the prostate or prostatic bed. The ability to detect or exclude local recurrence within the prostate by multiparametric magnetic resonance (MR) imaging could facilitate salvage treatment or potentially facilitate systemic therapy in patients with presumed distant failure based on biochemical failure in the absence of detectable local recurrence, ultimately improving the care and lives of patients with prostate cancer.

This review discusses the role of MR imaging in patients experiencing recurrent prostate cancer.

IMAGING TECHNIQUE

T2-weighted MR imaging demonstrates intrinsic, high soft tissue contrast on MR imaging and allows for the differentiation between healthy tissue and cancer within the untreated prostate. Furthermore, it provides the best depiction of the prostate's zonal anatomy and capsule. Prostate cancer is defined as an area of low signal intensity on T2-weighted imaging. The imaging protocol consists of at least 2 planes (Table 1). Preferably, an axial and coronal plane should be obtained. These T2-weighted planes must cover the prostate and seminal vesicles and is preferable orthogonal to the rectum. To reduce bowel- and motion-related artifacts, the phase-encoding direction is left to right.[25] The use of an endorectal coil provides an excellent signal-to-noise ratio. Depending on the local availability, it could be used for optimal signal reception. However, the endorectal coil has drawbacks in terms of cost and patient acceptability, especially in patients treated with EBRT who are prone to rectal complications as a result of radiotherapy toxicity. These complications may make the insertion of the endorectal coil even more cumbersome.

Diffusion-weighted MR imaging (DWI) can quantify the water motion in an indirect manner.[26,27] DWI is able to estimate the mean distance traveled by all hydrogen nuclei in every voxel of imaged tissue. The greater this mean distance, the more self-diffusion of water molecules has taken place in a certain time interval. From this estimate, an apparent diffusion coefficient (ADC) as a reflection of the self-diffusion of water in tissue in a certain direction can be calculated. Axial echo planar imaging sequence with at least 2 b-values (≥ 50 and 800–1000) using parallel imaging is applied. Motion-probing gradients in 3 orthogonal directions are acquired with enough averages to obtain an acceptable signal-to-noise ratio. Preferably, a high b-value sequence should be applied (ie, ≥ 1000 s/mm^2). Prostate cancer demonstrates typically high signal intensity on the DWI at high b-values (ie, >800 s/mm^2) and low signal intensity/value on the ADC map in the untreated prostate.

MR spectroscopic imaging measures spectral profiles in 2 or 3 spatial dimensions. These spectral profiles reflect resonance frequencies that are unique for protons in different metabolites present at the sampled location. The dominant spectral peaks observed in the prostate are from protons in citrate ($\sim$2.60 ppm), creatine (3.04 ppm), and choline compounds ($\sim$3.20 ppm). Polyamine signals (mostly from spermine) may be observed ($\sim$3.15 ppm). The signals of citrate are reduced

Table 1			
Local recurrence protocol: multiparametric MR imaging parameters at 3T			
	T2W	DWI	DCE-MR Imaging[a]
TR (ms)	5000	3000	32
TE (ms)	110.0	64.0	1.41
Flip angle (degrees)	160	NA	14
Slice thickness (mm)	3	3	3
b-values (s/mm^2)	—	0, 50, 500, 800	—
Matrix	192 × 192	256 × 256	192 × 192
Field of view (mm)	320	128	128 × 128
Temporal resolution (s)	—	—	4

Abbreviations: DCE, dynamic contrast-enhanced; DWI, diffusion-weighted MR imaging; NA, not applicable; TE, echo time; TR, repetition time; T2W, T2-weighted MR imaging.
 [a] Three-dimensional gradient echo sequence.

and those of choline compounds are often increased in prostate cancer tissue in the untreated prostate.

Dynamic contrast-enhanced (DCE) MR imaging is a noninvasive method to probe tumor angiogenesis. DCE-MR imaging following the administration of a low-molecular-weight contrast media is the most common imaging method for evaluating human tumor vascular function in situ.[28] A series of fast T1-weighted sequences covering the prostate and seminal vesicles before and after bolus injection ($\geq$4 mL/s) of a gadolinium chelate contrast agent is acquired during at least 3 to 4 minutes. Assessment of signal-intensity changes on DCE-MR imaging to detect recurrent prostate cancer can be performed qualitatively, semiquantitatively, or quantitatively. Qualitative analysis includes subtraction images and analysis of signal-intensity changes by assessing the shape of these curves. Semiquantitatively or quantitatively assessment of the signal-intensity curves is, in general, performed using either commercially available software packages or in-house made software (mostly academic sites).

IMAGING FINDINGS
Systemic Recurrence

Lymph node staging has a significant role in the work-up of patients with suspected recurrent disease. A noninvasive, reliable method for detecting and staging nodal metastasis is of utmost importance. Because normal and abnormal lymph nodes have similar signal intensities on T1- and T2-weighted images, metastatic lymph nodes are identified based on size and, to a lesser extent, on shape criteria. Computed tomography and MR imaging might be used to detect lymph node metastases, but the sensitivity of these techniques is only 36% and subsequent specificity is about 82%.[29,30]

For nodal involvement, capromab pendetide, a monoclonal antibody, which reacts with glycoprotein on the surface of normal and abnormal prostatic epithelium, seems promising. Sensitivity and specificity for the detection of extraprostatic disease are 75% and 86%, respectively. Compared with computed tomography and MR imaging, this may be a better option.[31] Wider availability and more experience are needed to use it as a standard staging tool.

Even though fluorodeoxyglucose–positron emission tomography (PET) has, in general, excellent results in other malignancies, its use in prostate cancer is limited. Other tracers, such as 11C-choline, may be more useful (eg, in detecting lymph node metastases).[32,33] The 11C-choline–PET is able to detect lymph node metastases as small as 5 mm. If less than this size, false negativity is an important issue. False positivity may be caused by bowel motion, bowel uptake, reactive lymph nodes, or nonspecific uptake in lymph nodes.[33,34] In a preliminary study in recurrence patients, 11C-choline–PET revealed promising results with a positive predictive value and negative predictive value of 86% and 72%, respectively.[35]

Metastatic bone disease: The assessment of distant recurrence is most frequently done by performing a technetium-99m-diphosphonate bone scan, which is positive in only 9.4% of patients after Radical prostatectomy (RP) with biochemical recurrence.[36] A meta-analysis of 23 prostate cancer studies deducted detection rates of 2.3%, 5.3%, and 16.2% for patients with PSA levels less than 10 ng/mL, between 10.0 and 19.9 ng/mL, and between 20.0 to 49.9 ng/mL, respectively.[37] Bone scintigraphy lacks specificity; thus, primary skeletal diseases may cause false positive findings.

Whole-body MR imaging seems to be a very sensitive tool to determine bone marrow metastases. The main advantages of MR imaging are the absence of radiation exposure and the ability to also detect nonskeletal metastases. Whole-body MR imaging combined with DWI performed superior to skeletal scintigraphy in the detection of osseus metastases in a small population of 30 patients, 9 of which had primary prostate cancer.[38] However, in breast cancer, the detection of lymph node metastasis and monitoring osseous metastases after therapy with DCE-MRI has shown reasonable accuracy. However, this has not been used in the identification of lymphogenic and osseous metastases of prostate cancer yet.

Local Recurrence

Following radical prostatectomy or radiation therapy, prostate evaluation with MR imaging is much more challenging. In a retrospective study, anatomic T2-weighted MR images were retrospectively examined in patients who were clinically validated of having postprostatectomy recurrence.[39] Clinical validation criteria for local recurrence were a positive biopsy result from the postprostatectomy fossa, a reduction in PSA level after salvage radiotherapy, or serial MR images that showed at least a 20% increase in size of a suspicious pelvic soft tissue mass. Sensitivity and specificity for MR imaging detection of postprostatectomy recurrence were 95% and 100%, respectively.

After external beam radiotherapy, prostatic tissue demonstrates diffuse low signal intensity on *T2-weighted MR images*, with indistinct zonal

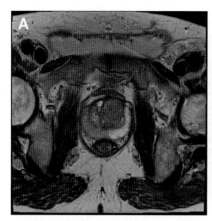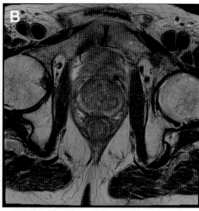

Fig. 1. (*A*) Axial T2-weighted MR imaging of a 66-year-old patient with a histopathologically proven prostate cancer (Gleason 4 + 3 = 7) in the right peripheral zone. The healthy left peripheral zone has a higher signal intensity compared with the transition zone. (*B*) Axial T2-weighted MR imaging of a 79-year-old man. The peripheral and transition zone is more difficult to distinct compared with (*A*).

anatomy and diffuse low T2 signal, which hinder tumor detection (**Fig. 1**). The untreated prostate gland has a clear zonal distinction whereas the irradiated gland has almost no differences in signal intensity between the zones. The contrast between benign irradiated tissues and recurrent cancer is, therefore, decreased, which makes the detection of recurrence more difficult. For this reason, T2-weighted MR imaging is less helpful in localizing recurrence of prostate cancer. An interesting finding in a small study that compared preradiotherapy MR imaging with postradiotherapy MR imaging using salvage radical prostatectomy specimens as the standard of reference is that postradiotherapy recurrence with a volume less than 0.2 cm³ is inclined to occur at the site of the primary tumor.[40]

Endorectal anatomic MR imaging revealed a moderate accuracy for the detection (area under the curve of 0.61–0.75), prediction of extracapsular extension (area under the curve of 0.76–0.87), and seminal vesicle invasion (area under the curve of 0.70–0.76) for local radiotherapy recurrence.[41,42] The number of studies using salvage radical prostatectomy specimens as the standard of reference is scarce.

Anatomic MR imaging in patients with clinically localized disease and local recurrent disease might have clinical consequences. The presence of postradiotherapy seminal vesicle invasion on endorectal MR imaging has been shown to result in earlier PSA failure. This finding may suggest the presence of locally advanced and/or occult micrometastatic prostate cancer.[43]

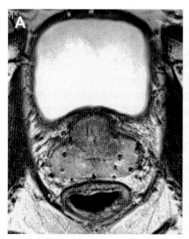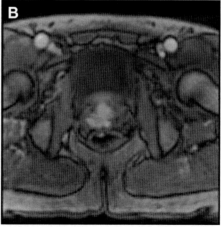

Fig. 2. Axial T2-weighted MR imaging of a 77-year-old patient with a histopathologically proven prostate cancer (Gleason 9) 25 months after external radiotherapy. (*A*) The tumor is located in the right peripheral zone, however, not visible. (*B*) Axial T1-weighted fat-saturated MR imaging demonstrates an abnormal enhancement in the right peripheral zone, which was MR imaging–guided biopsy-proven recurrent prostate cancer.

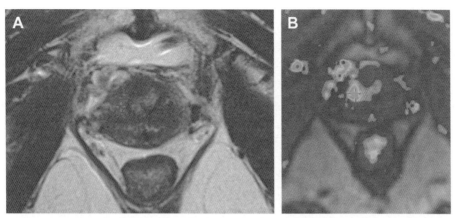

Fig. 3. A 71-year-old man with a local recurrent prostate cancer in the right transition zone, which is not visible (*A*) on T2-weighted MR imaging. (*B*) Postcontrast MR imaging shows abnormal enhancement in the treated right transition zone. MR imaging–guided biopsy showed recurrent prostate cancer with Gleason 7.

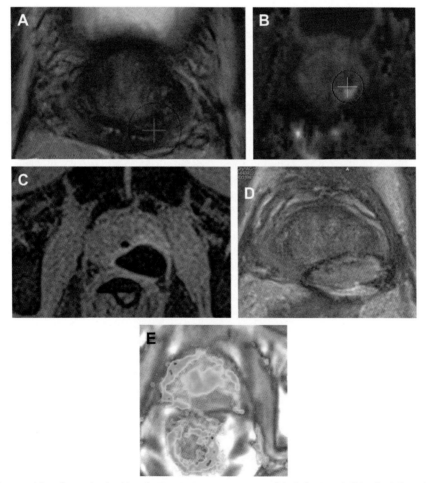

Fig. 4. A 67-year-old patient who had local recurrent prostate cancer (circle in *A* and *B*) in the left peripheral zone (Gleason 8) 4 years after internal low-dose brachytherapy. (*A*) Axial T2-weighted MR imaging shows no abnormalities other than postradiation effects. (*B*) Axial 1400 b-value MR imaging shows an abnormal high signal in the left peripheral zone. Patient underwent MR imaging–guided cryosurgery (*C*) in the biopsy-proven recurrent site, signal void is visible on the T1-weighted axial MR imaging. (*D*) Postcryo axial T2-weighted MR imaging demonstrating postcryosurgery changes in the left peripheral zone. (*E*) Postcryo axial contrast-enhanced, T1-weighted, fat-saturated MR imaging showing lack of enhancement in the treated area.

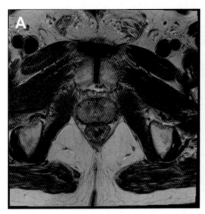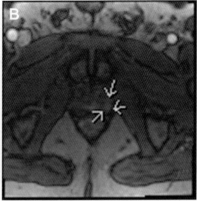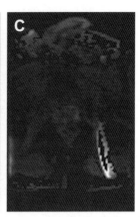

Fig. 5. A 78-year-old patient with a local recurrent prostate cancer in the left peripheral zone. (A) T2-weighted MR imaging shows posttreatment effects of external radiotherapy. The left peripheral zone shows suspicious signal intensities. (B) Postcontrast T1-weighted MR imaging demonstrates abnormal enhancement in this area (arrows), which is confirmed with MR imaging–guided biopsy. (C) Abnormal signal intensities on the high b-1400 MR imaging in the left peripheral zone.

A more prominent role for *MR spectroscopic imaging* could be in the planning and assessment of various prostate cancer treatments and in the detection of recurrence after treatment.[44–49] In a small retrospective study, MR spectroscopy was claimed to be more accurate for prostate cancer recurrence detection than endorectal T2-weighted MR imaging.[46] MR spectroscopy was performed in 23 patients with biochemical failure after external beam radiotherapy. Although this study used transrectal ultrasound-guided biopsy as a suboptimal standard of reference, the presence of 3 or more suspicious voxels in a hemi prostate had a sensitivity of 89% and a specificity of 82% for the detection of local recurrence. In a more recent study, the addition of MR spectroscopic imaging to T2-weighted MR imaging significantly improved the diagnostic accuracy (area under the curve of 0.67–0.79; $P = .001$) of endorectal MR imaging in the detection of locally recurrent prostate cancer after definitive EBRT.

Dynamic contrast-enhanced MR imaging is of added value in the detection of locally recurrent prostate cancer in either postradiotherapy or prostatectomy patients. Initial results show a promising value for DCE-MR imaging to depict postradiotherapy tumor recurrence, especially in the peripheral zone (**Figs. 2** and **3**).[50] Studies evaluating DCE-MR imaging after radiotherapy report sensitivities between 70% and 74% and a specificities between 73% and 85%.[50,51] Furthermore, the technique is valuable in detecting local recurrence occurring after radical prostatectomy, with a sensitivity and specificity of 71% and 94%, respectively.[52] Following other treatment options, such as high-intensity focused ultrasound and cryoablation, different investigators have also shown a superiority

of DCE-MR imaging over T2-weighted imaging in detecting recurrent disease (**Fig. 4**).

A significantly greater area under the receiver operating characteristics curve was determined for combined T2-weighed MR imaging (T2WI) and DWI (0.879) as compared with T2WI (0.612) (**Fig. 5**).[53] In more recent work, it was found that an ADC derived from DWI is a useful adjunct to T2-weighted MR imaging for detecting local tumor recurrence larger than 0.4 cm^2 within the prostate. A cutoff ADC of 1216 × 10(-6) mm(2)/s could predict tumor with 100% sensitivity and 96% specificity (area under the receiver operating characteristic curve = 0.992).[54] The incremental value of DWI and MR spectroscopic imaging in localizing prostate cancer (PCa) after radiotherapy (RT) has also shown to be useful.[25,26]

As in primary prostate cancer, also in recurrent prostate cancer, multiparametric MR imaging is of additional value. DCE-MR imaging is even better in combination with spectroscopic MR imaging resulting in area under the curve values of 0.94 to 0.96 for the detection of local recurrence against area under the curve values of 0.81 to 0.94 when either DCE-MR imaging or MR spectroscopic imaging was used.

SUMMARY

Although T2-weighted MR imaging plays an important role in localizing prostate cancer in the untreated gland, the evaluation of local recurrence in the radiated prostate gland by T2-weighted MR imaging is limited by treatment-induced relaxation time changes. Several reports suggest MR spectroscopic imaging, which detects abnormal metabolism, is accurate in this setting. Other functional

MR techniques, such as DWI and dynamic contrast-enhanced MR imaging, yield similar promising results. The ability to detect or exclude local recurrence within the prostate by multiparametric MR imaging can, thus, facilitate salvage treatment or systemic therapy in patients with presumed local recurrence based on biochemical failure.

REFERENCES

1. Siegel R, Naishadham D, Jemal A. Cancer statistics, 2012. CA Cancer J Clin 2012;62:10–29.

2. Djavan B, Moul JW, Zlotta A, et al. PSA progression following radical prostatectomy and radiation therapy: new standards in the new millennium. Eur Urol 2003;43:12–27.

3. Khan MA, Han M, Partin AW, et al. Long-term cancer control of radical prostatectomy in men younger than 50 years of age: update 2003. Urology 2003; 62:86–91 [discussion: 91–2].

4. Stephenson AJ, Kattan MW, Eastham JA, et al. Defining biochemical recurrence of prostate cancer after radical prostatectomy: a proposal for a standardized definition. J Clin Oncol 2006;24:3973–8.

5. Pound CR, Partin AW, Eisenberger MA, et al. Natural history of progression after PSA elevation following radical prostatectomy. JAMA 1999;281:1591–7.

6. Freedland SJ, Humphreys EB, Mangold LA, et al. Risk of prostate cancer-specific mortality following biochemical recurrence after radical prostatectomy. JAMA 2005;294:433–9.

7. Jhaveri FM, Zippe CD, Klein EA, et al. Biochemical failure does not predict overall survival after radical prostatectomy for localized prostate cancer: 10-year results. Urology 1999;54:884–90.

8. Stanford JL, Stephenson RA, Coyle LM, et al. Prostate cancer trends 1973-1995, SEER Program, National Cancer Institute. Bethesda (MD): NIH Pub; 1999.

9. Vulto JC, Lybeert ML, Louwman MW, et al. Population-based study of trends and variations in radiotherapy as part of primary treatment of cancer in the southern Netherlands between 1988 and 2006, with an emphasis on breast and rectal cancer. Int J Radiat Oncol Biol Phys 2009;74:464–71.

10. Cooperberg MR, Grossfeld GD, Lubeck DP, et al. National practice patterns and time trends in androgen ablation for localized prostate cancer. J Natl Cancer Inst 2003;95:981–9.

11. Zietman AL, DeSilvio ML, Slater JD, et al. Comparison of conventional-dose vs high-dose conformal radiation therapy in clinically localized adenocarcinoma of the prostate: a randomized controlled trial. JAMA 2005;294:1233–9.

12. Shipley WU, Thames HD, Sandler HM, et al. Radiation therapy for clinically localized prostate cancer: a multi-institutional pooled analysis. JAMA 1999; 281:1598–604.

13. Jabbari S, Weinberg VK, Shinohara K, et al. Equivalent biochemical control and improved prostate-specific antigen nadir after permanent prostate seed implant brachytherapy versus high-dose three-dimensional conformal radiotherapy and high-dose conformal proton beam radiotherapy boost. Int J Radiat Oncol Biol Phys 2010;76:36–42.

14. Abramowitz MC, Li T, Buyyounouski MK, et al. The Phoenix definition of biochemical failure predicts for overall survival in patients with prostate cancer. Cancer 2008;112:55–60.

15. Horwitz EM, Bae K, Hanks GE, et al. Ten-year follow-up of radiation therapy oncology group protocol 92-02: a phase III trial of the duration of elective androgen deprivation in locally advanced prostate cancer. J Clin Oncol 2008;26:2497–504.

16. Horwitz EM, Vicini FA, Ziaja EL, et al. The correlation between the ASTRO Consensus Panel definition of biochemical failure and clinical outcome for patients with prostate cancer treated with external beam irradiation. American Society of Therapeutic Radiology and Oncology. Int J Radiat Oncol Biol Phys 1998;41:267–72.

17. Pound CR, Brawer MK, Partin AW. Evaluation and treatment of men with biochemical prostate-specific antigen recurrence following definitive therapy for clinically localized prostate cancer. Rev Urol 2001; 3:72–84.

18. Moul JW. Prostate specific antigen only progression of prostate cancer. J Urol 2000;163:1632–42.

19. Stephenson AJ, Scardino PT, Bianco FJ Jr, et al. Salvage therapy for locally recurrent prostate cancer after external beam radiotherapy. Curr Treat Options Oncol 2004;5:357–65.

20. Catton C, Milosevic M, Warde P, et al. Recurrent prostate cancer following external beam radiotherapy: follow-up strategies and management. Urol Clin North Am 2003;30:751–63.

21. Letran JL, Brawer MK. Management of radiation failure for localized prostate cancer. Prostate Cancer Prostatic Dis 1998;1:119–27.

22. Crook J, Malone S, Perry G, et al. Postradiotherapy prostate biopsies: what do they really mean? Results for 498 patients. Int J Radiat Oncol Biol Phys 2000; 48:355–67.

23. Roehl KA, Antenor JA, Catalona WJ. Serial biopsy results in prostate cancer screening study. J Urol 2002;167:2435–9.

24. Pollack A, Zagars GK, Antolak JA, et al. Prostate biopsy status and PSA nadir level as early surrogates for treatment failure: analysis of a prostate cancer randomized radiation dose escalation trial. Int J Radiat Oncol Biol Phys 2002;54:677–85.

25. Barentsz JO, Richenberg J, Clements R, et al. ESUR prostate MR guidelines 2012. Eur Radiol 2012;22: 746–57.

26. Stejskal EO, Tanner JE. Spin diffusion measurements: spin echoes in the presence of a time-dependent field-gradient. J Chem Phys 1965;42: 288–92.

27. Basser PJ, Mattiello J, LeBihan D. Estimation of the effective self-diffusion tensor from the NMR spin echo. J Magn Reson 1994;103:247–54.

28. Collins DJ, Padhani AR. Dynamic magnetic resonance imaging of tumor perfusion. IEEE Eng Med Biol Mag 2004;23:65–83.

29. Wolf JS Jr, Cher M, Dall'era M, et al. The use and accuracy of cross-sectional imaging and fine needle aspiration cytology for detection of pelvic lymph node metastases before radical prostatectomy. J Urol 1995;153:993–9.

30. Hövels AM, Heesakkers RA, Adang EM, et al. The diagnostic accuracy of CT and MRI in the staging of pelvic lymph nodes in patients with prostate cancer: a meta-analysis. Clin Radiol 2008;63:387–95.

31. Hinkle GH, Burgers JK, Neal CE, et al. Multicenter radioimmunoscintigraphic evaluation of patients with prostate carcinoma using indium-111 capromab pendetide. Cancer 1998;83(4):739–47.

32. Picchio M, Messa C, Landoni C, et al. Value of [11C]-choline-positron emission tomography for restaging prostate cancer: a comparison with [18F]-fluorodeoxyglucose-positron emission tomography. J Urol 2003;169:1337–40.

33. de Jong IJ, Pruim J, Elsinga PH, et al. 11C-choline positron emission tomography for the evaluation after treatment of localized prostate cancer. Eur Urol 2003;44:32–8.

34. de Jong IJ, Pruim J, Elsinga PH, et al. Preoperative staging of pelvic lymph nodes in prostate cancer by 11C-choline PET. J Nucl Med 2003;44:331–5.

35. Scattoni V, Picchio M, Suardi N, et al. Detection of lymph-node metastases with integrated [11C]-choline PET/CT in patients with PSA failure after radical retropubic prostatectomy: results confirmed by open pelvic-retroperitoneal lymphadenectomy. Eur Urol 2007;52:423–9.

36. Kane CJ, Amling CL, Johnstone PA, et al. Limited value of bone scintigraphy and computed tomography in assessing biochemical failure after radical prostatectomy. Urology 2003;61:607–11.

37. Lentle BC, McGowan DG, Dierich H. Technetium-99M polyphosphate bone scanning in carcinoma of the prostate. Br J Urol 1974;46:543–8.

38. Nakanishi K, Kobayashi M, Nakaguchi K, et al. Whole-body MRI for detecting metastatic bone tumor: diagnostic value of diffusion-weighted images. Magn Reson Med Sci 2007;6:147–55.

39. Sella T, Schwartz LH, Swindle PW, et al. Suspected local recurrence after radical prostatectomy: endorectal coil MR imaging. Radiology 2004;231:379–85.

40. Pucar D, Hricak H, Shukla-Dave A, et al. Clinically significant prostate cancer local recurrence after radiation therapy occurs at the site of primary tumor: magnetic resonance imaging and step-section pathology evidence. Int J Radiat Oncol Biol Phys 2007;69:62–9.

41. Arrayeh E, Westphalen AC, Kurhanewicz J, et al. Does local recurrence of prostate cancer after radiation therapy occur at the site of primary tumor? Results of a longitudinal MRI and MRSI study. Int J Radiat Oncol Biol Phys 2012;82: 787–93.

42. Sala E, Eberhardt SC, Akin O, et al. Endorectal MR imaging before salvage prostatectomy: tumor localization and staging. Radiology 2006;238: 176–83.

43. Nguyen PL, Whittington R, Koo S, et al. Quantifying the impact of seminal vesicle invasion identified using endorectal magnetic resonance imaging on PSA outcome after radiation therapy for patients with clinically localized prostate cancer. Int J Radiat Oncol Biol Phys 2004;59: 400–5.

44. Kurhanewicz J, Vigneron DB, Hricak H, et al. Prostate cancer: metabolic response to cryosurgery as detected with 3D H-1 MR spectroscopic imaging. Radiology 1996;200:489–96.

45. Parivar F, Hricak H, Shinohara K, et al. Detection of locally recurrent prostate cancer after cryosurgery: evaluation by transrectal ultrasound, magnetic resonance imaging, and three-dimensional proton magnetic resonance spectroscopy. Urology 1996; 48:594–9.

46. Coakley FV, Teh HS, Qayyum A, et al. Endorectal MR imaging and MR spectroscopic imaging for locally recurrent prostate cancer after external beam radiation therapy: preliminary experience. Radiology 2004;233:441–8.

47. Pickett B, Kurhanewicz J, Coakley F, et al. Use of MRI and spectroscopy in evaluation of external beam radiotherapy for prostate cancer. Int J Radiat Oncol Biol Phys 2004;60:1047–55.

48. Pucar D, Shukla-Dave A, Hricak H, et al. Prostate cancer: correlation of MR imaging and MR spectroscopy with pathologic findings after radiation therapy-initial experience. Radiology 2005;236: 545–53.

49. Zaider M, Zelefsky MJ, Lee EK, et al. Treatment planning for prostate implants using magnetic-resonance spectroscopy imaging. Int J Radiat Oncol Biol Phys 2000;47:1085–96.

50. Haider MA, Chung P, Sweet J, et al. Dynamic contrast-enhanced magnetic resonance imaging for localization of recurrent prostate cancer after external beam radiotherapy. Int J Radiat Oncol Biol Phys 2008;70:425–30.

51. Rouvière O, Valette O, Grivolat S, et al. Recurrent prostate cancer after external beam radiotherapy: value of contrast-enhanced dynamic MRI in localizing

intraprostatic tumor–correlation with biopsy findings. Urology 2004;63:922–7.

52. Sciarra A, Panebianco V, Salciccia S, et al. Role of dynamic contrast-enhanced magnetic resonance (MR) imaging and proton MR spectroscopic imaging in the detection of local recurrence after radical prostatectomy for prostate cancer. Eur Urol 2008;54:589–600.

53. Morgan VA, Riches SF, Giles S, et al. Diffusion-weighted MRI for locally recurrent prostate cancer after external beam radiotherapy. AJR Am J Roentgenol 2012;198:596–602.

54. Kim CK, Park BK, Lee HM. Prediction of locally recurrent prostate cancer after radiation therapy: incremental value of 3T diffusion-weighted MRI. J Magn Reson Imaging 2009;29:391–7.

MR Imaging of Urinary Bladder Carcinoma and Beyond

Syed Arsalan Raza, MBBS, FRCR[a,b], Kartik S. Jhaveri, MD[a,b],*

KEYWORDS

- Urinary bladder • Urothelial carcinoma of urinary bladder • Bladder carcinoma • Bladder cancer
- Magnetic resonance imaging • Nonneoplastic bladder abnormalities

KEY POINTS

- Urinary bladder cancer is the fourth most common cancer in males and the tenth most common cancer in females. Urothelial cancer accounts for most cases.
- MR imaging with its superior resolution and multiplanar capabilities supplemented with new emerging sequences (diffusion-weighted imaging) is the optimal imaging modality for accurate local staging of bladder cancer.
- Potential mimickers of bladder cancer may show characteristic MR imaging features and awareness of these features is important for radiologists reporting pelvic MR imaging.

INTRODUCTION

Advances in technology have greatly facilitated faster and high-resolution MR imaging leading to its increased use in a variety of pelvic indications. Urinary bladder is an important pelvic organ often requiring diagnostic assessment, with cancer being one of the most common pathologies. Although cystoscopic evaluation is considered first line and the preferred diagnostic modality, there is increasing interest in exploiting the advantages of MR imaging. MR imaging has the potential to offer accurate anatomic information, especially in the context of muscle invasion by bladder carcinoma, which has been increasingly recognized as the most critical determinant in long-term survival and thus selection of appropriate therapy. This article emphasizes the current status of MR imaging in assessment of bladder cancer and the other less common but nevertheless important clinical indications.

MR IMAGING TECHNIQUE
Patient Preparation

Patient preparation and positioning are essential in the acquisition of high-quality pelvic MR images. Moderate bladder distention is important for bladder wall assessment, particularly for carcinoma staging. Underdistention and overdistention can give erroneous false results.[1] Optimal bladder distention can be obtained by instructing the patient to void approximately 2 hours before MR examination (range, 1–3 hours) or by clamping an indwelling catheter (if any) for about 2 hours before MR examination. Adequately distended urinary bladder also helps in displacing the small intestine out of the pelvis, allowing better delineation of seminal vesicles. Patients are examined in the supine position, with the examination lasting around 30 minutes; they should be in a comfortable position with gentle restraining abdominal bands to minimize body movement. Bowel peristalsis artifact is

Dr. Raza is now with the Department of Diagnostic Imaging, Cape Breton Regional Hospital, 1482 George Street, Sydney, Nova Scotia B1P 1P3, Canada. Funding sources: None.
Conflict of interests: None.
[a] Department of Medical Imaging, University of Toronto, 150 College Street, Room 112, Toronto, Ontario M5S 3E2, Canada; [b] Abdominal Imaging, University Health Network, Mt. Sinai and Women's College Hospital, 610 University Avenue, 3-957, Toronto, Ontario M5G 2M9, Canada
* Corresponding author. Abdominal Imaging, University Health Network, Mt. Sinai and Women's College Hospital, 610 University Avenue, 3-957, Toronto, Ontario M5G 2M9, Canada.
E-mail address: kartik.jhaveri@uhn.ca

Radiol Clin N Am 50 (2012) 1085–1110
http://dx.doi.org/10.1016/j.rcl.2012.08.011

radiologic.theclinics.com

reduced with antiperistaltic agents; in the authors' institution they use 20–40 mg buscopan, intravenous (IV) or intramuscular, or 1 mg glucagon, administered on the table immediately before scanning.

Coils

Standard body coils, used in the past, have failed to demonstrate small bladder tumors. Pelvic phased-array multicoils achieve a high signal-to-noise ratio (SNR), which provides excellent image quality with superior spatial resolution. Although endorectal coils can produce high-quality images of the prostate, bladder neck, bladder base, and posterior wall, these are not used in the authors' practice because of higher cost, time efficacy, and patient tolerance. The use of phased-array coils may provide better anterior wall visibility and image quality compared with endorectal coils because of fewer artifacts.

MR Imaging Parameters and Sequences

The MR imaging sequences and the parameters applied for bladder imaging are described in **Table 1**. MR imaging at 3 T has the potential of offering higher SNR and better image contrast, especially in a contrast-enhanced scenario. Clinically, these favorable parameters can translate into higher spatial resolution images and faster acquisitions. The higher strength also brings challenges, such as exaggerated B1 field heterogeneity, increased susceptibility artifact, and increased SAR.[2] The 3-T MR imaging may overcome the diagnostic challenge of imaging early small tumors in the bladder wall with respect to accurate anatomic localization.

A combination of sequences that demonstrate high signal intensity urine (ie, T2 and delayed postgadolinium) and low signal intensity urine (precontrast T1 with or without fat suppression and immediate postgadolinium) allows effective evaluation of abnormalities in the bladder wall and lumen. Preliminary localizer sequence is used for optimal coil positioning and degree of bladder distention.

Non–fat-saturated fast-spin-echo (FSE) T2-weighted images (T2WI) with a small field of view and a large matrix in three standard orthogonal planes provide submillimeter in-plane resolution and are excellent to evaluate the depth of tumor invasion within detrusor muscle and invasion of the surrounding organs.[2,3] FSE sequences significantly reduce acquisition time by threefold to fivefold without compromising image quality (**Fig. 1**). T2WI are also used to differentiate tumor from the low-intensity fibrosis and characterization of osseous lesions seen on T1-weighted images (T1WI).

Technologic advances in MR imaging are helping to use isotropic three-dimensional T2 sequences (eg, SPACE) in clinical practice by virtue of shorter acquisition times, volumetric coverage without intersection gaps, and an improved SNR. Encouraging results have been reported in assessment of female pelvis, rectum, and prostate[4] showing substantial time savings with similar or improved image quality. However, its role in bladder imaging is yet to be evaluated. T1WI with a large field of view is the optimal sequence for evaluating tumor extension into the bright perivesical fat, lymphadenopathy detection, and bone marrow involvement. Dynamic gadolinium-enhanced images should be performed in a plane perpendicular to the tumor-wall interface to avoid partial volume averaging and potential overstaging. Contrast administration and fast dynamic imaging improves the ability of MR imaging to detect and stage bladder cancers. Most carcinomas enhance intensely after IV contrast material administration. Coronal images are particularly useful in seminal vesicles and lateral wall neoplasm assessment, whereas sagittal images are useful in the assessment of posterior and anterior wall tumors. Diffusion-weighted imaging (DWI) is increasingly being used for detection and characterization of genitourinary malignancies.[5,6] Its role in assessment of bladder abnormalities is evolving and promising results are being shown in recent studies.

Artifact Reduction

Relevant artifacts in pelvic MR imaging result from motion, degree of bladder distention, chemical shift, and occasionally abnormal mixing of IV contrast. Respiratory motion can be reduced by using tight abdominal bands. Intestinal peristalsis and bladder motion can be minimized with a combination of moderate bladder distention and antiperistalic agents, as explained previously. Saturation bands placed along the anterior abdominal wall are useful to eliminate significant respiratory artifacts, which are not usually corrected sufficiently by image intensity correction algorithms (**Fig. 2**). Chemical shift artifact results from misregistration of spatial information caused by the difference in the resonant frequencies of water and fat. This artifact is evident only in the frequency-encoding (readout) direction. In the bladder, it appears as a dark band along the lateral wall on one side and a bright band along the lateral wall on the opposite side and can potentially limit visualization of disease.[7] Increasing the bandwidth can reduce this artifact. Chemical shift artifact can also be reduced by changing the frequency-encoding gradient in the direction that least interferes with examination of the bladder wall adjacent to the tumor.[8]

Table 1
MR imaging sequences and parameters for assessment of urinary bladder (1.5 T)

Pulse Sequence	T2 Haste Localizer	T2 TSE Axial	T2 TSE Sagittal	T2 TSE Coronal	T1 FLASH 2D Axial	Diffusion-Weighted Imaging (B-values = 0,100,800)	T2 TSE Oblique Axial (high resolution)	T1 VIBE Axial Precontrast	T1 VIBE Axial Dynamic	T2 SPACE Transv Isotropic (optional)
Field of view (mm)	400 × 100	200 × 200	220 × 220	220 × 220	240 × 240	300 × 300	200 × 200	220 × 220	220 × 220	260 × 260
Frequency-encoding steps	256	320	320	320	256	128	320	320	320	320
Phase-encoding steps	192	256	256	256	205	128	320	240	240	320
Number of slices (n)	20	40	27	32	45	15	15	40	40	52
Slice thickness (mm)	8	4	4	4	5	4	3	4	4	1.5
Repetition time (TR)	1000	3450	4550	5830	178	2000	3500	5.41	5.41	1500
Echo time (TE)	84	94	94	87	4.76	71	98	1.93	1.93	120
Averages/NEX	1	2	2	2	1	8	4	1	1	2
ETL/turbo factor	192	17	16	16	—	—	13	—	—	67
Bandwidth (Hz/pixel)	444	161	161	130	140	1698	130	260	260	822
Parallel imaging factor	2	2	2	2	2	2	2	2	2	3
Acquisition time	50 s	3.5 min	2.3 min	3 min	1.5 min	1.6 min	5.5 min	50 s	2.3 min	4.6 min

Abbreviations: ETL, echo train length; FOV, field of view; NEX, number of excitations; SPACE, sampling perfection with application optimized contrasts using different flip angle evolution; TE, echo time or effective echo time; TR, repetition time; TSE, turbo spin echo; VIBE, volumetric interpolated breath-hold examination.

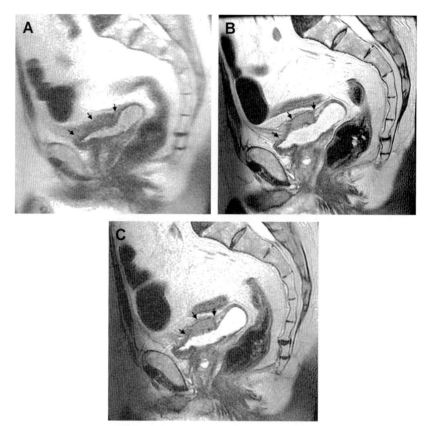

Fig. 1. Different T2W sequences used in assessment of bladder tumor (*arrows*). (*A*) Single Shot Fast Spin Echo / Half-Fourier Acquisition Single-Shot Turbo Spin-Echo (duration, 20 seconds). (*B*) Respiratory triggered Fast Relaxation Fast Spin Echo (driven equilibrium FSE T2) (duration, 90 seconds). (*C*) FSE T2W (duration, 300 seconds). The FSE sequence provides the highest degree of SNR with clear delineation of extent of tumor (*arrows*). However, note the change in T2 signal of urine on these sequences. Care should be taken when interpreting the T2 characteristics of tumor with different T2 parameters. Overall FSE type T2 provides most optimal tumor delineation.

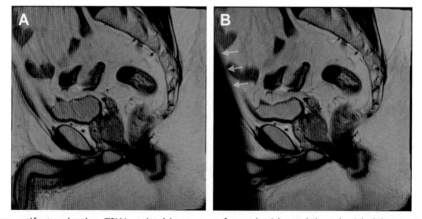

Fig. 2. Motion artifact reduction T2W sagittal images performed without (*A*) and with (*B*) anterior saturation band (*arrows* in *B*). Application of field-of-view anterior saturation band has significantly reduced the artifacts generated because of respiration-related motion of anterior abdominal wall.

NORMAL MR IMAGING ANATOMY OF BLADDER

The bladder is primarily an extraperitoneal organ. It consists of four layers: (1) an inner layer of mucosa, the urothelium; (2) a highly vascular lamina propria (submucosal connective tissue); (3) a nonstriated muscle layer (the detrusor muscle, consisting of outer and inner longitudinal fibers, enclosing a middle circular layer); and (4) an outer adventitial layer of connective tissue. A portion of the peritoneum serves as bladder serosa by reinforcing the bladder dome. The trigone has an extra layer of muscle, appears slightly thicker than does the adjacent bladder wall, and always remains smooth irrespective of bladder distention. The orifices of the ureters at the ureterovesical junction are joined by an elevated ridge covered by mucosa (the interureteric ridge).[7]

The normal bladder wall thickness ranges from 2 mm (with moderate distention) to 8 mm (when collapsed). On T1WI the muscular portion of the bladder wall has intermediate signal intensity similar to that of skeletal muscle, and the urine is dark. The perivesical fat is bright, when no fat saturation sequences are used, making perivesical tumor invasion conspicuous. The bladder wall may not be distinguished from the urine with this sequence. On T2WI the bladder wall also appears as a low signal intensity band, which represents the muscular layer (**Fig. 3**). At times, this band may be perceptible as two bands, of low signal intensity (inner) and intermediate signal intensity (outer), corresponding to the compact inner and looser outer smooth muscle layers. The thin serosal layer is not appreciated as a single layer; the outer aspect of the bladder wall may be delineated against the bright perivesical fat on T1W and T2W sequences. The normal bladder wall does not enhance substantially on early enhanced images, an important consideration in tumor imaging. However, there is delayed enhancement of normal bladder wall, best seen on fat-suppressed enhanced T1WI.

NEOPLASMS OF BLADDER

Bladder neoplasms can originate from any of the four layers with a classification scheme described

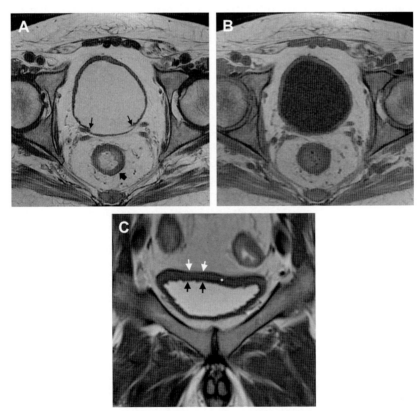

Fig. 3. Urinary bladder anatomy on 3-T MR imaging. (A) Axial T2WI shows T2 bright urine contrasting with T2 dark layers of bladder. The trigone area (*arrows*) is comprised of comparatively smooth and thin wall. Note the concentric mural thickening of rectum (*thick arrow*) and surrounding fat stranding consistent with acute inflammatory process. (B) Axial T1WI shows dark urine and wall layers. (C) Coronal T2WI in another patient shows better delineation of walls. The intermediate-to-dark signal of muscular layer (*asterisk*) can be readily distinguished from the much darker mucosal/submucosal (*black arrows*) and serosal (*white arrows*) interfaces.

in **Table 2**. Most bladder tumors are epithelial in origin (95%); most epithelial tumors are malignant (>95%); and most malignant tumors are urothelial in origin (90%–95%). Less common primary epithelial tumors include squamous cell carcinoma and adenocarcinoma. Epithelial tumors often appear as irregular, intraluminal filling defects. Mesenchymal tumors arise from the submucosal portion of the bladder wall and appear as smooth intramural lesions.[9] Malignant tumors include rhabdomyosarcoma, leiomyosarcoma, lymphoma, and osteosarcoma. Benign tumors include leiomyoma, paraganglioma, fibroma, plasmacytoma, hemangioma, solitary fibrous tumor, neurofibroma, and lipoma.

Urothelial Carcinoma

The term "urothelial carcinoma" is now preferred over "transitional carcinoma."[9] Urothelial bladder cancer is a common malignancy of the urinary tract, accounting for approximately 2% of all cancers. There are an estimated 70,530 new cases per year and it accounted for 14,680 cancer-related deaths in the United States in 2010.[10] It is the fourth most common malignancy in men (6%–8% of men) with a 4:1 male/female ratio and a peak age of occurrence in the sixth to seventh decade of life. There is rising incidence, especially in younger patients,[11] presumed

secondary to increased exposure to multiple environmental carcinogens, such as tobacco, artificial sweeteners, coffee, cyclophosphamides, and various aromatic amines.[12]

Pathology and genetics

Urothelial tumors exhibit a spectrum of neoplasia ranging from a benign papilloma through carcinoma in situ to invasive carcinoma. Up to one-quarter of urothelial carcinomas have mixed histology that includes small cell neuroendocrine, micropapillary (resembling serous papillary cancer of the ovary), sarcomatoid, and plasmacytoid components. These variants carry substantially worse prognoses than the pure urothelial cancers.

Urothelial carcinoma can be classified as either muscle invasive (nonpapillary) or non–muscle invasive (superficial or papillary). Superficial lesions are confined to mucosa and lamina propria. Invasive tumors extend into the detrusor muscle. Carcinoma in situ is a noninvasive high-grade lesion. Non–muscle invasive superficial papillary lesions account for approximately 80% to 85% of urothelial tumors. These are low-grade lesions that can be multifocal, and arise from a hyperplastic epithelium. These tumors usually carry good prognosis with a 5-year survival rate of 81%. These rarely transform into an invasive cancer, although urothelial recurrence rates are about 50%.[13] If left

Table 2		
Neoplasms of the urinary bladder		
Epithelial neoplasms	Benign neoplasms	Papilloma PUNLMP[a]
	Malignant neoplasms	Urothelial carcinoma Squamous cell carcinoma Adenocarcinoma Metastases Small cell or neuroendocrine
Nonepithelial neoplasms	Benign neoplasms	Leiomyoma Paraganglioma Fibroma Plasmacytoma Hemangioma Solitary fibrous tumor Neurofibroma Lipoma
	Malignant neoplasms	Rhabdomyosarcoma Leiomyosarcoma Lymphoma Osteosarcoma Angiosarcoma Malignant fibrous histiocytoma

[a] PUNLMP, papillary urothelial neoplasm of low malignant potential.

untreated, they are a precursor of muscle-invasive tumors. Muscle-invasive lesions arise from severe dysplasia or carcinoma in situ, and have a higher histologic grade.[14] Invasive cancer initially spreads radially through the wall of the bladder and then circumferentially through the muscular layer. It may then invade the perivesical fat and, depending on the location of the neoplasm, may invade the adjacent pelvic organs.

The genetic composition of muscle-invasive and non–muscle invasive tumors is different, which explains their distinct clinical behavior and course. Non–muscle-invasive tumors are characterized by activating mutations in the HRAS gene and fibroblast growth factor (which play a role in modulating the RTK [receptor tyrosine kinase]/RAS signaling pathway), whereas the muscle-invasive tumors are characterized by structural and functional defects in the p53 and retinoblastoma tumor suppressor pathways.[7,15] Insight into the genetic defects of these tumors provides therapeutic options of pathway modulation and posttreatment disease surveillance with biomarkers.[16]

Staging and management

Being a heterogeneous and frequently multifocal disease, bladder cancer is associated with variable clinical course and outcome. The major prognostic factors in bladder cancer are the depth of invasion into the bladder wall and the degree of differentiation or pathologic grade of the tumor. The TNM system of the American Joint Committee on Cancer[17] (Table 3) is the most commonly used staging system that determines the patient's overall disease stage (Table 4). Cancer-specific survival is correlated highly with the tumor stage

---

Table 3
TNM staging table for bladder cancer

Primary Tumor (T)	
TX	Primary tumor cannot be assessed.
T0	No evidence of primary tumor.
Ta	Noninvasive papillary carcinoma.
Tis	Carcinoma in situ: "flat tumor."
T1	Tumor invades subepithelial connective tissue.
T2	Tumor invades muscularis propria.
pT2a	Tumor invades superficial muscularis propria (inner half).
pT2b	Tumor invades deep muscularis propria (outer half).
T3	Tumor invades perivesical tissue.
pT3a	Microscopically.
pT3b	Macroscopically (extravesical mass).
T4	Tumor invades any of the following: prostatic stroma, seminal vesicles, uterus, vagina, pelvic wall, abdominal wall.
T4a	Tumor invades prostatic stroma, uterus, vagina.
T4b	Tumor invades pelvic wall, abdominal wall.
Regional Lymph Nodes (N)	
NX	Lymph nodes cannot be assessed.
N0	No lymph node metastasis.
N1	Single regional lymph node metastasis in the true pelvis (hypogastric, obturator, external iliac or presacral lymph node).
N2	Multiple regional lymph node metastases in the true pelvis (hypogastric, obturator, external iliac or presacral lymph node).
N3	Lymph node metastases to the common iliac lymph nodes.
Distant Metastasis (M)	
M0	No distant metastasis.
M1	Distant metastasis.

From Edge SB. American Joint Committee on Cancer, American Cancer Society. AJCC cancer staging handbook: from the AJCC cancer staging manual. 7th edition. New York: Springer; 2010; with permission.

Table 4
Anatomic stage/prognostic groups in bladder cancer

Stage	T	N	M
0a	Ta	N0	M0
0is	Tis	N0	M0
I	T1	N0	M0
II	T2a	N0	M0
	T2b	N0	M0
III	T3a	N0	M0
	T3b	N0	M0
	T4a	N0	M0
IV	T4b	N0	M0
	Any T	N1–3	M0
	Any T	Any N	M1

From Edge SB, American Joint Committee on Cancer, American Cancer Society. AJCC cancer staging handbook: from the AJCC cancer staging manual. 7th edition. New York: Springer; 2010; with permission.

(**Table 5**). The commoner superficial tumors (ie, stage Ta, Tis, or T1) are mostly well-differentiated and often can be cured. Most muscle-invasive tumors ($\geq$T2) are high grade and are at high risk of disease progression. Precise differentiation of tumor stage (T1 vs T2) is crucial. Superficial tumors (stages Ta–T1) are managed with transurethral resection of bladder tumor (TURBT) and bladder-salvaging treatments. Tumors of stage T2 or T3 require partial or total cystectomy or adjuvant therapies, because TURBT for invasive tumors often results in local tumor recurrence. Because clinical staging often underestimates the extent of tumor[18] (particularly in cancers that are less differentiated and more deeply invasive), there is a role for staging by noninvasive diagnostics. The multiplanar capabilities of MR imaging together with the potential to resolve the bladder layers with superb anatomic detail make it an ideal

Table 5
Survival rates for bladder cancer by stage

Stage	Relative 5-Year Survival Rate
0	98%
I	88%
II	63%
III	46%
IV	15%

Data from the National Cancer Institute's Surveillance, Epidemiology and End Results (SEER) database.

candidate for staging bladder cancer noninvasively.[19,20] The treatment for stage T4a and T4b tumors is palliative radiation. Metastatic disease is usually treated by chemotherapy. The treatment algorithm is detailed in **Fig. 4**.

MR Imaging in Bladder Cancer Staging

Apart from incidentally detected masses, imaging is not usually used for primary detection of urinary bladder cancer. By virtue of its higher spatial resolution, computed tomography (CT) urography is generally the initial modality of choice in evaluating the upper urinary tract and in detecting metastasis. However, CT is usually inadequate for staging of local urothelial neoplasm.[21] Transabominal sonographic assessment is also limited in its ability to accurately detect muscle invasion and extravesical spread. The multiparametricmultiplanar approach to MR imaging, combining conventional and functional sequences in optimized planes, allows clear differentiation of bladder wall layers and is currently the most accurate method of local staging. It is superior to CT and ultrasound including transurethral ultrasound. Additionally, MR imaging has the advantage of involving no ionizing radiation. The overall accuracy of contrast-enhanced MR imaging in determining tumor stage is 52% to 93%,[22,23] 10% to 33% higher than accuracy of CT scan (**Fig. 5**).[2,21,22]

Bladder cancer may manifest various growth patterns including papillary, sessile, infiltrating, mixed, or flat intraepithelial growth.[2,9] Around 80% of urothelial tumors are located at the bladder base at initial diagnosis; up to 30% to 40% are multifocal, and more than 50% are less than 2.5 cm in size.[9]

T1 disease
Preservation of low-signal intensity muscle layer underneath the lesion indicates non–muscle-invasive lesion and represents stage Ta, Tis, or T1. Currently, it is not reliable to differentiate stage Ta from T1 by MR imaging.[2]

T2 disease
Preoperative information regarding invasive characteristic of bladder tumor is critical for optimal management and multiple investigators have directed their efforts using different MR imaging techniques to improve its detection. MR imaging is more accurate than CT in demonstrating the degree of bladder wall invasion (ie, differentiating stage T1 from T2 and subdifferentiation of T2a and T2b disease). Muscle invasion is suggested by interruption of low signal intensity muscle layer by intermediate signal intensity tumor on T2W images (**Figs. 6** and **7**).[2] Contrast-enhanced MR

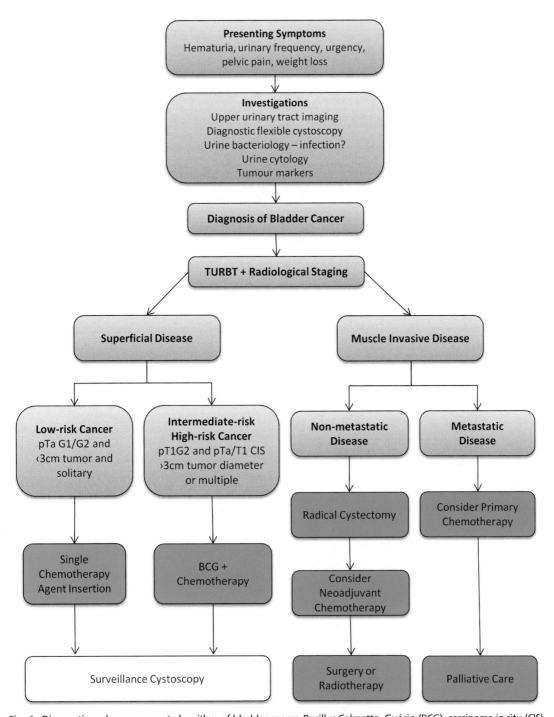

Fig. 4. Diagnostic and management algorithm of bladder cancer. Bacillus Calmette -Guérin (BCG), carcinoma in situ (CIS).

imaging has shown moderate efficacy in differentiating stage T1 and stage T2 or higher tumors, with an accuracy of 75% to 92%.[2,22]

Recently, DWI has shown promise as a complementary technique to other sequences in improving the diagnosis and staging of bladder cancer.[6,22,24] Takeuchi and colleagues[25] reported that a combination of three different MR imaging techniques (T2WI, contrast-enhanced, and DWI) resulted in an accuracy of 92% to differentiate stage T1 tumors from stage T2 and higher disease. Further details and application of DWI in the pelvis are discussed elsewhere in this issue.

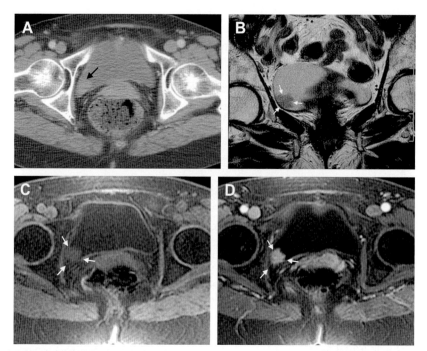

Fig. 5. (*A*) Axial CT image through pelvis shows a subtle mass in right posterolateral bladder wall (*arrow*). (*B*) FSE T2W coronal image shows mass lesion (*arrows*) with much improved soft tissue better defining the relationship with muscular layer. Pre–gadolinium-enhanced (*C*) and post–gadolinium-enhanced (*D*) T1 Fast spoiled gradient echo axial images show early enhancement of the tumor (*arrows*).

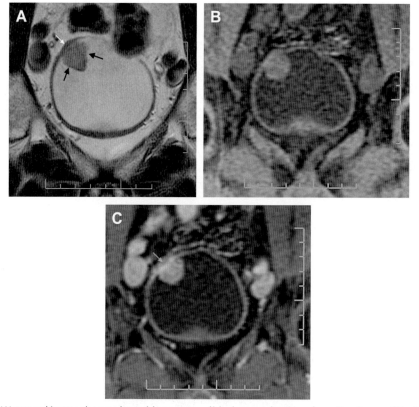

Fig. 6. (*A*) T2W coronal image shows a broad-base tumor (*black arrows*) arising from the dome of the bladder associated with wall thickening. The presence of muscularis invasion is difficult to ascertain (*white arrow*). (*B, C*) T1W fat-suppressed pre– and post–gadolinium-enhanced coronal images shows homogenous enhancement of tumor. There is partial invasion of muscularis with sparing of the outer half (*arrow*) in keeping with stage T2a disease.

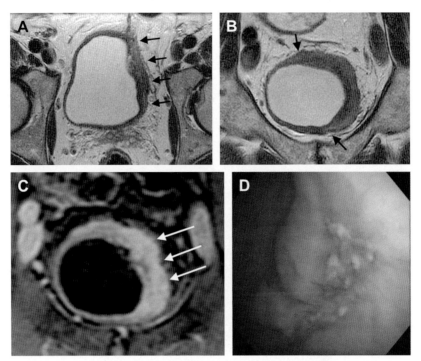

Fig. 7. (A) T2W axial image shows tumor involvement of the left lateral wall of the bladder (*arrows*) with a spiculated irregular margin along the serosal surface raising suspicion full length muscular involvement and possibly perivesical spread. (B) Coronal T2WI shows extent of tumor better with involvement of dome and base of the bladder (*arrows*). (C) T1W fat-suppressed gadolinium-enhanced image shows full-thickness bladder wall invasion (*white arrows*) in keeping with a stage T2b disease. (D) Cystoscopy shows the intraluminal view of tumor with surface papillary projections but does not provide information regarding muscular invasion.

T3 disease

Soft tissue extension of tumor into the perivesical fat can be seen on T1WI and T2WI (**Figs. 8** and **9**). Microscopic perivesical spread (T3a disease) is difficult to detect on imaging. Macroscopic perivesical disease (stage T3b) is more accurately assessed with MR imaging because CT is useful only in the presence of moderate tumor volume outside the bladder. There is potential of overstaging T3 disease because of perivesical soft tissue changes secondary to biopsy or treatment of bladder representing underlying edema, inflammation, or granulation tissue rather than tumor. Contrast-enhanced MR imaging may help differentiate perivesical tumor invasion from postbiopsy or posttreatment change, and better define invasion into adjacent organs.[26] Barentsz and colleagues[27] showed that tumor generally enhances earlier (average, 6.5 seconds ± 3.5) than postbiopsy granulation tissue (13.6 seconds ± 4.2) and using this parameter, their tumor staging accuracy improved significantly from 67% to 84%.

T4 disease

CT and MR imaging are accurate in staging advanced disease, although MR imaging offers better soft issue contrast resolution for assessing adjacent organ invasion, particularly the prostate and urethra. Tumors obstructing ureteral orifice cause hydronephrosis (**Fig. 8** and **Fig. 10**), signify a high probability of advanced tumors, and are considered an independent prognostic factor.[28] Diffuse spread to the ureterovesical junction and ureter may be seen (see **Fig. 10**). Because of a high propensity for multicentric disease, upper and lower urothelial tracts should be carefully evaluated (**Fig. 11**). The tumor may locally invade surrounding pelvic structures (**Fig. 12**).

Prostate invasion can occur either from extension of primary bladder tumor or noncontiguous from synchronous transitional cell carcinomas involving the prostate urethra (**Fig. 13**).[29,30] Noncontiguous tumor has significantly better prognosis (46%–55% 5-year survival rate vs 7%–21% 5-year survival for direct invasion) and its outcome differs with urethral mucosal involvement, ductal/acinar involvement, or stromal invasion. These facts had led to suggestions that noncontiguous prostate tumor should be staged separately according to the degree of invasion.[30]

N disease

Nodal metastasis occurs in approximately 30% of muscle-invasive bladder carcinomas and 60% of

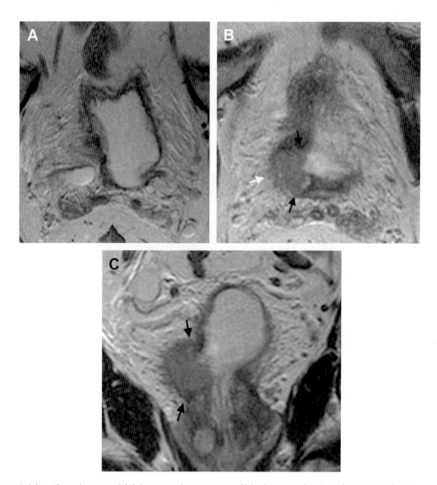

Fig. 8. T2W axial (*A*, *B*) and coronal (*C*) images show a mass (*black arrows*) arises from bladder base and inferior aspect of right lateral wall involving right ureterovesical junction (*white arrow*). Disruption of the muscular layer and infiltration of perivesical fat is demonstrated.

those with extravesical spread. Preoperative detection of lymph node metastases in bladder cancer is crucial for selection of the appropriate treatment strategy and thus for patient prognosis. Nodal disease requires treatment with cytotoxic chemotherapy and radiation after radical surgery. It implies adverse prognosis with significantly poor 5-year survival of 11% (vs 5-year survival rate of 28% in patients with no nodal involvement). The nodes that are involved in the spread of bladder cancer typically include the anterior paravesical, lateral paravesical, presacral, hypogastric, obturator, external iliac (**Fig. 14**), and subsequently common iliac and retroperitoneal nodes.[8]

Nodes are best seen on non–fat-saturated SE or FSE T1WI and T2WI. Additional upper abdominal imaging with body coil and fast T2 or T1WI can be performed easily at the time of pelvic MR imaging to assess upper abdomen retroperitoneal node status. Lymph nodes are considered pathologically enlarged if the short axis measures more that

10 mm for oval nodes and 8 mm in round nodes. Based on size criteria only, the accuracy of CT and MR imaging for staging nodal disease is comparable ranging from 73% to 90%.[27] However, size-based criteria can lead to false-positive (failure to distinguish[31] reactive enlarged nodes from metastatic nodes) and false-negative (inability to detect metastases in normal-sized nodes) results.

MR imaging with IV ferumoxtran-10 has shown potential for detecting metastases in normal size nodes and in differentiating reactive enlarged nodes from those with metastases.[32–34] The contrast agent is an ultra small super paramagnetic iron oxide (USPIO) particle, taken up by the macrophages resulting in signal loss in normal but not in metastatic lymph nodes on T2*WI. Recently, much effort has been dedicated to use DWI and USPIO-enhanced imaging to detect nodal involvement in pelvic malignancies.[31,33,35–37] Thoeny and colleagues[33] used a combination of USPIO-enhanced and DWI imaging, which yielded diagnostic accuracy of 90%

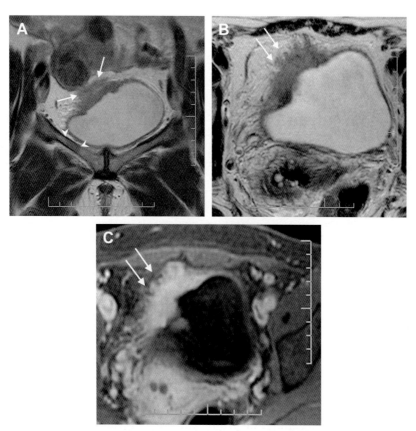

Fig. 9. T2W coronal (*A*) and axial (*B*) images demonstrate a mass arising from the anterior and right lateral wall of the bladder infiltrating the muscular layer (*arrows*) and extending into the perivesical fat in keeping with T3b disease. T1W FS gadolinium-enhanced image (*C*) shows enhancing spiculations within perivesical fat confirming invasion. Also note bony metastasis in the right ischiopubic ramus (*white arrowheads* in *A*).

for detecting nodal disease even in normal-sized nodes of patients with bladder or prostate cancer. The suspicious but indeterminate lymph nodes may need to undergo imaging-guided biopsy for a definitive diagnosis and appropriate treatment stratification.[38]

M disease

Distant metastasis are rare in bladder cancer; therefore, imaging is usually directed toward pertinent clinical signs and symptoms. The sites of metastasis, in decreasing order of frequency, include the lungs, liver, adrenal glands, and kidneys,

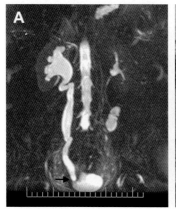
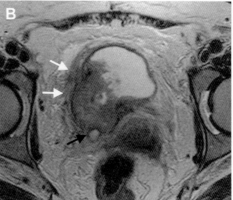

Fig. 10. Coronal T2W MR urography (*A*) and axial T2W (*B*) MR images show a right-sided bladder mass obstructing distal right ureter (*black arrow*) causing hydronephrosis. The bladder mass is associated with extensive perivesical spread along right lateral wall (*white arrows* in *B*) in keeping with T3b disease.

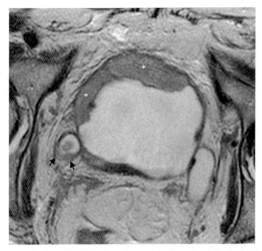

Fig. 11. Axial T2WI showing bladder mass (*asterisks*) arising from anterior and right lateral bladder wall. A further lesion in distal right ureter causing luminal expansion (*black arrows*) is seen. Appearances in keeping with synchronous urinary bladder and right ureteric urothelial neoplasms.

and even the peritoneal space. Occasionally, bony metastases occur in aggressive high-grade tumors at the time of presentation (see **Fig. 9**).

MR Imaging in Posttreatment Cancer

Non–muscle-invasive bladder cancer is followed-up because of high local recurrence rate and muscle-invasive tumor requires posttreatment surveillance because of high metastatic rate. Cystoscopy, urine cytology, and imaging of the upper tract with retrograde ureteroscopy are usually performed annually after bladder-conserving treatment for superficial

tumors.[39] The National Comprehensive Cancer Network guidelines for postcystectomy surveillance suggest urine cytology, chest radiography, and abdominopelvic imaging every 3 to 6 months for the first 2 years and subsequent surveillance based on clinical status.[7]

CT urography is more commonly used for evaluation of the urinary tract and assessment for complications related to various treatments. MR imaging is superior to detect local recurrence and can allow comprehensive evaluation of bladder and upper tract particularly for patients in whom contrast-enhanced CT is contraindicated because of reduced renal reserve. Imaging generally is challenging in posttreatment surveillance. Early inflammatory changes after intravesical medication or TURBT and late radiation therapy or surgery-related wall thickening all can mimic tumor recurrence. Presence of a mass with similar signal characteristics as treated tumor (especially enhancement pattern[26]) and interval progression may indicate the presence of tumor recurrence (**Fig. 15**). MR imaging has also shown promise for predicting early treatment response in the course of chemotherapy treatment for advanced bladder cancer, using changes in the time of start of tumor or lymph node enhancement at fast dynamic contrast-enhanced MR imaging.[40,41]

Bladder Cancer in Diverticula

There is a 2% to 10% incidence of carcinoma developing within bladder diverticula.[9] Increased risk is secondary to urine stasis in poorly contractile diverticulum leading to chronic inflammation

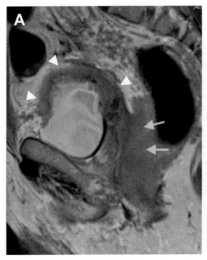
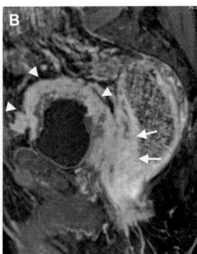

Fig. 12. T2W (*A*) and T1W FS gadolinium-enhanced (*B*) sagittal images showing extensive locally advanced bladder tumor (*white arrowheads*) involving the dome and posterior aspect with contiguous invasion of the anterior rectum (*white arrows*) in keeping with stage T4a disease.

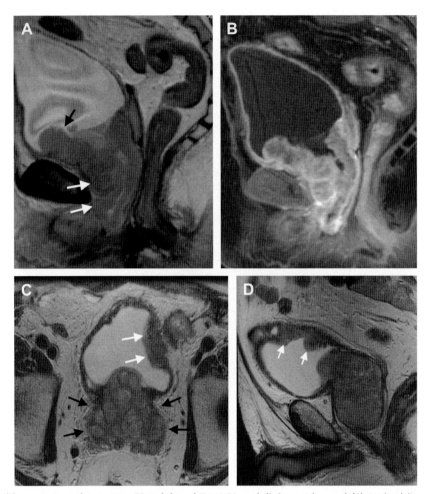

Fig. 13. Bladder cancer and prostate. T2W (*A*) and T1W FS gadolinium-enhanced (*B*) sagittal images showing a bladder mass (*black arrow*) extending contiguously within the urethra (*white arrows*) and prostate gland. Pathology confirmed urothelial high-grade neoplasm with invasion into perivesical fat and involvement of urethra and periurethral stroma. T2W axial (*C*) and sagittal (*D*) images in another patient show a mass along the left lateral bladder wall invading the muscle layer (*white arrows*). A separate mass is seen diffusely involving the urethra and prostate gland (*black arrows*). Pathology confirmed synchronous bladder and urethral urothelial malignancies.

and squamous metaplasia. These tumors may not be adequately seen at cystoscopy because of potentially difficult access in the narrow diverticular neck or unusual location. MR imaging plays an important role in identifying such occult neoplasm.[42,43] By definition the detrusor muscle is very thin to absent in diverticula. Therefore, tumors often have invaded the perivesical fat at the time of diagnosis leading to worse prognosis (Fig. 16). Most neoplasms of bladder diverticulum are of urothelial origin but all major epithelial types have been reported.

OTHER UROTHELIAL NEOPLASMS

Other tumors of urothelial origin include papilloma, inverted papilloma, and papillary urothelial neoplasm of low malignant potential (PUNLMP). Transitional cell papilloma constitutes 2% to 3% of all primary bladder tumors. It is histologically benign but may recur or become malignant. On MR imaging, papillomas are most evident on immediate postgadolinium images as small enhancing masses arising from lesser enhancing wall. Dynamic gadolinium-enhanced MR images (15–45 seconds) may be most useful to demonstrate the superficial nature of these lesions.

PUNLMP is a relatively recent entry to the World Health Organization classification.[44] It is a low-grade, small, solitary neoplasm with no invasive or metastasizing potential. Distinction from invasive low-grade carcinoma may be difficult. Because one-third of PUNLMPs recur and one-tenth progress in grade, surveillance is required.

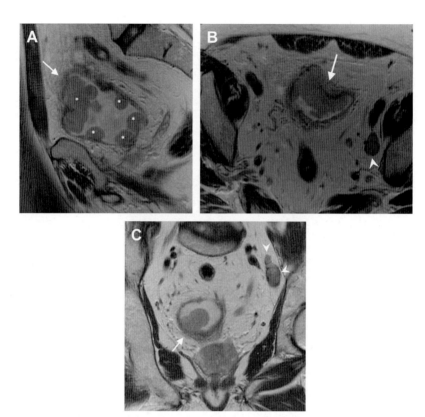

Fig. 14. T2W sagittal (*A*), axial (*B*), and coronal (*C*) images demonstrate multifocal tumors (*asterisks* in *A*) with extension through the muscular layer and invasion of perivesical fat (*white arrow*). Enlarged left obturator lymph node (*white arrowheads*) with heterogeneous T2 signal and abnormal morphology in keeping with metastatic involvement.

Squamous Cell Carcinoma

Squamous cell carcinoma accounts for less than 5% of bladder neoplasms in the western world but more than 50% of bladder cancers in parts of the world where schistosomiasis (bilharziasis) is endemic.[45] Nonbilharzial squamous bladder carcinoma occurs at peak age of 60 years, with slight male predilection. It is associated with chronic irritation from indwelling catheters, bladder calculi, or chronic infection (particular risk factors in paraplegics); smoking; cyclophosphamide; and intravesical Bacillus Calmette–Guérin therapy.

On MR imaging, a single enhancing bladder mass or diffuse or focal wall thickening may be noted (**Fig. 17**). Biopsy is essential to exclude underlying carcinoma. Muscle invasion is present in 80% of cases and extensive extravesical spread may be present.

Bilharzial squamous bladder carcinoma occurs in younger patients and is five times more common in males. Bladder wall thickening and calcification resulting from chronic inflammation or infection with *Bilharzia* may coexist and complicate the diagnosis of malignancy (**Fig. 18**). Some advocate

screening high-risk patients with urinary cytology and cystoscopy.

Adenocarcinoma

Adenocarcinoma constitutes less than 2% of bladder neoplasm and is subclassified into primary or secondary (metastatic). Primary adenocarcinoma is further subdivided into nonurachal and urachal types. It is classically associated with bladder exstrophy and a persistent urachus. Other associations include urinary diversions, such as enterocystoplasty and pelvic lipomatosis (caused by associated cystitis glandularis). Imaging findings include diffuse bladder wall thickening (75%); stranding of the perivesical fat (88%); lymphadenopathy (25%); direct invasion of the rectus muscle (25%); and a propensity to peritoneal metastases.[46]

Urachal adenocarcinoma arises from the juxtavesical segment of urachus. Diagnosis is often facilitated by the characteristic midline location of the mass anterosuperior to the bladder, best delineated in the sagittal plane (**Fig. 19**). T2WI shows focal areas of high signal intensity from mucin.[47] The solid components of the tumor are

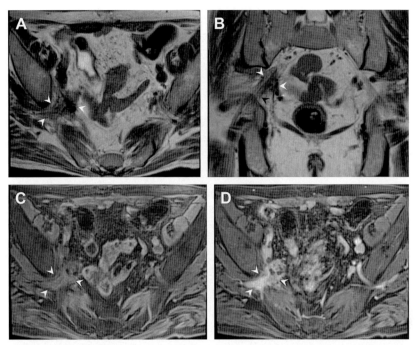

Fig. 15. Status post–radical cystectomy for muscle invasive bladder cancer. T2W axial (*A*) and coronal (*B*) images demonstrate infiltrative soft tissue (*white arrowheads*) along right pelvic sidewall, posterior to ileal conduit and in the vicinity of right internal iliac vessels and sciatic nerve (*black arrow* in *B*). T1W FS pre– (*C*) and post–gado-linium-enhanced (*D*) images shows early enhancement of the soft tissue mass (*white arrowheads*) in keeping with recurrent disease along ileal conduit.

isointense to soft tissue on T1WI and enhance with IV contrast material. Prominent extravesical component (88% of cases) and large size of tumor (mean size, 6 cm) help distinguish them from other nonurachal tumors of the bladder dome. Most tumors are high grade and advanced stage at diagnosis resulting in poor prognosis.

Metastatic or secondary adenocarcinoma is more common than primary adenocarcinoma of the bladder. It is the most common histologic type of secondary bladder neoplasms. The bladder can be directly invaded by adjacent pelvic neoplasms (most commonly from colon, prostate, and rectum).[48] Less frequently, blood-borne or lymphatic metastases from stomach, breast, or lung cancers can involve bladder. Evidence of a locally invasive primary pelvic neoplasm or signs of a distant primary neoplasm usually make diagnosis straightforward.

Leiomyosarcoma

Leiomyosarcoma is the most common nonepithelial malignant bladder tumor in adults (wide age range of 25–88 years; male/female ratio, 3:1), associated with radiation therapy or systemic chemotherapy with cyclophosphamide for another neoplasm. Leiomyoma and leiomyosarcoma can have relatively low signal intensity on T2WI. The findings of irregular margins, a size larger than 7 cm, and large areas of central necrosis (resulting in more heterogeneous T2 signal and nonenhancing necrotic areas) should suggest the more sinister diagnosis.[49]

Rhabdomyosarcomas

Rhabdomyosarcomas can occur anywhere in the body except bone. Bladder and prostate are the most common sites in the genitourinary tract. It is the most common bladder tumor in patients younger than age 10 years (mean age, 4 years; male/female ratio, 3:1). They can manifest as diffuse infiltrative lesion or masses (polypoid or "grape-like" sarcoma botryoides). Large, nodular filling defects or masses most commonly involve the bladder base and are often associated with urinary obstruction.[50] When large sized these are difficult to differentiate from tumor of prostatic origin. At MR imaging, rhabdomyosarcoma is T1 isointense and T2 bright with heterogeneous enhancement. Multiple grapelike intraluminal masses are highly suggestive of botryoid rhabdomyosarcoma.

OTHER MALIGNANT TUMORS

Metastases are commonly from breast, lung, and melanoma and less commonly from other

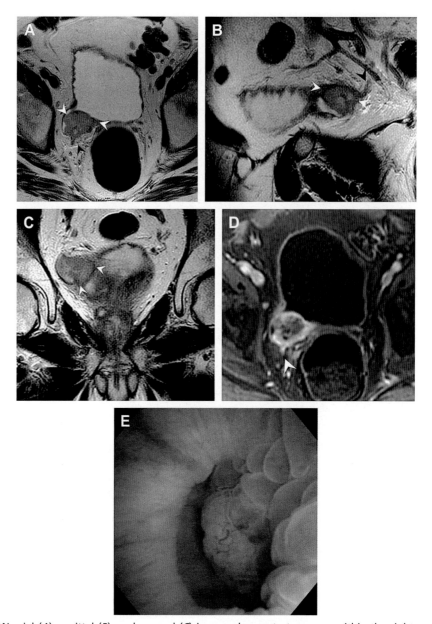

Fig. 16. T2W axial (*A*), sagittal (*B*), and coronal (*C*) images demonstrate a mass within the right posterolateral bladder diverticulum (*white arrowheads*). Along the posterior aspect of mass/diverticulum, there is a loss of T2 dark signal of muscular layer and nodularity within the perivesical fat (*black arrowheads*) in keeping with local invasion and spread. (*D*) T1W FS gadolinium-enhanced image shows heterogeneous enhancement within the tumor and enhancing spiculations within perivesical fat (*white arrowhead*). (*E*) Cystoscopy shows the diverticulum and polypoid mass with prominent superficial vessels.

malignancies (**Fig. 20**). Bladder metastases have no specific imaging findings.

Neuroendocrine Tumors

Small cell bladder tumor is a rare aggressive tumor, constituting less than 0.5% of bladder neoplasms. These typically manifest as large polypoid or nodular masses, most commonly involving lateral bladder walls. In contrast to urothelial tumors, enhancement is patchy.[51] Extensive local invasion and high incidence of nodal and distant metastases results in poor prognosis.

Primary carcinoid tumor of the bladder is an extremely rare variant of neuroendocrine tumor.[52] The imaging appearances are nonspecific but an intraluminal mass is most commonly seen.

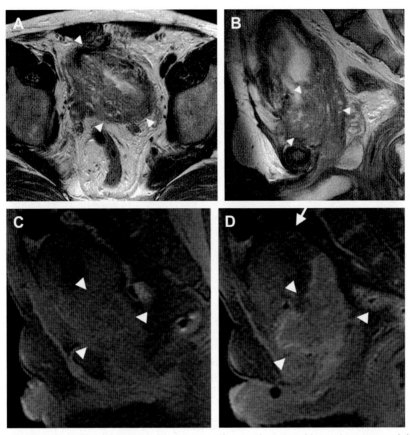

Fig. 17. T2W axial (*A*) and sagittal (*B*) images show intermediate to low signal intensity areas and diffuse bladder wall thickening (*white arrowheads*). Bladder thickening is more extensive and heterogeneous with intermediate T2 signal in the base of the bladder suggesting tumor tissue. T1W FS pre– (*C*) and post–gadolinium-enhanced (*D*) differentiate between enhancing tumor (*white arrowhead*) and nonenhancing inflammatory areas in the dome of bladder (*white arrow*). Pathology confirmed nonbilharzial squamous cell carcinoma.

Leiomyoma

Leiomyoma is the most common mesenchymal tumor of the bladder but represents less than 0.43% of all bladder tumors.[53] Most lesions are small (mean, 1.6 cm)[20] and occur equally in both genders with a wide age range of 22 to 78 years.[49] The MR imaging appearance of urinary bladder leiomyoma (**Fig. 21**) is similar to that of uterine leiomyoma, both seen as well-circumscribed lesions with areas of low-to-intermediate and high T2 signal corresponding to cellular and fluid components. Contrast enhancement is variable. MR imaging confirms submucosal location of leiomyoma but the growth pattern may be submucosal (7%); intravesical (63%); or extravesical (30%). Histologic evaluation is necessary to distinguish them from well-differentiated leiomyosarcoma. Focal excision of the mass is treatment of choice.

Lymphoma

Primary bladder lymphoma is rare (because there is no lymphoid tissue in bladder). MALT lymphomas (low grade B-cell type) are the most common primary bladder lymphoma and usually presents as well-defined masses that involve the trigone and less frequently the lateral walls.[54] It has also been reported to present as thickening of the bladder. MR imaging shows intermediate signal intensity on T1W and T2W sequences.[55] Secondary bladder involvement may occur in 10% to 25% of patients with lymphoma and leukemia.

Paraganglioma

Paraganglioma is a preferred term for pheochromocytomas arising outside the adrenal gland. Bladder paraganglioma accounts for 0.1% of all bladder tumors and 1% of all pheochromocytomas (age range, 10–78 years; female preponderance). Classical presentation of "micturition attack" occurs in 50% of patients. MR imaging is the best imaging modality to show the submucosal location. Imaging findings include a lobulated, well-marginated mass with low signal intensity on T1WI, heterogeneous high signal intensity on

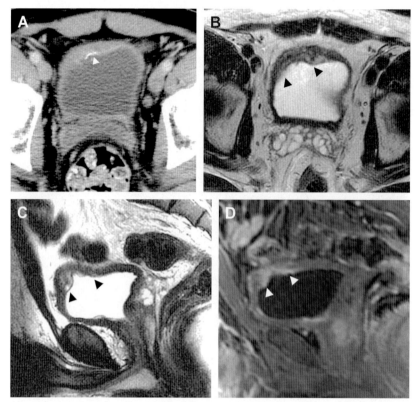

Fig. 18. Schistosomiasis. (*A*) Axial CT shows focal calcification (*white arrowhead*) and wall thickening. T2W axial (*B*) and sagittal image (*C*) shows focal wall thickening with intermediate-mixed signal (*black arrowheads*). (*D*) T1W FS gadolinium-enhanced image shows early enhancement of the thickened wall (*white arrowheads*). Biopsy revealed squamous cell carcinoma.

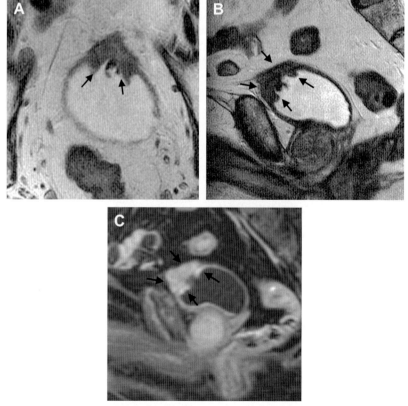

Fig. 19. Urachal carcinoma. T2W coronal (*A*) and sagittal (*B*) images show classic location of a mass in the anterosuperior aspect of the bladder (*black arrows*) with perivesical spread. (*C*) T1W FS gadolinium-enhanced image shows early intense tumoral enhancement.

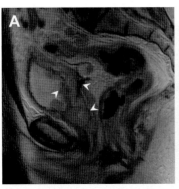
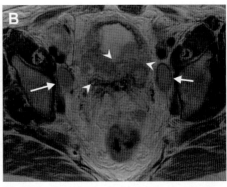

Fig. 20. Uterine sarcoma. T2W sagittal (*A*) and axial (*B*) images demonstrate extensive metastatic involvement of the bladder and urethra (*white arrowheads*). Bilateral pelvic sidewall lymphadenopathy (*white arrows* in *B*) is present.

T2WI, and intense contrast enhancement (**Fig. 22**). Occasionally, cystic change from necrosis or hemorrhage is seen.[56] Peripheral rim is a characteristic feature of paraganglioma, which may be difficult to appreciate on MR imaging. Preoperative tissue characterization is important to initiate pharmacologic adrenergic blockade before surgical removal.

NONNEOPLASTIC CONDITIONS MIMICKING BLADDER TUMOR
Cystitis Cystica or Cystitis Glandularis

This is a chronic inflammatory disorder that develops as a reaction to chronic irritation from infection, calculi, obstruction, or even tumor[57]

leading to cystic deposits (cystitis cystica) or intestinal columnar mucin-secreting glands (cystitis glandularis). It can also occur in association with pelvic lipomatosis or bladder exstrophy. There is predilection for the neck and trigone region of the bladder. At cystoscopy, these lesions usually have a cobblestone appearance but can also form papillary or polypoid mass (**Fig. 23**) mimicking carcinoma. On MR imaging, typically a T1 dark and T2 bright lesion with central branching high-intensity pattern is seen (see **Fig. 23**). The hyperintense central region shows most contrast enhancement and corresponds to the vascular stalk.[58] Intact muscle layer helps distinguish from urothelial carcinoma but often biopsy is required to establish diagnosis. Removing irritant sources

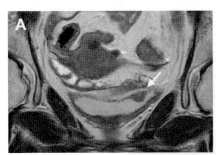
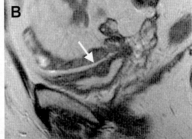
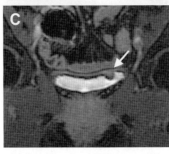

Fig. 21. Bladder leiomyoma. T2W coronal (*A*) and sagittal (*B*) images show a low signal intensity intramural lesion arising from the left dome wall of the bladder (*white arrows*). (*C*) Note the signal intensity of the mass is similar to bladder wall on T2 and T1W coronal delayed gadolinium-enhanced fat-suppressed images.

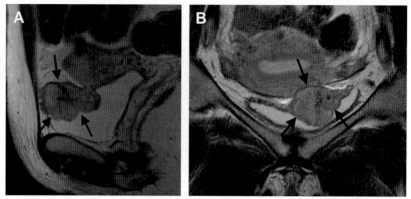

Fig. 22. Bladder paraganglioma. T2W sagittal (*A*) and coronal (*B*) images show a mass with well-defined margins, lobular contours, and intermediate T2 signal along the dome of the bladder (*black arrows*).

usually suffices for treatment but excision or even cystectomy may be required for severe cases.

Endometriosis

Urinary tract is the site of involvement in 1% to 2% of pelvic endometriosis, of which 84% affect the bladder. It mainly affects the posterior wall and dome of the bladder. The MR imaging appearance depends on the hemorrhagic and cystic nature of implants resulting in high-signal T1W and variably high or low T2W signal characteristics (**Fig. 24**). The extramucosal location of these lesions, along with MR imaging findings of typical endometriosis, should suggest this etiology when present in women of reproductive age.[59]

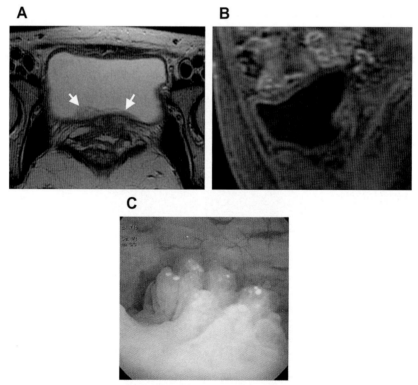

Fig. 23. Cystitis glandularis. (*A*) T2W axial image shows a subtle heterogeneous faintly hyperintense lesion with papillary projections arising from most of the surface of posterior wall of bladder (*white arrows*). Underlying muscular layer is intact. (*B*) T1W FS gadolinium-enhanced sagittal image shows enhancement. (*C*) Cystoscopy showed multiple translucent polypoid projections in the bladder lumen.

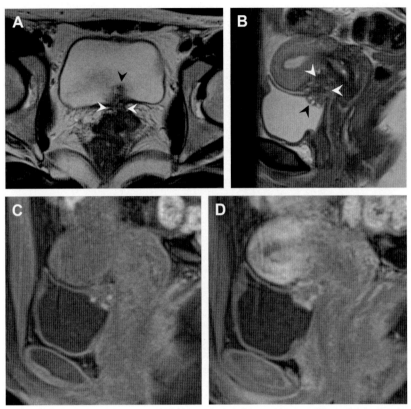

Fig. 24. Bladder endometriosis. T2W axial (*A*) and sagittal (*B*) images show hyperintense foci (*arrow*) within a predominantly hypointense plaque like soft tissue mass in the vesicouterine space (*white arrowheads*), projecting into the bladder lumen (*black arrowhead*). (*C*) T1W FS sagittal image shows hyperintense areas within the soft tissue plaque and bladder lesion in keeping with hemorrhagic foci. (*D*) T1W FS gadolinium-enhanced image shows enhancement within the lesion.

Inflammatory Pseudotumor/ Pseudosarcomatous Fibromyxoid Tumor

Inflammatory pseudotumor can occur in almost any organ of the body postulated to result from reaction to irritants, such as infection, inflammation, or malignancy, but a causative relation is not yet proved.[60] Within the bladder, it presents as a locally aggressive lesion with substantial extravesical component. It is more appropriately termed as "pseudosarcomatous fibromyxoid tumor." On MR imaging, a heterogeneous mass is seen on T2WI, with central hyperintensity and peripheral low signal intensity. The peripheral T2 dark area corresponds to edematous stromal and myxoid elements, which shows enhancement. The central T2 bright region corresponds to necrotic area and enhances poorly. Histologic confirmation is essential for establishing diagnosis. Treatment involves a variety of options including surgery, chemotherapy, radiotherapy, or conservative management with excellent prognosis.

Intravesical Blood Clot

Intraluminal clot within the bladder can mimic a bladder mass or calculi on different imaging modalities. Intraluminal clot can often be distinguished from bladder calculi. The calculi typically show high signal elements on T1WI, whereas the clot shows variable signal intensity depending on age of blood products. Urothelial tumor generally exhibits intermediate signal intensity on MR imaging and enhancement, which is absent in clot. Finally, change in position of clot within the bladder during examination or change in extent of mass with voiding can help in excluding true bladder mass.

Bladder Pseudomass

Surgical procedures involving the bladder that produce redundant uroepithelium may result in pseudomass formation.[61] Awareness of postsurgical appearances of the urinary bladder and related structures (**Fig. 25**) is important to differentiate benign pseudomass from true lesions.

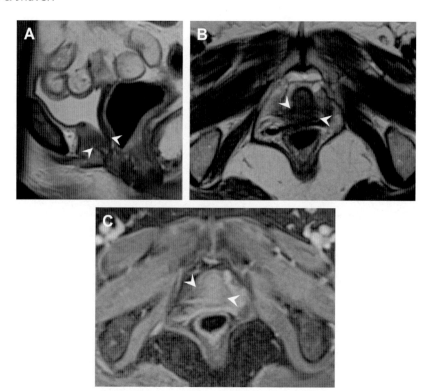

Fig. 25. Pseudomass. Status posthysterectomy. T2W sagittal (*A*) and axial (*B*) images show descent and mild prolapse of the bladder neck (*white arrowheads* in *A*) resulting in compaction of the bladder neck and urethral muscles, giving the impression of a mass within this region (*white arrowheads* in *B*). (*C*) T1W FS post–gadolinium-enhanced early phase axial image shows no enhancement confirming artifactual nature of this apparent mass.

SUMMARY

MR imaging with its superior resolution and multiplanar capabilities supplemented with new emerging sequences is the optimal imaging modality for accurate local staging of bladder cancer, particularly for the noninvasive assessment of muscle invasion, cornerstone to treatment decision making. Attention to patient preparation and protocol optimization is key to acquiring high-quality imaging data for appropriate interpretation. MR imaging also provides for useful noninvasive characterization of some benign neoplasms and mass-like nonneoplastic conditions from bladder carcinoma.

ACKNOWLEDGMENTS

Figs. 5–11, 16–19 and 21 are reproduced with permission from the article by Haider and colleagues.[19]

REFERENCES

1. Altu E, Deurdulian C, Elias J Jr, et al. Bladder. In: Semelka RC, editor. Abdominal-pelvic MRI, vol. 2. Hoboken (NJ): John Wiley & Sons; 2010. p. 1297–341.

2. Tekes A, Kamel I, Imam K, et al. Dynamic MRI of bladder cancer: evaluation of staging accuracy. AJR Am J Roentgenol 2005;184(1):121–7.

3. Maeda H, Kinukawa T, Hattori R, et al. Detection of muscle layer invasion with submillimeter pixel MR images: staging of bladder carcinoma. Magn Reson Imaging 1995;13(1):9–19.

4. Rosenkrantz AB, Neil J, Kong X, et al. Prostate cancer: comparison of 3D T2-weighted with conventional 2D T2-weighted imaging for image quality and tumor detection. Am J Roentgenol 2010;194(2):446–52.

5. Kim B, Semelka RC, Ascher SM, et al. Bladder tumor staging: comparison of contrast-enhanced CT, T1- and T2-weighted MR imaging, dynamic gadolinium-enhanced imaging, and late gadolinium-enhanced imaging. Radiology 1994;193(1):239–45.

6. Verma S, Rajesh A, Morales H, et al. Assessment of aggressiveness of prostate cancer: correlation of apparent diffusion coefficient with histologic grade after radical prostatectomy. Am J Roentgenol 2011; 196(2):374–81.

7. Verma S, Rajesh A, Prasad SR, et al. Urinary bladder cancer: role of MR imaging. Radiographics 2012; 32(2):371–87.

8. Lawler LP. MR imaging of the bladder. Radiol Clin North Am 2003;41(1):161–77.

9. Wong-You–Cheong JJ, Woodward PJ, Manning MA, et al. Neoplasms of the urinary bladder: radiologic-pathologic correlation1. Radiographics 2006;26(2): 553–80.

10. Jemal A, Siegel R, Xu J, et al. Cancer Statistics, 2010. CA Cancer J Clin 2010;60(5):277–300.

11. Jewett MA, Pereira G, Nijmeh P, et al. Increasing incidence, but stable mortality, of bladder cancer in Ontario. Analysis of a population sample. Urology 1991;37(Suppl 5):4–7.

12. Murta-Nascimento C, Schmitz-Dräger B, Zeegers M, et al. Epidemiology of urinary bladder cancer: from tumor development to patient's death. World J Urol 2007;25(3):285–95.

13. Sadow CA, Silverman SG, O'Leary MP, et al. Bladder cancer detection with CT urography in an academic medical center1. Radiology 2008;249(1): 195–202.

14. Pashos CL, Botteman MF, Laskin BL, et al. Bladder cancer. Cancer Pract 2002;10(6):311–22.

15. Wu XR. Urothelial tumorigenesis: a tale of divergent pathways. Nat Rev Cancer 2005;5(9):713–25.

16. Shariat SF, Karakiewicz PI, Ashfaq R, et al. Multiple biomarkers improve prediction of bladder cancer recurrence and mortality in patients undergoing cystectomy. Cancer 2008;112(2):315–25.

17. Edge SB. American Joint Committee on Cancer, American Cancer Society. AJCC cancer staging handbook: from the AJCC cancer staging manual. 7th edition. New York: Springer; 2010.

18. Hall TB, MacVicar AD. Imaging of bladder cancer. Imaging 2001;13(1):1–10.

19. Haider EA, Jhaveri KS, O'Malley ME, et al. Magnetic resonance imaging of the urinary bladder: cancer staging and beyond. Can Assoc Radiol J 2008; 59(5):241–58.

20. Zhang J, Gerst S, Lefkowitz RA, et al. Imaging of bladder cancer. Radiol Clin North Am 2007;45(1): 183–205.

21. Stenzl A, Cowan NC, De Santis M, et al. The up-dated EAU guidelines on muscle-invasive and metastatic bladder cancer. Eur Urol 2009;55(4):815–25.

22. Hayashi N, Tochigi H, Shiraishi T, et al. A new staging criterion for bladder carcinoma using gadolinium-enhanced magnetic resonance imaging with an endorectal surface coil: a comparison with ultrasonography. BJU Int 2000;85(1):32–6.

23. Scattoni V, Da Pozzo LF, Colombo R, et al. Dynamic gadolinium-enhanced magnetic resonance imaging in staging of superficial bladder cancer. J Urol 1996; 155(5):1594–9.

24. Hatano K, Tsuda K, Kawamura N, et al. Clinical value of diffusion-weighted magnetic resonance imaging for localization of prostate cancer–comparison with the step sections of radical prostatectomy. Nihon Hinyokika Gakkai Zasshi 2010;101(4):603–8 [in Japanese].

25. Takeuchi M, Sasaki S, Ito M, et al. Urinary bladder cancer: diffusion-weighted MR imaging—accuracy for diagnosing T stage and estimating histologic grade1. Radiology 2009;251(1):112–21.

26. Siegelman ES, Schnall MD. Contrast-enhanced MR imaging of the bladder and prostate. Magn Reson Imaging Clin N Am 1996;4(1):153–69.

27. Barentsz JO, Jager GJ, van Vierzen PB, et al. Staging urinary bladder cancer after transurethral biopsy: value of fast dynamic contrast-enhanced MR imaging. Radiology 1996;201(1):185–93.

28. Bartsch GC, Kuefer R, Gschwend JE, et al. Hydro-nephrosis as a prognostic marker in bladder cancer in a cystectomy-only series. Eur Urol 2007;51(3):690–8.

29. Pagano F, Bassi P, Ferrante GL, et al. Is stage pT4a (D1) reliable in assessing transitional cell carcinoma involvement of the prostate in patients with a concurrent bladder cancer? A necessary distinction for contiguous or noncontiguous involvement. J Urol 1996;155(1):244–7.

30. Esrig D, Freeman JA, Elmajian DA, et al. Transitional cell carcinoma involving the prostate with a proposed staging classification for stromal invasion. J Urol 1996;156(3):1071–6.

31. Lin G, Ho KC, Wang JJ, et al. Detection of lymph node metastasis in cervical and uterine cancers by diffusion-weighted magnetic resonance imaging at 3T. J Magn Reson Imaging 2008;28(1):128–35.

32. Deserno WM, Harisinghani MG, Taupitz M, et al. Urinary bladder cancer: preoperative nodal staging with ferumoxtran-10-enhanced MR imaging. Radiology 2004;233(2):449–56.

33. Thoeny HC, Triantafyllou M, Birkhaeuser FD, et al. Combined ultrasmall superparamagnetic particles of iron oxide–enhanced and diffusion-weighted magnetic resonance imaging reliably detect pelvic lymph node metastases in normal-sized nodes of bladder and prostate cancer patients. Eur Urol 2009;55(4):761–9.

34. Laurent S, Mahmoudi M. Superparamagnetic iron oxide nanoparticles: promises for diagnosis and treatment of cancer. Int J Mol Epidemiol Genet 2011;2(4):367–90.

35. Kim MY, Kim AY, Ha HK, et al. MRI in rectal cancer: added value of diffusion-weighted imaging (DWI) for discrimination of metastatic lymph nodes. Presented at the 93rd Scientific Assembly and Annual Meeting of the Radiological Society of North America: 2007. Chicago, November 25–30, 2007.

36. Lahaye MJ, Engelen SM, Kessels AG, et al. USPIO-enhanced MR imaging for nodal staging in patients with primary rectal cancer: predictive criteria1. Radiology 2008;246(3):804–11.

37. Koh DM, Brown G, Collins DJ. Nanoparticles in rectal cancer imaging. Cancer Biomark 2009;5(2):89–98.

38. Barentsz JO, Jager GJ, Witjes JA. MR imaging of the urinary bladder. Magn Reson Imaging Clin N Am 2000;8(4):853–67.

39. Bradford TJ, Montie JE, Hafez KS. The role of imaging in the surveillance of urologic malignancies. Urol Clin North Am 2006;33(3):377–96.

40. Barentsz JO, Berger-Hartog O, Witjes JA, et al. Evaluation of chemotherapy in advanced urinary bladder cancer with fast dynamic contrast-enhanced MR imaging. Radiology 1998;207(3):791–7.

41. Barentsz JO, Engelbrecht M, Jager GJ, et al. Fast dynamic gadolinium-enhanced MR imaging of urinary bladder and prostate cancer. J Magn Reson Imaging 1999;10(3):295–304.

42. Dondalski M, White EM, Ghahremani GG, et al. Carcinoma arising in urinary bladder diverticula: imaging findings in six patients. AJR Am J Roentgenol 1993;161(4):817–20.

43. Durfee SM, Schwartz LH, Panicek DM, et al. MR imaging of carcinoma within urinary bladder diverticulum. Clin Imaging 1997;21(4):290–2.

44. Montironi R, Lopez-Beltran A. The 2004 WHO classification of bladder tumors: a summary and commentary. Int J Surg Pathol 2005;13(2):143–53.

45. Shokeir AA. Squamous cell carcinoma of the bladder: pathology, diagnosis and treatment. BJU Int 2004;93(2):216–20.

46. Hughes MJ, Fisher C, Sohaib SA. Imaging features of primary nonurachal adenocarcinoma of the bladder. AJR Am J Roentgenol 2004;183(5):1397–401.

47. Rafal RB, Markisz JA. Urachal carcinoma: the role of magnetic resonance imaging. Urol Radiol 1991; 12(4):184–7.

48. Bates AW, Baithun SI. Secondary neoplasms of the bladder are histological mimics of nontransitional cell primary tumours: clinicopathological and histological features of 282 cases. Histopathology 2000; 36(1):32–40.

49. Martin SA, Sears DL, Sebo TJ, et al. Smooth muscle neoplasms of the urinary bladder: a clinicopathologic comparison of leiomyoma and leiomyosarcoma. Am J Surg Pathol 2002;26(3):292–300.

50. Agrons GA, Wagner BJ, Lonergan GJ, et al. From the archives of the AFIP. Genitourinary rhabdomyosarcoma in children: radiologic-pathologic correlation. Radiographics 1997;17(4):919–37.

51. Kim JC. CT features of bladder small cell carcinoma. Clin Imaging 2004;28(3):201–5.

52. Martignoni G, Eble JN. Carcinoid tumors of the urinary bladder. Immunohistochemical study of 2 cases and review of the literature. Arch Pathol Lab Med 2003;127(1):e22–4.

53. Binsaleh S, Corcos J, Elhilali MM, et al. Bladder leiomyoma: report of two cases and literature review. Can J Urol 2004;11(5):2411–3.

54. Bates AW, Norton AJ, Baithun SI. Malignant lymphoma of the urinary bladder: a clinicopathological study of 11 cases. J Clin Pathol 2000;53(6):458–61.

55. Yeoman LJ, Mason MD, Olliff JF. Non-Hodgkin's lymphoma of the bladder — CT and MRI appearances. Clin Radiol 1991;44(6):389–92.

56. Chen M, Lipson SA, Hricak H. MR imaging evaluation of benign mesenchymal tumors of the urinary bladder. AJR Am J Roentgenol 1997;168(2): 399–403.

57. Thrasher JB, Rajan RR, Perez LM, et al. Cystitis glandularis. Transition to adenocarcinoma of the urinary bladder. N C Med J 1994;55(11):562–4.

58. Kim SH, Yang DM, Kim NR. Polypoid and papillary cystitis mimicking a large transitional carcinoma in a patient without a history of catheterization: computed tomography and magnetic resonance findings. J Comput Assist Tomogr 2004;28(4):485–7.

59. Umaria N, Olliff JF. MRI appearances of bladder endometriosis. Br J Radiol 2000;73(871):733–6.

60. Narla LD, Newman B, Spottswood SS, et al. Inflammatory pseudotumor1. Radiographics 2003;23(3): 719–29.

61. Markle BM, Catena L. Bladder pseudomass following cystography-related bladder trauma. Radiology 1986;159(1):265.

Pelvic Nodal Imaging

Sandeep S. Hedgire, MD[a,*], Vivek K. Pargaonkar, MD[a],
Azadeh Elmi, MD[a], Alpana M. Harisinghani, MD[b],
Mukesh G. Harisinghani, MD[c,d]

KEYWORDS

- Lymph node • Metastasis • Testicular cancer • Prostate cancer • Penile cancer • Bladder cancer

KEY POINTS

- Understanding the relevant anatomy and pathways of lymphatic spread of male pelvic malignancies.
- To review imaging features, diagnostic criteria and newer advances in male pelvic nodal imaging.
- To illustrate differential diagnosis of lymph nodes in the male pelvis.

INTRODUCTION

In patients with known pelvic malignancies, presence of nodal disease signifies adverse prognosis. The location of nodal metastases is governed by site of the primary tumor (bladder, prostate, testes, and penis) and integrity of the draining lymphatics. It is important to assign node regional or nonregional categories because this localization changes the staging (eg, a metastatic inguinal node is considered regional for penile cancer but nonregional for prostate cancer).[1] Currently, computed tomography (CT) and magnetic resonance (MR) imaging are routinely used for preoperative staging of these patients. These techniques rely on inaccurate and nonspecific features such as size and morphologic criteria to distinguish a benign from a malignant lymph node.[2,3] Emerging functional imaging techniques like positron emission tomography (PET), diffusion-weighted (DW) MR imaging, and lymphotrophic nanoparticle-enhanced MR (LNMR) imaging have shown promising results in surmounting these limitations and may have important implications in the future.[3]

ANATOMY

Nodal groups that drain the male pelvis can be broadly divided into 5 groups (common, internal and external iliac, inguinal, and retroperitoneal nodes) (**Fig. 1**). Knowledge of the relevant clinical anatomy is essential to assign the node into a particular group that, in turn, affects the staging and prognosis.

Common Iliac Nodes

This group is in close proximity to the common iliac vessels and comprises 3 chains: lateral, middle, and medial (**Fig. 2**). Nodes in the medial chain lie in the triangular area formed by both common iliac arteries between their origins in the aortic bifurcation and their bifurcation into external and internal iliac arteries. Nodes at the sacral promontory are also included in this chain. The lumbosacral fossa contains middle chain nodes. The fossa is the area bordered by the psoas muscle anterolaterally, the lower lumbar or upper sacral vertebral bodies posteromedially, and by the common iliac vessels anteromedially (between the common iliac artery and common iliac vein).[4]

Internal Iliac Nodes

The internal iliac or hypogastric nodes are nodal chains that are distributed along the visceral branches of the internal iliac artery.[5] Those located at the junction between the internal and external iliac nodal are also called the junctional nodes.[4]

[a] Division of Abdominal Imaging and Intervention, Massachusetts General Hospital-Harvard Medical School, 55 Fruit Street, White 270, Boston, MA 02114, USA; [b] Perceptive Informatics, 2 Federal Street, Billerica, MA 01821, USA; [c] Harvard Medical School, Boston, MA 02114, USA; [d] Massachusetts General Hospital, Boston, MA 02114, USA
* Corresponding author.
E-mail address: hedgire.sandeep@mgh.harvard.edu

Radiol Clin N Am 50 (2012) 1111–1125
http://dx.doi.org/10.1016/j.rcl.2012.08.002

radiologic.theclinics.com

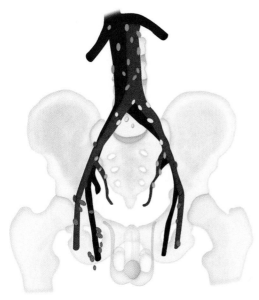

Fig. 1. Lymph nodal groups pertinent to male pelvis. Para-aortic and aortocaval (*blue*), common iliac (*yellow*), external iliac (*purple*), internal iliac (*green*), and inguinal (*red*).

External Iliac Nodes

Similar to the common iliac nodes, there are 3 chains of the external iliac nodes: lateral, middle, and medial. The lateral chain nodes are those located along the lateral aspect of the external iliac artery. Middle chain nodes are located between

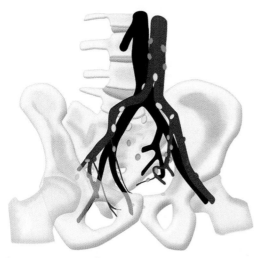

Fig. 2. Common iliac lymph nodes (*yellow*). The common iliac nodal group consists of 3 chains: lateral chain, which is located lateral to the common iliac artery; medial chain, which occupies the triangular area bordered by both common iliac arteries and includes nodes at the sacral promontory; and the middle chain, which consists of nodes within the lumbosacral fossa.

the external iliac artery and vein. The medial chain nodes, which are also known as the obturator nodes (**Fig. 3**), are located posteromedial to the external iliac vein.[4,6]

Inguinal Nodes

Inguinal nodes can be superficial or deep.[4,7] Nodes located subcutaneously along superficial femoral vessels are part of superficial inguinal nodes. The sentinel node for this group is at the saphenous-femoral junction providing easy access to biopsy. The deep inguinal nodes lie along the common femoral vessels. The inguinal ligament and origins of the inferior epigastric and circumflex iliac vessels serve as a landmark allowing differentiation between the medial chain of the external iliac nodes and the deep inguinal nodes.

Para-aortic Nodes

There are 7 subgroups of para-aortic nodes: lateroaortic, preaortic, retroaortic, laterocaval, aortocaval (**Fig. 4**), precaval, and retrocaval.[4]

In addition, there are perivisceral nodes (perirectal, perivesical, periprostatic) located adjacent to the pelvic viscera.[8]

IMAGING FINDINGS

In clinical practice, anatomic imaging techniques such as multidetector CT (MDCT) and MR imaging are the most commonly used for staging of pelvic malignancies. MDCT offers high spatial resolution, rapid image acquisition, and multiplanar reconstruction, allowing accurate measurements. MR imaging is helpful in the staging of pelvic malignancies by virtue of its superior soft tissue resolution and is more robust in nodal detection than CT.[9]

Metastatic Lymph Node Imaging Criteria

Size
MDCT and MR imaging allow visualization of lymph nodes and use enlargement as a criteria to identify metastatic nodes. According to Response Evaluation Criteria In Solid Tumors (RECIST) 1.1, a lymph node is considered a target lesion only if the short-axis measurement is greater than or equal to 15 mm.[10] However, these techniques overlook normal-sized nodes that may harbor metastatic foci and may include enlarged reactive benign nodes. Also there is a lack of consensus on the upper limit of maximum short-axis diameter for each nodal group in the pelvis. **Table 1** summarizes the normal upper limits of short-axis diameter of various nodal groups in the pelvis.[5,11,12]

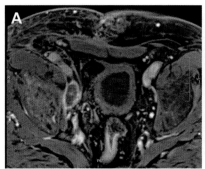
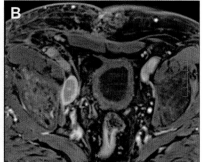

Fig. 3. (*A*, *B*) Axial gadolinium-enhanced T1-weighted image shows a necrotic right obturator lymph node (*green*) metastatic from primary penile cancer.

Multiple studies using various size thresholds in to increase the detection rate of malignancy in the lymph nodes have previously been published. The results from these studies show that there is no ideal size criterion that produces optimal sensitivity and specificity. With decrease in size threshold, the sensitivity tends to increase at the expense of reduced specificity.[5,13–17]

Location
Each tumor type in the male pelvis tends to spread to lymph nodes along its drainage pathway and, while evaluating for the nodal disease, these regions must be evaluated metastatic adenopathy into regional and nonregional nodes. **Table 2** elaborates distribution of each nodal group as regional or nonregional with respect to the site of primary tumors.[1]

There are various other secondary features (**Table 3**) to distinguish benign and malignant nodes; however, these are not specific and are unreliable.[5,18–22]

PATHWAYS

The pattern of nodal metastasis of male genitourinary tumors depends on site of the primary tumor. These pathways are shown in **Figs. 5–8**.[1,4,23–25]

PEARLS, PITFALLS, AND MIMICS

In patients with genitourinary malignancies, when an imaging test is ordered, the oncologist is seeking answers to pertinent questions. This article highlights important considerations that may have prognostic implications.

Prostate Cancer

Nodal involvement is noted in 5% to 10% of patients with prostate carcinoma (**Algorithm 1**). Probability of the nodal disease is as high as 50% in high-risk groups (prostate-specific antigen [PSA] level ≥20 ng/mL, Gleason score ≥7, clinical stage T3/T4), compared with 4% in the low-risk group (PSA level <20 ng/mL, Gleason score <7, clinical stage T1/T2). The 5-year survival rates depend on total number of lymph nodes involved and vary from 75% to 80% in patients with solitary nodal metastasis to only 20% to 30% in those with more than 5 nodal metastases. Hence it is prudent to mention the total number of nodes involved.[26]

The categorization of an involved lymph node into N or M stage is not determined by laterality but by the level of the node. The lymph nodes below the level of bifurcation of common iliac

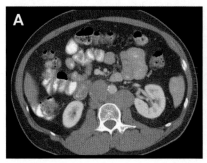
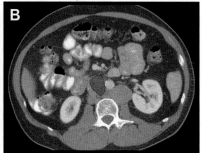

Fig. 4. (*A*, *B*) Axial contrast-enhanced CT image shows metastatic aortocaval lymph node (*red*) in a patient with prostate cancer.

Table 1
Summary of the normal upper limits of short-axis diameter of various nodal groups in the pelvis

Location of the Node	Size (mm)
Common iliac	9
Internal iliac	7
External iliac	10
Obturator	8
Inguinal	15
Upper para-aortic	9
Lower para-aortic	11

vessels are classified into N stage (**Figs. 9** and **10**), whereas the lymph nodes situated above this level are classified into M stage (**Fig. 11**).[27] In the setting of radical prostatectomy and radiation therapy, extrapelvic nodes are the usual site of recurrence.[28]

In the detection of nodal disease, CT and MR imaging have shown comparable results. It has been suggested that decreasing the threshold value for measuring the lymph node size to 6 mm yields higher sensitivity (78%) and specificity (98%) in the detection of nodal metastases.[14]

Penile Cancer

The importance of detection of lymph node metastasis is manifold (**Algorithm 2**). Penile carcinoma is an example in which regional lymphadenectomy can be curative. Up to 45% of patients have nodal metastases at the time of diagnosis.

An enlarged inguinal lymph node in penile cancer should not always be considered malignant because 50% of enlarged nodes are reactive[29] and 20% of small nodes show malignancy.[24] Antibiotic therapy often precedes the resection to distinguish reactive nodes from metastatic nodes.

Persistent enlargement of such nodes even after antibiotic therapy is considered malignant until proved otherwise. Imaging is important in identifying metastatic lymph nodes, because clinical examination is often inadequate and leads to false-positive and false-negative results.[30]

Similar to prostate cancer, in patients with penile cancers, the nodal staging is not affected by laterality of the tumor. Enlarged contralateral nodes may also be seen in addition to ipsilateral nodes owing to abundant lymphatics crossing over at the base of penis. Such bilateral involvement is common in penile cancer compared with other tumors of the male pelvis (**Fig. 12**).[31] A greater number of metastatic nodes, bilateral disease, deep pelvic nodal metastases, and extranodal extensions adversely affect prognosis. The 5-year survival rate decreases from 82% to 88% (in patients with only 1 or 2 involved nodes) to 7% to 50% (among those with more than 2 nodes).[29]

Testicular Cancer

When enlarged retroperitoneal/para-aortic lymph nodes are seen in a young male patient, testicular cancer should always be suspected (**Fig. 13**, **Algorithm 3**). Lymphatics are a major route of cancer spread for testicular malignancies because the tunica albuginea forms a barrier for local extension. Hence, the main role of imaging is to accurately detect the nodal spread of the cancer because it determines the therapeutic approach.

In testicular malignancies, nodal involvement of the inguinal, external iliac, and the pelvic nodes is usually considered as distant spread. Prior surgical procedures alter drainage of this area and these nodes are considered as regional (**Fig. 14**).

While determining the nodal burden in testicular malignancies, the lymph nodes should be measured by calculating the maximum diameter of the lymph node, as opposed to many other malignancies in

Table 2
Distribution of each nodal group into regional or nonregional with respect to the site of primary tumors

Nodal Group	Prostate	Penile	Testes	Bladder
Common iliac	Nonregional	Nonregional	Nonregional	Nonregional
Internal ILIAC	Regional	Regional	Nonregional	Regional
External iliac	Regional	Regional	Regional (in the context of previous scrotal/inguinal surgery)	Regional
Inguinal	Nonregional	Regional	Regional (in the context of previous scrotal/inguinal surgery)	Nonregional
Para-aortic	Nonregional	Nonregional	Regional	Nonregional
Perivisceral	Regional	Regional	Regional	Regional

Table 3
Secondary features to distinguish benign from malignant nodes

Criteria	Benign	Malignant
Shape	Ovoid or elongated	Round or spherical
Margin	Smooth	Irregular/speculated/lobulated
Perinodal fat	Clear	Infiltrated
Internal architecture	Preserved central fatty hilum Homogenous on T2WI Necrosis (in tuberculosis, fungal infection and cavitating node syndrome, after therapy)	Loss of central fatty hilum Heterogeneous on T2WI Central necrosis
Enhancement	Homogeneous	Heterogeneous Similar to the primary tumor

Abbreviation: T2WI, T2-weighted imaging.

which the short-axis of the lymph nodes is measured.[3] This difference is important because it has major implications in the staging of the malignancy.

It is possible to speculate about the histologic type of testicular malignancy from the imaging characteristics of the involved lymph nodes. Lymph node metastases from seminoma usually show soft tissue attenuation on CT, whereas lymph node metastases from nonseminomatous germ cell tumors are heterogeneous and show cystic changes within.

Bladder Carcinoma

Presence of nodal metastases influences therapy in patients with bladder cancer.[32] Presence of any lymph node involvement by bladder cancer is regarded as stage 4 disease.[33] Also, as the number of nodes involved increases, the survival rate decreases (**Fig. 15**). In patients with bladder cancer, the maximum diameter of the largest node is measured while categorizing the N staging. In patients with bladder cancer, the involved lymph nodes often show similar contrast enhancement features and calcifications as are seen in the primary tumor. It is important to report the distribution of involved lymph nodes, because lymph nodes below the level of the common iliac vessels are regional nodes, and above the level of common iliac vessels they are considered nonregional.

Differential Diagnosis

False-positive interpretation of a finding as a metastatic node may alter the staging in pelvic malignancies. At times, anatomic variants, approximation of various anatomic structures, or imaging technique limitations create a diagnostic dilemma by making delineation of lymph nodes difficult. This article lists the commonly encountered lymph node mimics in the male pelvis.[34–39]

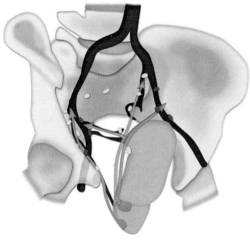

Fig. 5. Common pathways of metastasis of prostate cancer. The obturator nodes in the external iliac (*purple*) nodal group are the lateral route (*yellow arrows*), and the junctional nodes in the internal iliac (*yellow*) nodal group are the hypogastric route (*blue arrows*).

Serial numbers	Lymph node mimic
1	Nonopacified bowel loops (**Fig. 16A, B**)
2	Phleboliths (especially on MR imaging)
3	Extramedullary hematopoiesis
4	Poorly opacified or nonenhanced vessels (see **Fig. 16C, D**)
5	Localized hemorrhage, especially when focal
6	Undescended testes (see **Fig. 16E**)

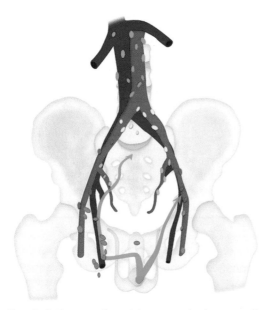

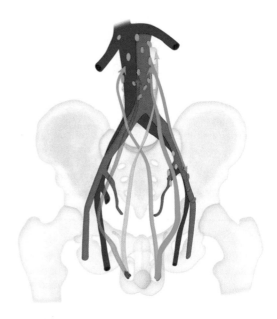

Fig. 6. Pathways of nodal metastasis from penile cancer: the superficial inguinal lymphatic drainage pathway for which the sentinel node is the saphenofemoral node (*red*). The second pathway is direct involvement of the external iliac nodes (*purple*). Involvement of common iliac (*yellow*) nodes indicates M1 disease.

Fig. 7. Common routes of nodal metastasis from testicular cancer along the para-aortic pathway. In metastases from the right testis (*purple arrow*), the sentinel nodes are in the aortocaval chain at the level of the second lumbar vertebral body. In metastases from the left testis (*green arrow*), the sentinel nodes are usually the left para-aortic nodes located just inferior to the left renal vein. Involvement of a nodal group of the opposite side is also known. External iliac nodes may subsequently be involved (*dark green arrow on right*).

RECENT ADVANCES

As discussed previously, CT and MR imaging, which are the most commonly used imaging techniques for staging pelvic malignancies, are not sensitive or specific. These techniques use size and morphology criteria to identify metastatic lymph nodes and thus normal-sized malignant lymph nodes and micrometastases are missed and enlarged reactive lymph nodes are vulnerable to false-positive interpretation.[40] It has been shown in recent studies that cautious lymph node dissection in prostate and bladder cancer reveal a higher rate of metastases in patients with negative preoperative radiological staging studies.[41–44] These challenges have led to the development of newer imaging techniques designed to increase metastatic lymph node detection and help in accurate staging and better treatment planning.

PET/CT

PET is a technique that uses metabolic characteristics to distinguish benign from malignant tissue. It has increasingly been used in staging of various malignancies.

The basic principle of PET/CT involves the use of a radiopharmaceutical agent. The most commonly used agent is [^{18}F]fluorodeoxyglucose (FDG). FDG is a glucose analogue and is taken up and retained by tissues that have high metabolic activity, such as most malignant tumors. FDG uptake by tumor is analyzed by PET/CT in terms of standard uptake value (SUV). However, because FDG is excreted via the kidneys and bowel, it limits optimum assessment of the pelvis. Hence, FDG PET/CT is not considered useful for pelvic nodal staging in cases of male pelvic malignancies.

To surpass this limitation of FDG, many other radiotracers were analyzed for their efficacy in male pelvic malignancy staging. [^{11}C]Acetate or [^{11}C]choline is one such radiotracer that has shown promising results in the detection of lymph node metastases in patients with prostate and bladder cancer.[45,46] Studies with these newer agents have shown increased sensitivity, specificity, positive predictive value, negative predictive value, and percentage of correctly identified nodes compared with CT alone. However, PET/CT is unable to identify lymph nodes smaller than 5 mm because of image resolution limitations.

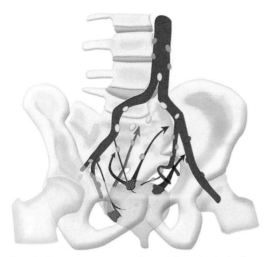

Fig. 8. Common routes of nodal metastasis from bladder cancer. Cancers in the bladder fundus metastasize mainly via an anterior route (*pink arrows*), whereas those in upper or lower lateral parts of the bladder can metastasize via a lateral route (*blue arrow*) directly to the external iliac (*purple*) nodes. Cancer in the bladder neck metastasizes via the presacral route (*red arrow*).

DW MR Imaging

DW MR imaging is a noninvasive imaging technique that characterizes molecular diffusion. It determines the brownian motion of water molecules within a tissue.[47] The degree of restriction to water diffusion in biologic tissue is inversely correlated to the tissue cellularity and the integrity of cell membranes.[48–51] High cellularity and cell membrane integrity restrict diffusion. DW imaging

is quick to perform, does not require the use of intravenous contrast material and enables the characterization of tissue at a microscopic level, highlighting a mechanism that is different from T1 and T2 relaxations. It aids in early detection and localization of tumor, and prediction of tumor response and recurrence by virtue of its ability to detect microstructural changes in the cells. Multiple b values are used to change the diffusion sensitivity during image acquisition. DW MR imaging also provides quantitative analysis of diffusion characteristics and tissue perfusion by acquiring the apparent diffusion coefficient (ADC) maps.

Malignant lymph nodes tend to be hypercellular, have enlarged hyperchromatic nuclei, with an abundance of macromolecular proteins leading to a reduction of both the intracellular and the extracellular matrix space. Benign lymph nodes are hypocellular, have small nuclei and lower nucleus/cytoplasm ratios, leading to more extracellular space. Thus, benign lymph nodal architecture facilitates better water diffusion and higher ADCs than malignant lymph nodes (**Fig. 17**).[52–54]

In a study conducted by Eiber and colleagues[55] in patients with prostate cancer with lymph node metastases, DW imaging differentiated malignant from benign lymph nodes with an accuracy of 86%, a sensitivity of 86%, and a specificity of 85% when a cutoff ADC value of 1.30×10^{-3} mm^2/s was used.

Although DW imaging is a promising technique, it has potential limitations. All studies done to distinguish benign from malignant lymph node showed a certain level of overlap and no studies

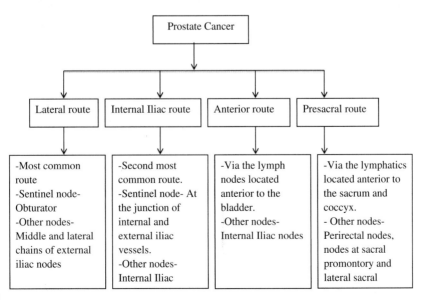

Algorithm 1.

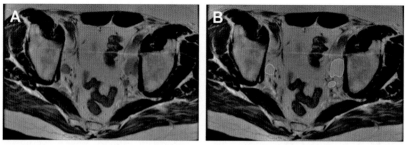

Fig. 9. (A, B) Lymph node involvement in prostate cancer. Axial T2-weighted image shows bilateral metastatic obturator lymph nodes (*green*) and a left internal iliac lymph node (*orange*).

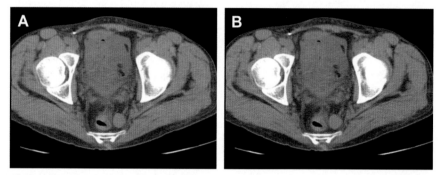

Fig. 10. (A, B) Lymph node involvement in prostate cancer. Axial CT image shows an enlarged left perirectal lymph node (*blue*) that was pathologically proved to be metastatic from primary prostatic cancer.

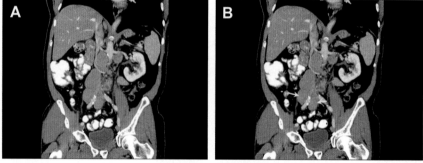

Fig. 11. (A, B) Lymph node involvement in prostate cancer. Coronal reformatted CT image shows metastatic retroperitoneal (*red arrows*) and right common iliac (*yellow arrows*) lymph nodes.

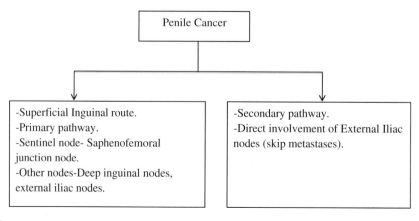

Algorithm 2.

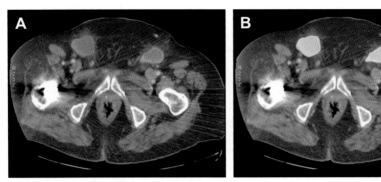

Fig. 12. (*A, B*) Lymph node involvement in penile cancer. Axial CT image shows bilateral necrotic, metastatic inguinal lymph nodes (*yellow*).

could ascertain the negative predictive value of this technique. Also, limited spatial resolution and morphologic information and frequent artifacts make image interpretation difficult. Mir and colleagues[56] showed that fusion of diffusion-weighted MR with T2-weighted images improves identification of pelvic lymph nodes compared with T2-weighted images alone. A recent study by Theony and colleagues[57] in patients with prostate and bladder cancers showed that ultrasmall particles of iron oxide (USPIO combined with DW MR imaging is a fast and accurate method for detecting pelvic lymph node metastases, even in normal-sized nodes.

Lymphotropic Nanoparticle-Enhanced MR Imaging

Lymphotropic nanoparticle-enhanced MR imaging is an investigational molecular imaging technique for lymph node characterization. Its role has been studied in various malignancies including malignancies of the prostate, rectum, bladder, testes, kidney, penis, female gynecologic system, stomach, lung, esophagus, breast, and head and neck.[58–69]

Ferumoxtran-10 and ferumoxytol are lymphotropic contrast agents that consist of ultrasmall superparamagnetic iron oxide nanoparticles targeted at the reticuloendothelial system. After

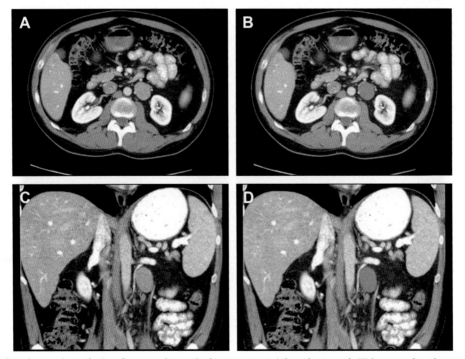

Fig. 13. (*A–D*) Lymph node involvement in testicular cancer. Axial and coronal CT images showing metastatic lymph node below the left renal hilum in a patient with testicular cancer (*red*).

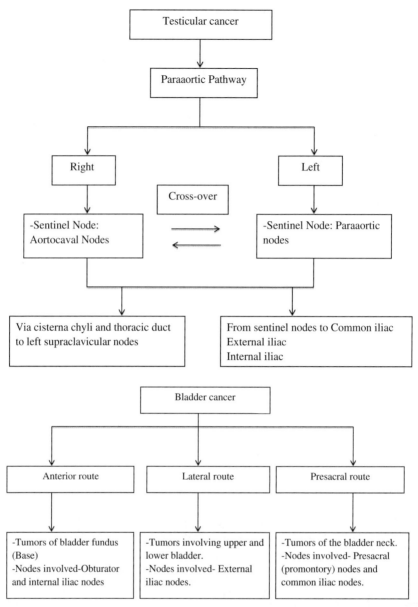

Testicular cancer

↓

Paraaortic Pathway

Right | Cross-over | Left

-Sentinel Node: Aortocaval Nodes → ← -Sentinel Node: Paraaortic nodes

Via cisterna chyli and thoracic duct to left supraclavicular nodes

From sentinel nodes to Common iliac
External iliac
Internal iliac

Bladder cancer

Anterior route | Lateral route | Presacral route

-Tumors of bladder fundus (Base)
-Nodes involved-Obturator and internal iliac nodes

-Tumors involving upper and lower bladder.
-Nodes involved- External iliac nodes.

-Tumors of the bladder neck.
-Nodes involved- Presacral (promontory) nodes and common iliac nodes.

Algorithm 3.

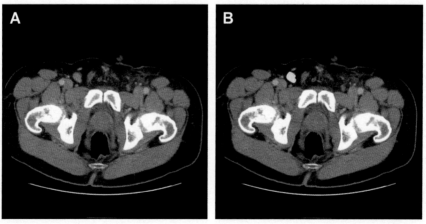

Fig. 14. (*A*, *B*) Metastatic right inguinal lymph node in testicular cancer in a patient with a history of inguinal hernia repair (*yellow*).

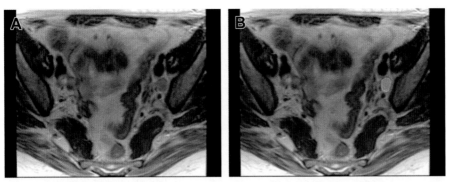

Fig. 15. (*A*, *B*) Lymph node involvement in bladder cancer. Axial T2-weighted image shows metastatic left external iliac lymph node (*green*).

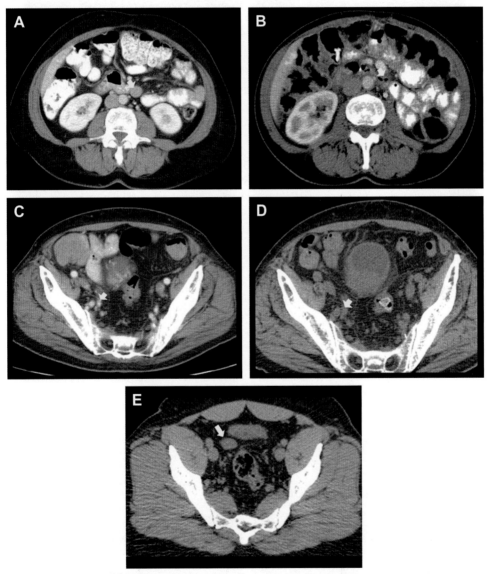

Fig. 16. (*A*) Nonopacified bowel loop mimicking a lymph node in left periaortic location (*yellow arrow*); follow-up images (*B*) in the same patient shows gas in the bowel loop. (*C*) Axial CT image shows what looks like an enlarged right internal iliac lymph node (*arrow*) in a patient with bladder cancer. (*D*) The structure enhances on the post-contrast images and is in continuity with the right internal iliac vein. (*E*) Axial CT image shows right undescended testis (*arrow*) that can be mistaken for right pelvic lymph node.

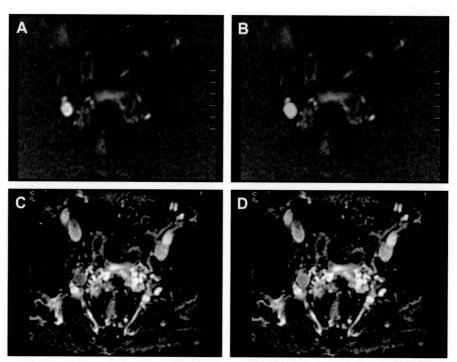

Fig. 17. (*A–D*) Axial DW (b = 1000) image (*A, B*) and ADC map (*C, D*) in a patient with prostate cancer showing metastatic right internal iliac node (*orange*) with restricted diffusion appearing bright on DW imaging and dark on ADC map.

intravenous injection, these particles are extravasated from the capillaries and engulfed by the macrophages, which subsequently enter the node. Abnormal patterns of uptake are seen when the lymph node architecture is altered by metastases or when the normal lymphatic drainage is disturbed. MR imaging can detect these abnormal accumulation patterns by use of T2 and T2*, which are shortened by the susceptibility effects of iron oxide. Metastatic nodes lack uptake of these particles, enabling detection of even partial or micrometastases (**Fig. 18**).[70] Many

recent trials have shown increased sensitivity, specificity, and negative predictive value of LNMR imaging in the detection of lymph node metastases in prostate, testicular, bladder, and penile cancers.

Although LNMR imaging seems promising, it has a few limitations. False-positive results may be seen in cases of benign conditions like granulomatous diseases causing necrosis of the lymph nodes, reactive nodal hyperplasia, nodal fibrosis, and lipomatosis in which normal macrophages are replaced from the lymph node, leading to abnormal uptake

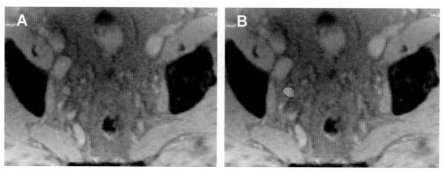

Fig. 18. (*A, B*) Axial T2* images following administration of superparamagnetic iron oxide nanoparticles showing metastatic right posterior obturator (*green*) lymph node in patients with prostate cancer. Lack of iron oxide uptake characterizes the node as malignant.

patterns on imaging. Also, LNMR imaging may lead to false-negative results in cases of lymph node metastases less than 3 mm because they cannot be adequately assessed because of spatial limitations of the current MR imaging systems.[71]

SUMMARY

Knowledge of relevant clinical anatomy, drainage pathways, and alterations in the drainage patterns after intervention is the key to accurate interpretation of imaging studies performed on the male pelvis for nodal staging. In the realm of emerging functional imaging techniques, the coming decades may bring a paradigm shift from the current size-based criteria as understanding of nodal metastasis evolves.

REFERENCES

1. Greene FL. American Joint Committee on Cancer, American Cancer Society. AJCC cancer staging manual. New York: Springer-Verlag; 2002.
2. Roy C, Bierry G, Matau A, et al. Value of diffusion-weighted imaging to detect small malignant pelvic lymph nodes at 3 T. Eur Radiol 2010;20(8):1803–11.
3. Paño B, Sebastià C, Buñesch L, et al. Pathways of lymphatic spread in male urogenital pelvic malignancies. Radiographics 2011;31(1):135–60.
4. Park JM, Charnsangavej C, Yoshimitsu K, et al. Pathways of nodal metastasis from pelvic tumors: CT demonstration. Radiographics 1994;14(6):1309–21.
5. Koh DM, Hughes M, Husband JE. Cross-sectional imaging of nodal metastases in the abdomen and pelvis. Abdom Imaging 2006;31(6):632–43.
6. Walsh JW, Amendola MA, Konerding KF, et al. Computed tomographic detection of pelvic and inguinal lymph-node metastases from primary and recurrent pelvic malignant disease. Radiology 1980;137(1 Pt 1):157–66.
7. Saksena MA, Kim JY, Harisinghani MG. Nodal staging in genitourinary cancers. Abdom Imaging 2006;31(6):644–51.
8. Gray H. The lymphatics of abdomen and pelvis [Internet]. In: Gray's anatomy. 1918. Available at: http://www.bartleby.com/107/180.html. Accessed September 5, 2012.
9. Saokar A, Islam T, Jantsch M, et al. Detection of lymph nodes in pelvic malignancies with computed tomography and magnetic resonance imaging. Clin Imaging 2010;34(5):361–6.
10. Chalian H, Töre HG, Horowitz JM, et al. Radiologic assessment of response to therapy: comparison of RECIST versions 1.1 and 1.0. Radiographics 2011;31(7):2093–105.
11. Grubnic S, Vinnicombe SJ, Norman AR, et al. MR evaluation of normal retroperitoneal and pelvic lymph nodes. Clin Radiol 2002;57(3):193–200 [discussion: 201–4].
12. Vinnicombe SJ, Norman AR, Nicolson V, et al. Normal pelvic lymph nodes: evaluation with CT after bipedal lymphangiography. Radiology 1995;194(2):349–55.
13. Hilton S, Herr HW, Teitcher JB, et al. CT detection of retroperitoneal lymph node metastases in patients with clinical stage I testicular nonseminomatous germ cell cancer: assessment of size and distribution criteria. AJR Am J Roentgenol 1997;169(2):521–5.
14. Oyen RH, Van Poppel HP, Ameye FE, et al. Lymph node staging of localized prostatic carcinoma with CT and CT-guided fine-needle aspiration biopsy: prospective study of 285 patients. Radiology 1994;190(2):315–22.
15. Fukuda H, Nakagawa T, Shibuya H. Metastases to pelvic lymph nodes from carcinoma in the pelvic cavity: diagnosis using thin-section CT. Clin Radiol 1999;54(4):237–42.
16. Brown G, Richards CJ, Bourne MW, et al. Morphologic predictors of lymph node status in rectal cancer with use of high-spatial-resolution MR imaging with histopathologic comparison. Radiology 2003;227(2):371–7.
17. Grey AC, Carrington BM, Hulse PA, et al. Magnetic resonance appearance of normal inguinal nodes. Clin Radiol 2000;55(2):124–30.
18. Som PM. Detection of metastasis in cervical lymph nodes: CT and MR criteria and differential diagnosis. AJR Am J Roentgenol 1992;158(5):961–9.
19. Lien HH, Lindsköld L, Stenwig AE, et al. Shape of retroperitoneal lymph nodes at computed tomography does not correlate to metastatic disease in early stage non-seminomatous testicular tumors. Acta Radiol 1987;28(3):271–3.
20. Dooms GC, Hricak H, Moseley ME, et al. Characterization of lymphadenopathy by magnetic resonance relaxation times: preliminary results. Radiology 1985;155(3):691–7.
21. Choi HJ, Kim SH, Seo SS, et al. MRI for pretreatment lymph node staging in uterine cervical cancer. AJR Am J Roentgenol 2006;187(5):W538–43.
22. Magnusson A, Andersson T, Larsson B, et al. Contrast enhancement of pathologic lymph nodes demonstrated by computed tomography. Acta Radiol 1989;30(3):307–10.
23. Morisawa N, Koyama T, Togashi K. Metastatic lymph nodes in urogenital cancers: contribution of imaging findings. Abdom Imaging 2006;31(5):620–9.
24. Pandey D, Mahajan V, Kannan RR. Prognostic factors in node-positive carcinoma of the penis. J Surg Oncol 2006;93(2):133–8.
25. Abol-Enein H, El-Baz M, Abd El-Hameed MA, et al. Lymph node involvement in patients with bladder cancer treated with radical cystectomy: a pathoanatomical study–a single center experience. J Urol 2004;172(5 Pt 1):1818–21.

26. Daneshmand S, Quek ML, Stein JP, et al. Prognosis of patients with lymph node positive prostate cancer following radical prostatectomy: long-term results. J Urol 2004;172(6 Pt 1):2252–5.

27. Mattei A, Fuechsel FG, Bhatta Dhar N, et al. The template of the primary lymphatic landing sites of the prostate should be revisited: results of a multimodality mapping study. Eur Urol 2008;53(1):118–25.

28. Spencer JA, Golding SJ. Patterns of lymphatic metastases at recurrence of prostate cancer: CT findings. Clin Radiol 1994;49(6):404–7.

29. Misra S, Chaturvedi A, Misra NC. Penile carcinoma: a challenge for the developing world. Lancet Oncol 2004;5(4):240–7.

30. Horenblas S. Lymphadenectomy for squamous cell carcinoma of the penis. Part 1: diagnosis of lymph node metastasis. BJU Int 2001;88(5):467–72.

31. Solsona E, Algaba F, Horenblas S, et al. EAU guidelines on penile cancer. Eur Urol 2004;46(1):1–8.

32. Simms MS, Mann G, Kockelbergh RC, et al. The management of lymph node metastasis from bladder cancer. Eur J Surg Oncol 2005;31(4):348–56.

33. AJCC cancer staging manual [Internet]. [date unknown]. Available at: http://www.springer.com/medicine/surgery/book/978-0-387-88440-0. Accessed May 22, 2012.

34. Feuerbach S, Lukas P, Gmeinwieser J. False interpretations of computed tomograms in malignant lymph node diseases of the pelvis and abdomen. Digitale Bilddiagn 1984;4(4):176–80 [in German].

35. Sáenz-Santamaría J, Catalina-Fernandez I. Fine needle aspiration diagnosis of extramedullary hematopoiesis resembling mediastinal and paravesical tumors. A report of 2 cases. Acta Cytol 2004;48(1):95–8.

36. Siewert B, Sosna J, McNamara A, et al. Missed lesions at abdominal oncologic CT: lessons learned from quality assurance. Radiographics 2008;28(3):623–38.

37. Koehler PR, Mancuso AA. Pitfalls in the diagnosis of retroperitoneal adenopathy. J Can Assoc Radiol 1982;33(3):197–201.

38. Carmody E, Klotz L, Leonhardt C. Bilateral retrovesical testes: an unusual location for impalpable undescended testes. Abdom Imaging 1993;18(3):301–3.

39. Ko SW, Ko KS. Undescended testis appearing as a cecal mass in an adult. AJR Am J Roentgenol 2002;179(6):1646–7.

40. Studer UE, Scherz S, Scheidegger J, et al. Enlargement of regional lymph nodes in renal cell carcinoma is often not due to metastases. J Urol 1990;144(2 Pt 1):243–5.

41. Bader P, Burkhard FC, Markwalder R, et al. Disease progression and survival of patients with positive lymph nodes after radical prostatectomy. Is there a chance of cure? J Urol 2003;169(3):849–54.

42. Fleischmann A, Thalmann GN, Markwalder R, et al. Extracapsular extension of pelvic lymph node metastases from urothelial carcinoma of the bladder is an independent prognostic factor. J Clin Oncol 2005;23(10):2358–65.

43. Schumacher MC, Burkhard FC, Thalmann GN, et al. Good outcome for patients with few lymph node metastases after radical retropubic prostatectomy. Eur Urol 2008;54(2):344–52.

44. Mills RD, Fleischmann A, Studer UE. Radical cystectomy with an extended pelvic lymphadenectomy: rationale and results. Surg Oncol Clin N Am 2007;16(1):233–45.

45. Schiavina R, Scattoni V, Castellucci P, et al. 11C-choline positron emission tomography/computerized tomography for preoperative lymph-node staging in intermediate-risk and high-risk prostate cancer: comparison with clinical staging nomograms. Eur Urol 2008;54(2):392–401.

46. Picchio M, Treiber U, Beer AJ, et al. Value of 11C-choline PET and contrast-enhanced CT for staging of bladder cancer: correlation with histopathologic findings. J Nucl Med 2006;47(6):938–44.

47. Vargas HA, Akin O, Franiel T, et al. Diffusion-weighted endorectal MR imaging at 3 T for prostate cancer: tumor detection and assessment of aggressiveness. Radiology 2011;259(3):775–84.

48. Guo Y, Cai YQ, Cai ZL, et al. Differentiation of clinically benign and malignant breast lesions using diffusion-weighted imaging. J Magn Reson Imaging 2002;16(2):172–8.

49. Gauvain KM, McKinstry RC, Mukherjee P, et al. Evaluating pediatric brain tumor cellularity with diffusion-tensor imaging. AJR Am J Roentgenol 2001;177(2):449–54.

50. Sugahara T, Korogi Y, Kochi M, et al. Usefulness of diffusion-weighted MRI with echo-planar technique in the evaluation of cellularity in gliomas. J Magn Reson Imaging 1999;9(1):53–60.

51. Lang P, Wendland MF, Saeed M, et al. Osteogenic sarcoma: noninvasive in vivo assessment of tumor necrosis with diffusion-weighted MR imaging. Radiology 1998;206(1):227–35.

52. Sumi M, Van Cauteren M, Nakamura T. MR microimaging of benign and malignant nodes in the neck. AJR Am J Roentgenol 2006;186(3):749–57.

53. Holzapfel K, Duetsch S, Fauser C, et al. Value of diffusion-weighted MR imaging in the differentiation between benign and malignant cervical lymph nodes. Eur J Radiol 2009;72(3):381–7.

54. Abdel Razek AA, Soliman NY, Elkhamary S, et al. Role of diffusion-weighted MR imaging in cervical lymphadenopathy. Eur Radiol 2006;16(7):1468–77.

55. Eiber M, Beer AJ, Holzapfel K, et al. Preliminary results for characterization of pelvic lymph nodes in patients with prostate cancer by diffusion-weighted MR-imaging. Invest Radiol 2010;45(1):15–23.

56. Mir N, Sohaib SA, Collins D, et al. Fusion of high b-value diffusion-weighted and T2-weighted MR images improves identification of lymph nodes in the pelvis. J Med Imaging Radiat Oncol 2010; 54(4):358–64.

57. Thoeny HC, Triantafyllou M, Birkhaeuser FD, et al. Combined ultrasmall superparamagnetic particles of iron oxide-enhanced and diffusion-weighted magnetic resonance imaging reliably detect pelvic lymph node metastases in normal-sized nodes of bladder and prostate cancer patients. Eur Urol 2009;55(4):761–9.

58. Harisinghani MG, Barentsz J, Hahn PF, et al. Noninvasive detection of clinically occult lymph-node metastases in prostate cancer. N Engl J Med 2003;348(25):2491–9.

59. Koh DM, Brown G, Temple L, et al. Rectal cancer: mesorectal lymph nodes at MR imaging with USPIO versus histopathologic findings–initial observations. Radiology 2004;231(1):91–9.

60. Deserno WM, Harisinghani MG, Taupitz M, et al. Urinary bladder cancer: preoperative nodal staging with ferumoxtran-10-enhanced MR imaging. Radiology 2004;233(2):449–56.

61. Harisinghani MG, Saksena M, Ross RW, et al. A pilot study of lymphotrophic nanoparticle-enhanced magnetic resonance imaging technique in early stage testicular cancer: a new method for noninvasive lymph node evaluation. Urology 2005;66(5): 1066–71.

62. Guimaraes AR, Tabatabei S, Dahl D, et al. Pilot study evaluating use of lymphotrophic nanoparticle-enhanced magnetic resonance imaging for assessing lymph nodes in renal cell cancer. Urology 2008; 71(4):708–12.

63. Tabatabaei S, Harisinghani M, McDougal WS. Regional lymph node staging using lymphotropic nanoparticle enhanced magnetic resonance imaging with ferumoxtran-10 in patients with penile cancer. J Urol 2005;174(3):923–7 [discussion: 927].

64. Rockall AG, Sohaib SA, Harisinghani MG, et al. Diagnostic performance of nanoparticle-enhanced magnetic resonance imaging in the diagnosis of lymph node metastases in patients with endometrial and cervical cancer. J Clin Oncol 2005; 23(12):2813–21.

65. Tatsumi Y, Tanigawa N, Nishimura H, et al. Preoperative diagnosis of lymph node metastases in gastric cancer by magnetic resonance imaging with ferumoxtran-10. Gastric Cancer 2006;9(2):120–8.

66. Nguyen BC, Stanford W, Thompson BH, et al. Multicenter clinical trial of ultrasmall superparamagnetic iron oxide in the evaluation of mediastinal lymph nodes in patients with primary lung carcinoma. J Magn Reson Imaging 1999;10(3):468–73.

67. Nishimura H, Tanigawa N, Hiramatsu M, et al. Preoperative esophageal cancer staging: magnetic resonance imaging of lymph node with ferumoxtran-10, an ultrasmall superparamagnetic iron oxide. J Am Coll Surg 2006;202(4):604–11.

68. Memarsadeghi M, Riedl CC, Kaneider A, et al. Axillary lymph node metastases in patients with breast carcinomas: assessment with nonenhanced versus USPIO-enhanced MR imaging. Radiology 2006; 241(2):367–77.

69. Sigal R, Vogl T, Casselman J, et al. Lymph node metastases from head and neck squamous cell carcinoma: MR imaging with ultrasmall superparamagnetic iron oxide particles (Sinerem MR) – results of a phase-III multicenter clinical trial. Eur Radiol 2002;12(5):1104–13.

70. Islam T, Harisinghani MG. Overview of nanoparticle use in cancer imaging. Cancer Biomark 2009;5(2): 61–7.

71. Boughanim M, Leboulleux S, Rey A, et al. Histologic results of para-aortic lymphadenectomy in patients treated for stage IB2/II cervical cancer with negative [18F]fluorodeoxyglucose positron emission tomography scans in the para-aortic area. J Clin Oncol 2008;26(15):2558–61.

Diffusion-Weighted Imaging of the Male Pelvis

Dow-Mu Koh, MD, MRCP, FRCR*, Aslam Sohaib, MRCP, FRCR

KEYWORDS

- Diffusion-weighted MR imaging • MR imaging • Male pelvis • Pelvic malignancies

KEY POINTS

- Diffusion-weighted magnetic resonance (MR) imaging (DWI) is now widely incorporated as a standard MR imaging sequence for the assessment of the male pelvis.
- DWI can improve the detection, characterization, and staging of pelvic malignancies, such as prostate, bladder, and rectal cancers.
- There is growing interest in applying quantitative DWI for the assessment of tumor treatment response.
- The technique seems promising for the evaluation of metastatic nodal and bone disease in the pelvis.

INTRODUCTION

Diffusion-weighted magnetic resonance (MR) imaging (DWI) is an MR imaging technique that is increasingly applied for disease evaluation in the pelvis. The imaging contrast is based on differences in the mobility of water, which differs according to the cellular density, cell membrane integrity, structural organization, and microcapillary perfusion of the tissues.[1] In general, pathologic processes such as tumors (increased cellular proliferation) and inflammation (increased cellular infiltration) will show greater impeded water diffusion compared with normal tissues and return higher signal intensity on diffusion-weighted images.

By performing DWI using at least two different diffusion-weightings (b-values), typically ranging between 0 and 1000 s/mm², it is possible to calculate the apparent diffusion coefficient (ADC) of each imaging voxel on an image section to yield an ADC map. By drawing a region of interest (ROI) over diseased tissue on the ADC map, the mean or median ADC value can be recorded. Not surprisingly, tumor tissues usually return lower ADC values compared with normal tissues, reflecting their lower water diffusivity. Thus, DWI is a unique imaging technique that informs on tissue cellularity which can be assessed both qualitatively (by reviewing the b-value images and ADC maps) and quantitatively (by recording the mean or median ADC values of tissues).

TECHNICAL CONSIDERATIONS

DWI can be successfully executed on most modern 1.5-T or 3.0-T MR scanners. The technique most widely applied is single-shot fat-suppressed spin-echo echo-planar DWI. The echo-planar–based technique is widely used because it is quick to perform (typically 3–4 minutes) and thus can be easily appended to existing imaging protocols. However, the sequence is prone to ghosting artifacts and image distortion, which requires careful optimization.[1,2]

Imaging is typically performed in quiet respiration. Multiple signal averaging technique is used to average out the effects of bulk motion. Intravenous spasmolytic agents (eg, buscopan or glucagon) are

Department of Radiology, Royal Marsden Hospital, Royal Marsden NHS Foundation Trust, Downs Road, Sutton SM2 5PT, UK
* Corresponding author.
E-mail address: dowmukoh@icr.ac.uk

Radiol Clin N Am 50 (2012) 1127–1144
http://dx.doi.org/10.1016/j.rcl.2012.08.008

generally not required for DWI but may be administered to reduce motion artifacts that may degrade the T1- or T2-weighted anatomic imaging.

One possible imaging protocol for performing DWI in the male pelvis includes an initial large field of view sequence (eg, 430–450 mm) using two b-values (eg, 0 and 900–1400 s/mm^2) with 5-7 mm section thickness as a survey sequence, to localize any area of abnormally impeded diffusion in the pelvis. A higher b-value may be considered in the male pelvis; several studies have shown that this can be helpful to detect prostate cancer[3–5] because of the high signal appearance of the normal prostate peripheral zone on DWI (T2 shine-through effects), which can reduce the contrast between the normal gland and malignant tissue. However, the application of a high b-value, greater than1000 s/mm^2, should be judicious, and consideration should be given to adequate image signal-to-noise ratio, because noisy images may not confer any advantages.[4]

A dedicated smaller field-of-view DWI sequence (200–240 mm) is usually performed over the area of suspected anatomy (eg, prostate gland, rectum, or urinary bladder), and image sections may be angled and ranged to match those of the small field-of-view T2-weighted imaging. These may be acquired using thinner slice thickness (eg, 3–5 mm) and also using more b-values (eg, 3 or 4 b-values between 0 and 1000 s/mm^2) to optimize ADC calculation. Examples of scan parameters for imaging the male pelvis on a 1.5-T and 3.0-T MR system are presented in **Table 1**.

There are several other noteworthy features of DWI sequences. First, the fat-suppression technique used in the pelvis should be robust over a large field-of-view to minimize chemical shifts and ghosting artifacts. For this reason, fat suppression is usually performed using a short-tau inversion recovery (STIR) technique, although an optimized spectral attenuated inversion recovery (SPAIR) technique may be adopted. Second, the receiver bandwidth used is typically higher than those used for the morphologic T1- and T2-weighted sequences. This helps to minimize image distortion. Third, a simultaneous gradient application scheme (eg, 3 scan-trace, 3-in-1, tetrahedral encoding) is usually instituted, which helps to minimize the echo-time and improve image quality and signal-to-noise ratio. The reader should also be aware of and familiar with the range of imaging artifacts that may arise from DWI studies using the echo-planar imaging technique, which is beyond the scope of this article to discuss.

IMAGE INTERPRETATION

The DWI and ADC maps should not be interpreted in isolation but should be combined with conventional T1- and T2-weighted images to allow the best assessment.

In oncologic practice, the high b-value image and/or ADC map can be used to improve tumor detection and characterization. Typically, a solid tumor will show impeded diffusion as bright signal intensity on the high b-value diffusion-weighted images and appear relatively dark on the ADC map. The ADC value of a lesion is measured by drawing regions of interest on the ADC map; this can aid lesion characterization or assessment of treatment response.

Table 1
Examples of imaging parameters used for echo-planar spin-echo DWI in the pelvis at 1.5 T and 3.0 T

Imaging Sequence	1.5 T		3.0 T	
	Larger FOV	Smaller FOV	Larger FOV	Smaller FOV
FOV, cm	430–240	200–240	430–240	200–240
Matrix size, pixels	180	180	256	256
Repetition time, ms	7400	3200	6700	3600
Echo time, ms	66	72	79	80
Slice thickness, mm	6	5	5	5
b values, s/mm^2	0 and 900–1400	0, 350, 750	1500	0, 300, 800
No. of averages	4	8	15	6
Receiver bandwidth, Hz/pixel	1812	1726	1653	1653
Fat suppression	SPAIR	SPAIR	SPAIR	SPAIR

Abbreviations: FOV, field of view; SPAIR, spectral attenuated inversion recovery.

However, radiologists should be aware of pitfalls that can confound interpretation. One of these is the T2 shine-through effect, where the high signal intensity observed within a tissue is not caused by impeded water diffusion but, instead, its long T2 relaxation time. This can, for example, be observed in the normal peripheral zone of the prostate gland, which may diminish the contrast between tumors and normal glandular tissue on DWI. To confirm T2 shine-through effects, one can review the corresponding ADC map to observe high ADC values in such areas, instead of the low ADC values typical of cellular disease (**Fig. 1**).

False-positive interpretation for malignancy may arise from benign cellular processes (eg, inflammation or abscess), which result in impeded diffusion. False-negative results can occur in cystic or mucinous tumors. Hence, DW-MR images should be read with some attention to these pitfalls, especially by individuals who are less experienced using the technique.

APPLICATIONS OF DWI IN THE MALE PELVIS

There is now substantial evidence for the use of DWI in the male pelvis. The published evidence is most compelling for suspected or known prostate carcinoma. However, the technique can be applied to assess the urinary bladder, rectum, and pelvic lymph nodes. Last, but not least, DWI appears to be highly sensitive for the diagnosis of metastases to the bony pelvis.

PROSTATE GLAND

Prostate cancer remains a major cause of mortality in men. Even though the disease is frequently multicentric in approximately 30% of individuals, patient outcome seems linked to the biologic behavior of the "index" lesion,[6] which is associated with a higher Gleason score and biologic aggressiveness. The accurate detection, localization, and staging of the index lesions are therefore important for management planning.

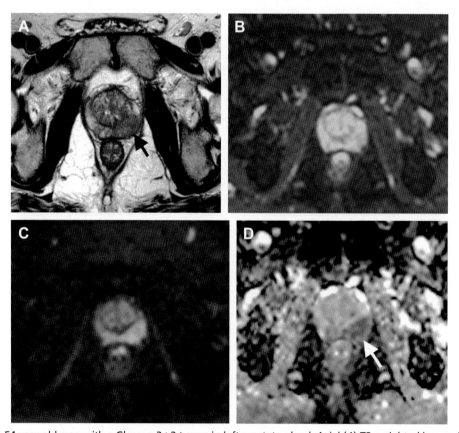

Fig. 1. A 54-year-old man with a Gleason 3+3 tumor in left prostate gland. Axial (*A*) T2-weighted image, (*B*) b = 0 s/mm^2 DWI, (*C*) b = 800 s/mm^2 DWI, and (*D*) ADC map. Tumor is seen as area of hypointensity on T2-weighted image (*black arrow*) but is less discernible on DWI images, as a result of high signal intensity returned from relatively normal contralateral right gland (T2 shine-through). By comparison, tumor is better appreciated on the ADC map (*white arrow*).

Active surveillance is a management policy currently adopted in patients with the appropriate low-risk profile. In these patients, treatment is offered at follow-up when the risk behavior of the tumor increases.[7–9] Thus, the ability to predict or detect a change in the tumor biologic behavior will have an impact on patient management.

In patients with organ-confined prostate cancer, radical prostatectomy is associated with significant morbidity and mortality. Thus, gland-preserving treatment for the index lesion is being investigated as a potential treatment strategy,[10,11] which puts into focus the need for an accurate noninvasive method of assessing treatment response.

There is no doubt that imaging plays an increasing role toward the management of patients with prostate cancer in the light of these evolving clinical practices. In particular, developments in DW MR imaging have enhanced the radiologist's role within the management team.

Tumor Detection and Localization

On MR imaging, the detection and localization of prostate cancer have been reliant on small field of view T2-weighted images, which has limited diagnostic sensitivity and specificity. In patients with an elevated serum prostate specific antigen (PSA) level, it has been shown that DWI can improve diagnostic performance.

Whether it is using ultrahigh b-value images (>1000 s/mm^2)[5] or the ADC map,[12–18] DWI can increase the diagnostic accuracy of lesion detection in the prostate gland when combined with T2-weighted imaging, compared with T2-weighted imaging alone. Tumor is recognized visually as an area of high signal impeded diffusion on the b-value images and returns low ADC values. Because of the variable high signal intensity of the normal peripheral zone of the prostate gland at DWI (T2 shine-through), tumors are usually more easily discernible

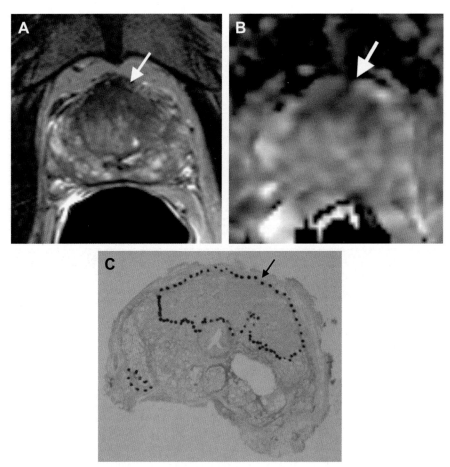

Fig. 2. A 57-year-old man with Gleason 4+3 tumor in anterior gland, which is easily missed on transrectal ultrasound biopsy. Axial (*A*) T2-weighted image shows ill-defined low signal intensity in anterior gland (*arrow*), which returns (*B*) correspondingly a low ADC value (*arrow*) on the ADC map. Following prostatectomy, (*C*) whole mount (hematoxylin and eosin stain) tissue section confirms tumor in anterior gland (*arrow, region outline in pink*).

on the ADC map compared with the b-value images.[19]

The diagnostic improvement using DWI for disease detection and localization seems greater for the peripheral zone compared with central gland tumors.[15,20,21] This is because normal benign glandular hyperplasia in the central gland may impede diffusion and return lower ADC values, resulting in an overlap with the features of prostate cancer. Nevertheless, Yoshimitsu and colleagues[22] showed contrary results in achieving diagnostic improvement in the transitional zone but not in the peripheral zone using the combination of T2-weighted imaging and DWI.

The diagnostic improvement using DWI has also been shown in studies in which conventional imaging techniques and transrectal ultrasound-guided biopsy have not been successful in revealing the presence of cancer in patients with rising serum PSA level.[23,24] On transrectal ultrasound-guided biopsy, lesions may be missed as a result of sampling errors or if the lesion is difficult to reach because of its location (eg, tumor in

the anterior prostate or at the glandular apex) (**Figs. 2** and **3**). Using DWI, it is possible to identify and localize apparently "occult" prostate cancer, and guide targeted or template biopsy to confirm the diagnosis.[23–26]

Once a cancer is diagnosed, DWI may also improve local disease staging. Studies have shown improved assessment of tumor invasion of the urinary bladder and seminal vesicles by DWI.[27,28] However, there is no current evidence that DWI contributes to the assessment of extracapsular disease extension compared with conventional T2-weighted MR imaging.

Disease Characterization: Benign Versus Malignant?

DWI can increase the diagnostic specificity for prostate cancer compared with T2-weighted imaging,[14,16,21,29–32] although this observation has not been universal.[5,15,19] One possible reason for false-positive results could be the misinterpretation of postbiopsy change or other benign

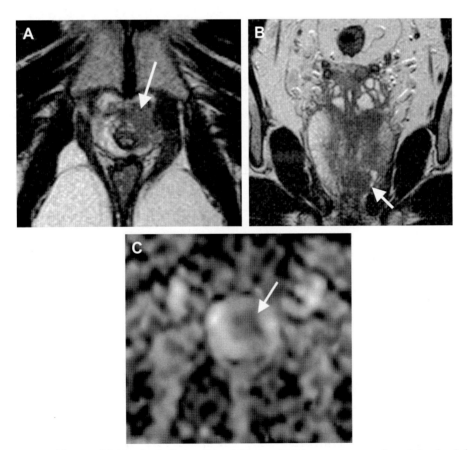

Fig. 3. A 64-year-old man with histologically confirmed Gleason 3+3 tumor at apex of prostate gland. (*A*) Axial and (*B*) coronal T2-weighted images show focal hypointensiy at left glandular apex (*arrows*). (*C*) Tumor returns lower ADC value compared with adjacent prostate gland.

processes (eg, prostatitis) as malignancy. For this reason, it is common practice to wait at least 4 weeks after the prostate biopsy to perform prostate imaging including DWI. However, Rosenkrantz and colleagues[33] found that even in the presence of acute postbiopsy hemorrhage, there was usually sufficient difference in the ADC values between hemorrhage and tumors for the two entities to be distinguished.

By ADC measurements, the highly glandular normal peripheral zone returns higher ADC values compared with the central gland. By contrast, prostate cancers return significantly lower ADC values compared with the normal peripheral zone or the central gland.[26,34–41] However, the averaged ADC values of the peripheral zone, central gland, and cancers reported across different series show variations across imaging platforms and institutions (Table 2). Values reported at 3.0 T seem slightly higher than at 1.5 T. There also seems to be greater variation to the reported values at 1.5 T. Thus, readers should verify the accuracy of quantitative ADC measurements on their own MR system (eg, using phantoms) and compare their results with ADC values derived from use of a similar MR system and technique.

A few studies have evaluated diffusion tensor imaging (DTI) for distinguishing between benign and malignant disease.[42–50] However, the reported results are inconsistent, presumably because of measurement variability associated with DTI measurements. For example, although some studies have shown that the normal peripheral zone has a lower fractional isotropy compared with the central gland,[43] others have found the reverse.[47,48,50] Likewise, there are conflicting reports as to whether the fractional anisotropy in tumors is higher or lower than in normal glandular tissue.[42,43,48,51] Clearly, the value of DTI in the characterization of prostate carcinoma warrants further evaluation.

By performing DWI using multiple b-values and biexponential data fitting (taking into account intravoxel incoherent motion), Dopfert and colleagues[52] showed that prostate cancers are characterized not only by their low water diffusivity but also by their lower perfusion fraction compared with normal tissue. However, in another study, Pang and colleagues[53] found the perfusion fraction in tumors to be higher than in normal tissues. Because biexponential analysis is highly sensitive to image signal-to-noise variations and may have

Table 2
Selected literature reported ADC values of the normal peripheral zone, central glands, and prostate cancers using echo-planar DWI

Study (Year)	No. of Patients	b Values, s/mm²	ADC Peripheral Zone (PZ)	ADC Central Gland (CG)	ADC of Tumor
Studies at 3.0 T					
Pickles et al,[40] 2006	49	0, 500	1.95 ± 0.50		1.38 ± 0.32
Gibbs et al,[51] 2006	62	0, 500	1.87 ± 0.47		1.33 ± 0.32
Kim et al,[106] 2007	35	0, 1000	1.97 ± 0.25	1.79 ± 0.19	1.32 ± 0.24 (PZ) 1.37 ± 0.29 (CG)
Zelhof et al,[107] 2009	32	0, 500	1.90 ± 0.33		1.45 ± 0.27 (PZ)
Kim et al,[108] 2010	48	0, 1000	2.04 ± 0.34	1.77 ± 0.30	1.19 ± 0.33 (PZ) 1.21 ± 0.23 (CG)
Studies at 1.5 T					
Kumar et al,[26] 2007	23	0, 250, 500, 750, 1000	1.34 ± 0.30	1.12 ± 0.15	0.98 ± 0.22 (PZ) 1.00 ± 0.25 (CG)
deSouza et al,[30] 2007	30	0, 300, 500, 800	1.71 ± 0.16	1.46 ± 0.14	1.30 ± 0.30
Reinsberg et al,[109] 2007	37	0, 300, 500, 800	1.51 ± 0.27	1.31 ± 0.20	1.03 ± 0.18
Tamada et al,[36] 2008	90 (125 controls*)	0, 1000	1.80 ± 0.27*	1.34 ± 0.14*	1.02 ± 0.25 (PZ) 0.94 ± 0.21 (CG)
Kitajima et al,[4] 2008	26	0, 1000	1.69 ± 0.23		0.82 ± 0.27 (PZ)
Woodfield et al,[63] 2010	57	0,1000	1.48 ± 0.29		0.74 ± 0.15 (PZ)
Sato et al,[110] 2005	23	0, 300, 600	1.80 ± 0.41	1.58 ± 0.37	1.08 ± 0.39 (PZ) 1.13 ± 0.42 (CG)

poor measurement repeatability, the reader should be aware of this when adopting the technique.

Characterizing and Predicting Tumor Aggressiveness and Biologic Behavior

Unique among MR techniques, DWI is able provide an assessment of tumor aggressiveness, and hence the potential to predict its biologic behavior. Several studies have clearly demonstrated a negative correlation between ADC values and the Gleason score in prostate cancer (ie, high-grade tumors typically have lower ADC values) (**Fig. 4**).[12,54–64] The corollary of this is that low-grade tumors may show less impeded diffusion, which is more likely to be missed on DWI.[18] Furthermore, irrespective of tumor grade, cancers that demonstrate a diffuse "loose" pattern of growth are also harder to detect on imaging.[65] However, given that patient prognosis seems to be linked to the most biologically adverse index lesion, nonvisualization of low-grade tumors

on imaging may not have a significant bearing on patient survival and outcome. Nonetheless, such a paradigm would have to be tested in prospective studies.

Because DWI has a generally high sensitivity for disease detection in the prostate, the ADC map can be used to direct biopsy toward the most biologically aggressive lesion detected on imaging.[66] In one study, MR assessment of the tumor aggressiveness of focal prostate cancer correlated better with the Gleason grade determined at histology following prostatectomy than with the Gleason grade determined by transrectal biopsy.[55] This attests to the ability of DWI to provide a global assessment across the whole gland. In another study, the ADC map was also found useful in predicting the likelihood of a positive biopsy at ultrasound-guided transrectal biopsy.[25]

In patients undergoing active surveillance, the baseline tumor ADC value is of prognostic value. In this cohort of patients, lesions with lower

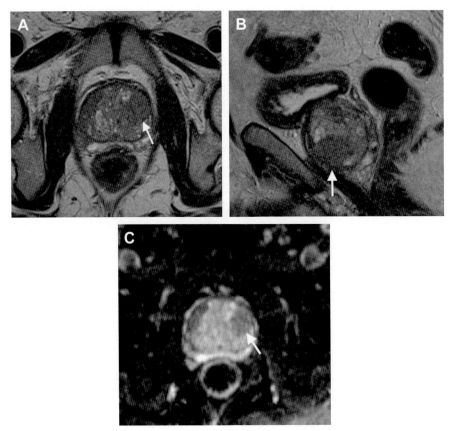

Fig. 4. A 47-year-old man with Gleason 4+3 tumor in central gland. (*A*) Axial and (*B*) sagittal T2-weighted images show low signal intensity focus in left gland (*arrows*), which is suspicious. This corroborates well with (*C*) focal area of lower ADC (*arrow*) on the ADC map, returning mean value of 0.73×10^{-3} mm^2/s, suggesting higher grade disease.

ADC values were found to have larger disease volumes and were more likely to show progression over time.[64] As tumors progressed, tumor and whole gland ADC values significantly decreased.[67] A lower tumor ADC baseline value was also found to predict for adverse repeat biopsy at follow-up and a shorter time to radical treatment.[68]

Assessment of Tumor Response to Treatment

Quantitative ADC values are being used to assess the response of prostate cancer to treatment. Cellular death and necrosis have been corroborated with an increase in ADC values in several tumor types.

With antiandrogen treatment, the ADC values of tumor have been shown to increase,[69] thus reducing the contrast between tumor and nontumor tissue. Antiandrogen treatment has also been shown to reduce tumor and glandular volume (**Fig. 5**). When external beam radiotherapy is administered, an increase in the mean ADC values of tumor is observed, but the normal peripheral and transitional zones show reduction in ADC values.[70] Interestingly, in an animal model, minimally invasive therapy using cryoablation results in an acute decrease in the tumor ADC value.[71] These studies suggest that quantitative ADC measurements may be used as a response biomarker to assess the effectiveness of antitumor treatment and possibly prostate-sparing minimally invasive treatment.

Multiparametric Imaging Paradigm

Prostate imaging is now often performed using a combination of imaging sequences, which includes T2-weighted imaging, DWI, dynamic contrast-enhanced MR imaging (DCE-MR imaging), and MR spectroscopy.

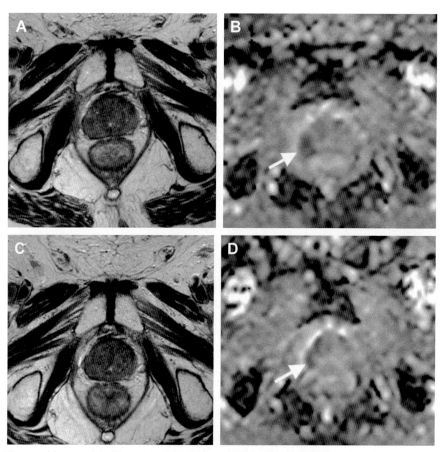

Fig. 5. An 83-year-old man with Gleason 4+5 prostate cancer. Pretreatment (*A*) T2-weighted image and (*B*) ADC map shows lesion in right prostate gland (*arrow*) on ADC map, which is less well defined on T2-weighted imaging because of reduced background T2-signal intensity in peripheral zone. Posttreatment (*C*) T2-weighted image and (*D*) ADC map show regression of low ADC area in right gland (*arrow*), but this is not appreciable on conventional T2-weighted image.

Key points

1. DWI improves the detection of tumor in the prostate gland.

2. The ADC value of prostate cancer reflects the tumor grade and aggressiveness.

3. ADC value may be used to monitor response to antitumor treatment.

Many studies have shown that of these imaging techniques, DWI seems to have a high diagnostic accuracy on its own, but combining DWI with DCE-MR imaging and/or MRS can further improve diagnostic performance.[20,32,72,73] In one study of patients with minimally elevated serum PSA levels, combining T2-weighted imaging, DWI, and DCE-MR imaging resulted in 80% sensitivity and 83% specificity for detecting prostate cancer.[74] Tanimoto and colleagues[75] and Langer and colleagues[73] also showed that the highest diagnostic accuracy

for detecting prostate cancer was achieved by combining T2-weighted MR imaging with DWI and DCE-MR imaging. Multiparametric MR imaging was also found to be the most accurate approach for diagnosing local recurrence of prostate cancer[76,77] after radiotherapy treatment (**Fig. 6**).

URINARY BLADDER

There are now several studies confirming the value of DWI for assessing bladder tumors.

Disease Detection and Staging

DWI can aid detection of bladder carcinoma because tumors show impeded diffusion compared with the normal bladder wall. In one study evaluating patients presenting with hematuria, there was excellent agreement between DWI results and cystoscopy ($\kappa = .94$) for the identification of bladder neoplasm.[78] DW MR imaging had a sensitivity and positive predictive value of 98.5% and 100%, respectively.[78]

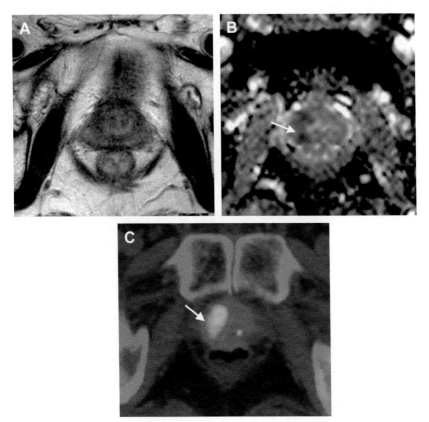

Fig. 6. A 73-year-old man with Gleason 3+4 prostate cancer, previously treated with neoadjuvant bicalutamide and radical radiotherapy. Patient now presents with rising serum PSA levels. (*A*) Axial T2-weighted imaging shows no definite focal abnormality. (*B*) Axial ADC map shows focal areas of low ADC value within right gland toward glandular apex (*arrow*), which shows (*C*) intense tracer uptake on ¹⁸F-chone PET-CT, in keeping with disease relapse (*arrow*).

Using the ADC map may also improve the differentiation of tumor from the normal bladder wall and, in so doing, assess the depth of local tumor invasion in relation to the bladder wall.[79] DWI was shown to have greater diagnostic confidence compared with T2-weighted MR imaging in diagnosing patients with organ confined bladder tumors,[79–81] as well as in distinguishing between muscle invasive versus non–muscle invasive tumors (**Fig. 7**).[82] By performing DWI over the entire pelvis, DWI is also helpful in detecting metastatic or synchronous pelvic disease.

Disease Aggressiveness and Prognostication

Not dissimilar to prostate cancer, studies have found an inverse relationship between tumor grade and the measured ADC values.[83] High-grade tumors were found to return lower ADC values compared with the lower-grade tumors.[83] The pretreatment ADC value may also have prognostic value in bladder cancers. Tumors with lower pretreatment ADC values have been shown to predict for better or complete response to chemoradiotherapy.

RECTUM

Rectal cancer continues to be an important cause of mortality and morbidity in the adult population.

DWI has been shown to aid tumor detection in the pelvis[84] and may identify occult tumors when imaging is performed for other clinical indications. However, local disease staging is still largely reliant on small field of view high spatial resolution

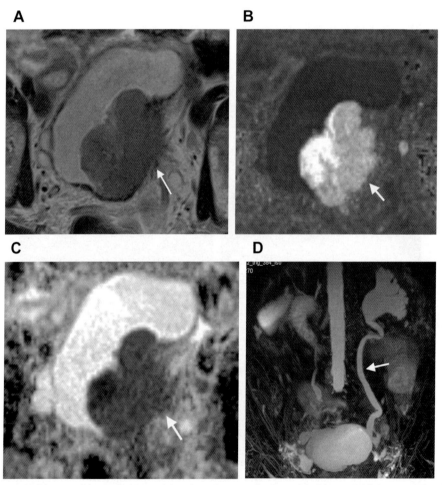

Fig. 7. A 62-year-old man with grade III transitional carcinoma of urinary bladder. Axial (*A*) T2-weighted, (*B*) high b-value (b = 1000 s/mm²), and (*C*) ADC map, clearly showing a large polypoidal bladder mass (*arrow*), which extends through muscle wall (stage T3 disease). (*D*) MR urography shows left hydronephrosis (*arrow*) as a result of tumor infiltration of distal ureter.

T2-weighted MR imaging. Nevertheless, one of the emerging applications of DWI for rectal imaging is for the assessment of treatment response.

Studies have demonstrated that after chemotherapy and radiotherapy, an increase in tumor ADC is observed in responding disease (**Fig. 8**).[85–87] Kim and colleagues[88] demonstrated that complete responders to chemoradiotherapy showed a higher post treatment tumor ADC and higher percentage ADC increase compared with noncomplete responders. Interestingly, several studies showed that a lower pretreatment ADC seems to predict for better tumor volume regression following treatment,[89–91] although this observation is not universal.[86,88] More recently, it has been suggested that the change in tumor volume may also be a sensitive indicator of complete disease response compared with the ADC value.[92] In addition, one study found good correlation between tumor volume derived by DWI with the tumor regression grade assessed at histopathology.[93]

Key points

1. ADC maps in bladder cancer can aid local disease staging and provide prognostic information.

2. In rectal cancer, ADC value is being evaluated as a potential response and prognostic quantitative marker.

NODAL DISEASE

One ongoing diagnostic challenge in imaging is the accurate identification of metastatic lymph node disease. Although size measurement criteria are widely applied to CT and MR imaging to distinguish between malignant and nonmalignant lymph nodes, there are inherent limitations. In pelvic cancers, nodal metastases are not uncommon to lymph nodes that are smaller than the conventional threshold (ie, 10-mm short-axis diameter)

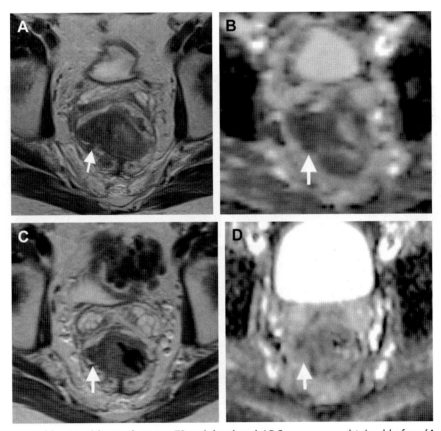

Fig. 8. A 58-year-old man with rectal cancer. T2-weighted and ADC maps were obtained before (A and B) and after (C and D) at 12 weeks following neoadjuvant chemoradiation. On T2-weighted image, note slight reduction in tumor diameter (<30%) after treatment. However, by ADC measurements, there was significant increase in mean ADC value within tumor (arrows) (1.13×10^{-3} mm^2/s to 1.47×10^{-3} mm^2/s).

used to classify lymph nodes as being benign or malignant.

Because lymph nodes are highly cellular structures composed of lymphoid elements, they show significant impeded diffusion on DWI. The technique can be used to visualize the distribution of lymph nodes (both normal and abnormal) within the pelvis.[94] However, distinguishing between benign and malignant nodes on DWI can still be challenging because lymph nodes, whether benign or malignant, will show varying degrees of high signal intensity on DWI (**Fig. 9**).

Some studies have shown that malignant nodes return lower ADC values compared with benign lymph nodes[95,96] and may be superior to size criteria for nodal classification.[97] In one study,[96] DWI was found to have a low sensitivity (18.8%) but high specificity (97.6%) for the detection of nodal metastases in patients with prostate cancer. However, one of the problems encountered is the substantial overlap in ADC values between malignant and benign nodes, making it difficult to confidently classify any single node prospectively as being benign or malignant. Furthermore, it may be difficult to reliably obtain a quantitative ADC value for a small node because of partial volume effects.

For these reasons, nodal assessment in the pelvis by radiologists is currently made using a combination of size measurement criteria, morphologic appearances, and diffusion characteristics. One promising technology is the combination of DWI with the administration of a lymphotropic contrast media (ultrasmall iron oxide particles).[98] These iron particles are taken up by normal lymph nodes and the presence of iron results in nodal signal suppression on DWI. Using such a technique, one study showed a very high diagnostic accuracy (90%) for identifying malignant infiltration in a cohort of normal size (<10-mm short-axis diameter) lymph nodes in men with pelvic urologic malignancies.[98]

METASTASES TO THE BONY PELVIS

It is not uncommon to find metastases to the bony pelvis in patients with prostate or bladder carcinoma. On conventional imaging, T1-weighted sequences are generally more useful than T2-weighted imaging in depicting these lesions as low signal intensity foci against the high signal intensity fatty marrow. However, using DWI can enhance metastatic detection (**Fig. 10**).

Studies have shown that DWI is similar or superior to skeletal scintigraphy for detecting bone

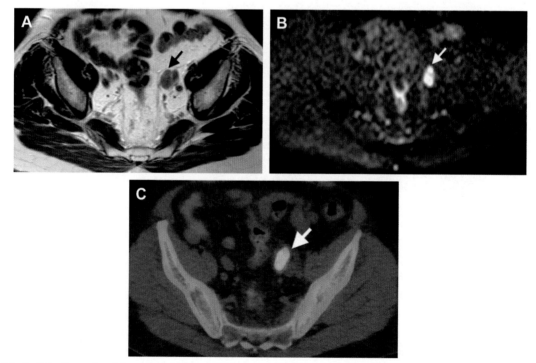

Fig. 9. Detection of pelvic nodes. A 46-year-old man with Gleason 4+5 grade prostate cancer. Axial (*A*) T2-weighted image, (*B*) b = 1000 s/mm² DWI image, and (*C*) ¹⁸F-choline PET-CT image. T2-weighted imaging shows 1.2-cm (maximum short-axis diameter) lymph node at left pelvic side wall, which also shows strong impeded diffusion. The lymph node also demonstrates intense tracer uptake consistent with nodal involvement (*arrows*).

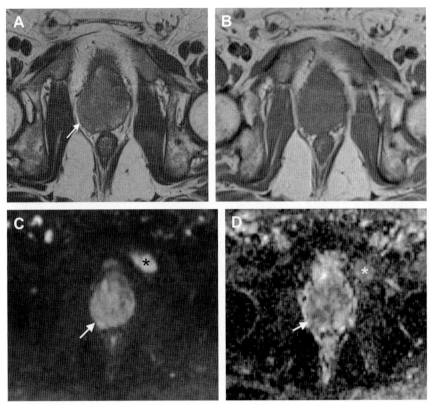

Fig. 10. Unsuspected bone metastases. A 60-year-old man with Gleason 4+4 prostate cancer. Axial (A) T2-weighted image, (B) T1-weighted image, (C) b = 1000 s/mm² DWI image, and (D) ADC map. Images show a large lesion in the right peripheral zone, which extends into central gland (arrows). However, note high signal intensity on DWI in left pubic ramus as a result of malignant infiltration (asterisk). Area returns relatively low ADC values.

metastases. In patients with bone metastases arising from prostate cancer, lesions appear more conspicuous on the high b-value DWI compared with a short-tau inversion recovery sequence.[99] In other studies, DWI was found to have similar or higher diagnostic accuracy for the detection of bone metastases compared with skeletal scintigraphy and at least equal to choline PET-CT.[100–103]

More importantly, conventional imaging techniques are unable to provide an assessment of disease response to treatment. ADC measurements in bone seem to be a promising response biomarker, which shows an increase in value in response to antiandrogen or chemotherapy treatment.[104,105]

Key points

1. ADC value on its own may not reliably discriminate between malignant and benign lymph nodes because of significant overlap.

2. DWI is highly sensitive for detecting metastatic bone disease, and the ADC value could also be used to assess treatment response.

SUMMARY

DWI is evolving as an important imaging sequence for the evaluation of the male pelvis. In particular, DWI provides important diagnostic and prognostic information for the assessment of the patient with prostate cancer. The role of DWI in the assessment of rectal and urinary bladder tumors will continue to evolve. The technique shows substantial promise for the evaluation of metastatic bone disease and may also enhance nodal assessment in the pelvis.

REFERENCES

1. Koh DM, Collins DJ. Diffusion-weighted MRI in the body: applications and challenges in oncology. AJR Am J Roentgenol 2007;188(6):1622–35.

2. Koh DM, Takahara T, Imai Y, et al. Practical aspects of assessing tumors using clinical diffusion-weighted imaging in the body. Magn Reson Med Sci 2007;6(4):211–24.

3. Kitajima K, Takahashi S, Ueno Y, et al. Clinical utility of apparent diffusion coefficient values obtained using high b-value when diagnosing prostate

cancer using 3 tesla MRI: comparison between ultra-high b-value (2000 s/mm(2)) and standard high b-value (1000 s/mm(2)). J Magn Reson Imaging 2012;36(1):198–205.

4. Kitajima K, Kaji Y, Kuroda K, et al. High b-value diffusion-weighted imaging in normal and malignant peripheral zone tissue of the prostate: effect of signal-to-noise ratio. Magn Reson Med Sci 2008; 7(2):93–9.

5. Katahira K, Takahara T, Kwee TC, et al. Ultra-high-b-value diffusion-weighted MR imaging for the detection of prostate cancer: evaluation in 201 cases with histopathological correlation. Eur Radiol 2011;21(1):188–96.

6. Ahmed HU. The index lesion and the origin of prostate cancer. N Engl J Med 2009;361(17): 1704–6.

7. Dall'Era MA, Cooperberg MR, Chan JM, et al. Active surveillance for early-stage prostate cancer: review of the current literature. Cancer 2008;112(8):1650–9.

8. Klotz L. Active surveillance for favorable-risk prostate cancer: who, how and why? Nat Clin Pract Oncol 2007;4(12):692–8.

9. Parker C. Active surveillance of early prostate cancer: rationale, initial results and future developments. Prostate Cancer Prostatic Dis 2004;7(3): 184–7.

10. Williams SB, Lei Y, Nguyen PL, et al. Comparative effectiveness of cryotherapy vs brachytherapy for localised prostate cancer. BJU Int 2012;110(2 Pt B): E92–8.

11. Ward JF, Jones JS. Focal cryotherapy for localized prostate cancer: a report from the national Cryo On-Line Database (COLD) Registry. BJU Int 2012;109(11):1648–54.

12. Vargas HA, Akin O, Franiel T, et al. Diffusion-weighted endorectal MR imaging at 3 T for prostate cancer: tumor detection and assessment of aggressiveness. Radiology 2011;259(3):775–84.

13. Yagci AB, Ozari N, Aybek Z, et al. The value of diffusion-weighted MRI for prostate cancer detection and localization. Diagn Interv Radiol 2011; 17(2):130–4.

14. Lim HK, Kim JK, Kim KA, et al. Prostate cancer: apparent diffusion coefficient map with T2-weighted images for detection: a multireader study. Radiology 2009;250(1):145–51.

15. Haider MA, van der Kwast TH, Tanguay J, et al. Combined T2-weighted and diffusion-weighted MRI for localization of prostate cancer. AJR Am J Roentgenol 2007;189(2):323–8.

16. Morgan VA, Kyriazi S, Ashley SE, et al. Evaluation of the potential of diffusion-weighted imaging in prostate cancer detection. Acta Radiol 2007;48(6): 695–703.

17. Miao H, Fukatsu H, Ishigaki T. Prostate cancer detection with 3-T MRI: comparison of diffusion-weighted and T2-weighted imaging. Eur J Radiol 2007;61(2):297–302.

18. Doo KW, Sung DJ, Park BJ, et al. Detectability of low and intermediate or high risk prostate cancer with combined T2-weighted and diffusion-weighted MRI. Eur Radiol 2012;22(8):1812–9.

19. Rosenkrantz AB, Mannelli L, Kong X, et al. Prostate cancer: utility of fusion of T2-weighted and high b-value diffusion-weighted images for peripheral zone tumor detection and localization. J Magn Reson Imaging 2011;34(1):95–100.

20. Delongchamps NB, Rouanne M, Flam T, et al. Multiparametric magnetic resonance imaging for the detection and localization of prostate cancer: combination of T2-weighted, dynamic contrast-enhanced and diffusion-weighted imaging. BJU Int 2011;107(9):1411–8.

21. Hatano K, Tsuda K, Kawamura N, et al. Clinical value of diffusion-weighted magnetic resonance imaging for localization of prostate cancer– comparison with the step sections of radical prostatectomy. Nihon Hinyokika Gakkai Zasshi 2010; 101(4):603–8 [in Japanese].

22. Yoshimitsu K, Kiyoshima K, Irie H, et al. Usefulness of apparent diffusion coefficient map in diagnosing prostate carcinoma: correlation with stepwise histopathology. J Magn Reson Imaging 2008;27(1):132–9.

23. Roy C, Pasquali R, Matau A, et al. The role of diffusion 3-Tesla MRI in detecting prostate cancer before needle biopsy: multiparametric study of 111 patients. J Radiol 2010;91(11 Pt 1):1121–8 [in French].

24. Park BK, Lee HM, Kim CK, et al. Lesion localization in patients with a previous negative transrectal ultrasound biopsy and persistently elevated prostate specific antigen level using diffusion-weighted imaging at three Tesla before rebiopsy. Invest Radiol 2008;43(11):789–93.

25. Chen YJ, Pu YS, Chueh SC, et al. Diffusion MRI predicts transrectal ultrasound biopsy results in prostate cancer detection. J Magn Reson Imaging 2011;33(2):356–63.

26. Kumar V, Jagannathan NR, Kumar R, et al. Apparent diffusion coefficient of the prostate in men prior to biopsy: determination of a cut-off value to predict malignancy of the peripheral zone. NMR Biomed 2007;20(5):505–11.

27. Ren J, Huan Y, Li F, et al. Combined T2-weighted and diffusion-weighted MRI for diagnosis of urinary bladder invasion in patients with prostate carcinoma. J Magn Reson Imaging 2009;30(2):351–6.

28. Ren J, Huan Y, Wang H, et al. Seminal vesicle invasion in prostate cancer: prediction with combined T2-weighted and diffusion-weighted MR imaging. Eur Radiol 2009;19(10):2481–6.

29. Chen M, Dang HD, Wang JY, et al. Prostate cancer detection: comparison of T2-weighted imaging,

diffusion-weighted imaging, proton magnetic reso-nance spectroscopic imaging, and the three tech-niques combined. Acta Radiol 2008;49(5):602–10.

30. deSouza NM, Reinsberg SA, Scurr ED, et al. Magnetic resonance imaging in prostate cancer: the value of apparent diffusion coefficients for iden-tifying malignant nodules. Br J Radiol 2007;80(950): 90–5.

31. Jeong IG, Kim JK, Cho KS, et al. Diffusion-weighted magnetic resonance imaging in patients with unilateral prostate cancer on extended pros-tate biopsy: predictive accuracy of laterality and implications for hemi-ablative therapy. J Urol 2010; 184(5):1963–9.

32. Kitajima K, Kaji Y, Fukabori Y, et al. Prostate cancer detection with 3 T MRI: comparison of diffusion-weighted imaging and dynamic contrast-enhanced MRI in combination with T2-weighted imaging. J Magn Reson Imaging 2010;31(3):625–31.

33. Rosenkrantz AB, Kopec M, Kong X, et al. Prostate cancer vs. post-biopsy hemorrhage: diagnosis with T2- and diffusion-weighted imaging. J Magn Reson Imaging 2010;31(6):1387–94.

34. Oto A, Kayhan A, Jiang Y, et al. Prostate cancer: differentiation of central gland cancer from benign prostatic hyperplasia by using diffusion-weighted and dynamic contrast-enhanced MR imaging. Radiology 2010;257(3):715 23.

35. Kim JH, Kim JK, Park BW, et al. Apparent diffusion coefficient: prostate cancer versus noncancerous tissue according to anatomical region. J Magn Re-son Imaging 2008;28(5):1173–9.

36. Tamada T, Sone T, Jo Y, et al. Apparent diffusion coefficient values in peripheral and transition zones of the prostate: comparison between normal and malignant prostatic tissues and correlation with histologic grade. J Magn Reson Imaging 2008; 28(3):720–6.

37. Shi H, Kong X, Feng G, et al. Diffusion-weighted single-shot echo planar MR imaging of normal human prostate using different b values. J Huazhong Univ Sci Technolog Med Sci 2008;28(6):737–40.

38. Ren J, Huan Y, Wang H, et al. Diffusion-weighted imaging in normal prostate and differential diag-nosis of prostate diseases. Abdom Imaging 2008; 33(6):724–8.

39. Kozlowski P, Chang SD, Goldenberg SL. Diffusion-weighted MRI in prostate cancer: comparison between single-shot fast spin echo and echo planar imaging sequences. Magn Reson Imaging 2008;26(1):72–6.

40. Pickles MD, Gibbs P, Sreenivas M, et al. Diffusion-weighted imaging of normal and malignant pros-tate tissue at 3.0T. J Magn Reson Imaging 2006; 23(2):130–4.

41. Gibbs P, Tozer DJ, Liney GP, et al. Comparison of quantitative T2 mapping and diffusion-weighted imaging in the normal and pathologic prostate. Magn Reson Med 2001;46(6):1054–8.

42. Reischauer C, Wilm BJ, Froehlich JM, et al. High-resolution diffusion tensor imaging of prostate cancer using a reduced FOV technique. Eur J Ra-diol 2011;80(2):e34–41.

43. Li C, Chen M, Li S, et al. Diffusion tensor imaging of prostate at 3.0 Tesla. Acta Radiol 2011;52(7):813–7.

44. Kim CK, Jang SM, Park BK. Diffusion tensor imaging of normal prostate at 3T: effect of number of diffusion-encoding directions on quantitation and image quality. Br J Radiol 2012;85(1015):e279–83.

45. Kozlowski P, Chang SD, Meng R, et al. Combined prostate diffusion tensor imaging and dynamic contrast enhanced MRI at 3T: quantitative correla-tion with biopsy. Magn Reson Imaging 2010; 28(5):621–8.

46. Xu J, Humphrey PA, Kibel AS, et al. Magnetic reso-nance diffusion characteristics of histologically defined prostate cancer in humans. Magn Reson Med 2009;61(4):842–50.

47. Gurses B, Kabakci N, Kovanlikaya A, et al. Diffu-sion tensor imaging of the normal prostate at 3 Tesla. Eur Radiol 2008;18(4):716–21.

48. Manenti G, Carlani M, Mancino S, et al. Diffusion tensor magnetic resonance imaging of prostate cancer. Invest Radiol 2007;42(6):412–9.

49. Gibbs P, Pickles MD, Turnbull LW. Repeatability of echo-planar-based diffusion measurements of the human prostate at 3 T. Magn Reson Imaging 2007;25(10):1423–9.

50. Sinha S, Sinha U. In vivo diffusion tensor imaging of the human prostate. Magn Reson Med 2004;52(3): 530–7.

51. Gibbs P, Pickles MD, Turnbull LW. Diffusion imaging of the prostate at 3.0 tesla. Invest Radiol 2006;41(2):185–8.

52. Dopfert J, Lemke A, Weidner A, et al. Investigation of prostate cancer using diffusion-weighted intra-voxel incoherent motion imaging. Magn Reson Imaging 2011;29(8):1053–8.

53. Pang Y, Turkbey B, Bernardo M, et al. Intravoxel incoherent motion MR imaging for prostate cancer: an evaluation of perfusion fraction and diffusion coefficient derived from different b-value combina-tions. Magn Reson Med 2012. http://dx.doi.org/10.1002/mrm.24277.

54. Nagarajan R, Margolis D, Raman S, et al. Correla-tion of Gleason scores with diffusion-weighted imaging findings of prostate cancer. Adv Urol 2012;2012:374805.

55. Hambrock T, Hoeks C, Hulsbergen-van de Kaa C, et al. Prospective assessment of prostate cancer aggressiveness using 3-T diffusion-weighted mag-netic resonance imaging-guided biopsies versus a systematic 10-core transrectal ultrasound pros-tate biopsy cohort. Eur Urol 2012;61(1):177–84.

56. Bittencourt LK, Barentsz JO, de Miranda LC, et al. Prostate MRI: diffusion-weighted imaging at 1.5T correlates better with prostatectomy Gleason grades than TRUS-guided biopsies in peripheral zone tumours. Eur Radiol 2012;22(2):468–75.

57. Yamamura J, Salomon G, Buchert R, et al. Magnetic resonance imaging of prostate cancer: diffusion-weighted imaging in comparison with sextant biopsy. J Comput Assist Tomogr 2011; 35(2):223–8.

58. Verma S, Rajesh A, Morales H, et al. Assessment of aggressiveness of prostate cancer: correlation of apparent diffusion coefficient with histologic grade after radical prostatectomy. AJR Am J Roentgenol 2011;196(2):374–81.

59. Turkbey B, Shah VP, Pang Y, et al. Is apparent diffusion coefficient associated with clinical risk scores for prostate cancers that are visible on 3-T MR images? Radiology 2011;258(2):488–95.

60. Oto A, Yang C, Kayhan A, et al. Diffusion-weighted and dynamic contrast-enhanced MRI of prostate cancer: correlation of quantitative MR parameters with Gleason score and tumor angiogenesis. AJR Am J Roentgenol 2011;197(6): 1382–90.

61. Itou Y, Nakanishi K, Narumi Y, et al. Clinical utility of apparent diffusion coefficient (ADC) values in patients with prostate cancer: can ADC values contribute to assess the aggressiveness of prostate cancer? J Magn Reson Imaging 2011;33(1): 167–72.

62. Hambrock T, Somford DM, Huisman HJ, et al. Relationship between apparent diffusion coefficients at 3.0-T MR imaging and gleason grade in peripheral zone prostate cancer. Radiology 2011; 259(2):453–61.

63. Woodfield CA, Tung GA, Grand DJ, et al. Diffusion-weighted MRI of peripheral zone prostate cancer: comparison of tumor apparent diffusion coefficient with Gleason score and percentage of tumor on core biopsy. AJR Am J Roentgenol 2010;194(4): W316–22.

64. deSouza NM, Riches SF, Vanas NJ, et al. Diffusion-weighted magnetic resonance imaging: a potential non-invasive marker of tumour aggressiveness in localized prostate cancer. Clin Radiol 2008;63(7): 774–82.

65. Langer DL, van der Kwast TH, Evans AJ, et al. Intermixed normal tissue within prostate cancer: effect on MR imaging measurements of apparent diffusion coefficient and T2-sparse versus dense cancers. Radiology 2008;249(3):900–8.

66. Somford DM, Hambrock T, Hulsbergen-van de Kaa CA, et al. Initial experience with identifying high-grade prostate cancer using diffusion-weighted MR imaging (DWI) in patients with a Gleason score </= 3 + 3 = 6 upon schematic TRUS-guided biopsy: a radical prostatectomy correlated series. Invest Radiol 2012;47(3):153–8.

67. Morgan VA, Riches SF, Thomas K, et al. Diffusion-weighted magnetic resonance imaging for monitoring prostate cancer progression in patients managed by active surveillance. Br J Radiol 2011; 84(997):31–7.

68. van As NJ, de Souza NM, Riches SF, et al. A study of diffusion-weighted magnetic resonance imaging in men with untreated localised prostate cancer on active surveillance. Eur Urol 2009;56(6):981–7.

69. Nemoto K, Tateishi T, Ishidate T. Changes in diffusion-weighted images for visualizing prostate cancer during antiandrogen therapy: preliminary results. Urol Int 2010;85(4):421–6.

70. Song I, Kim CK, Park BK, et al. Assessment of response to radiotherapy for prostate cancer: value of diffusion-weighted MRI at 3 T. AJR Am J Roentgenol 2010;194(6):W477–82.

71. Chen J, Daniel BL, Diederich CJ, et al. Monitoring prostate thermal therapy with diffusion-weighted MRI. Magn Reson Med 2008;59(6):1365–72.

72. Iwazawa J, Mitani T, Sassa S, et al. Prostate cancer detection with MRI: is dynamic contrast-enhanced imaging necessary in addition to diffusion-weighted imaging? Diagn Interv Radiol 2011; 17(3):243–8.

73. Langer DL, van der Kwast TH, Evans AJ, et al. Prostate cancer detection with multi-parametric MRI: logistic regression analysis of quantitative T2, diffusion-weighted imaging, and dynamic contrast-enhanced MRI. J Magn Reson Imaging 2009;30(2): 327–34.

74. Tamada T, Sone T, Higashi H, et al. Prostate cancer detection in patients with total serum prostate-specific antigen levels of 4-10 ng/mL: diagnostic efficacy of diffusion-weighted imaging, dynamic contrast-enhanced MRI, and T2-weighted imaging. AJR Am J Roentgenol 2011;197(3):664–70.

75. Tanimoto A, Nakashima J, Kohno H, et al. Prostate cancer screening: the clinical value of diffusion-weighted imaging and dynamic MR imaging in combination with T2-weighted imaging. J Magn Reson Imaging 2007;25(1):146–52.

76. Akin O, Gultekin DH, Vargas HA, et al. Incremental value of diffusion weighted and dynamic contrast enhanced MRI in the detection of locally recurrent prostate cancer after radiation treatment: preliminary results. Eur Radiol 2011;21(9):1970–8.

77. Tamada T, Sone T, Jo Y, et al. Locally recurrent prostate cancer after high-dose-rate brachytherapy: the value of diffusion-weighted imaging, dynamic contrast-enhanced MRI, and T2-weighted imaging in localizing tumors. AJR Am J Roentgenol 2011;197(2):408–14.

78. Abou-El-Ghar ME, El-Assmy A, Refaie HF, et al. Bladder cancer: diagnosis with diffusion-weighted

MR imaging in patients with gross hematuria. Radiology 2009;251(2):415–21.

79. El-Assmy A, Abou-El-Ghar ME, Refaie HF, et al. Diffusion-weighted MR imaging in diagnosis of superficial and invasive urinary bladder carcinoma: a preliminary prospective study. SciWorld J 2008;8: 364–70.

80. El-Assmy A, Abou-El-Ghar ME, Mosbah A, et al. Bladder tumour staging: comparison of diffusion- and T2-weighted MR imaging. Eur Radiol 2009; 19(7):1575–81.

81. Watanabe H, Kanematsu M, Kondo H, et al. Preoperative T staging of urinary bladder cancer: does diffusion-weighted MRI have supplementary value? AJR Am J Roentgenol 2009;192(5):1361–6.

82. Giannarini G, Petralia G, Thoeny HC. Potential and limitations of diffusion-weighted magnetic resonance imaging in kidney, prostate, and bladder cancer including pelvic lymph node staging: a critical analysis of the literature. Eur Urol 2012;61(2): 326–40.

83. Takeuchi M, Sasaki S, Ito M, et al. Urinary bladder cancer: diffusion-weighted MR imaging–accuracy for diagnosing T stage and estimating histologic grade. Radiology 2009;251(1):112–21.

84. Shinya S, Sasaki T, Nakagawa Y, et al. The efficacy of diffusion-weighted imaging for the detection of colorectal cancer. Hepatogastroenterology 2009; 56(89):128–32.

85. Hein PA, Kremser C, Judmaier W, et al. Diffusion-weighted magnetic resonance imaging for monitoring diffusion changes in rectal carcinoma during combined, preoperative chemoradiation: preliminary results of a prospective study. Eur J Radiol 2003;45(3):214–22.

86. Barbaro B, Vitale R, Valentini V, et al. Diffusion-weighted magnetic resonance imaging in monitoring rectal cancer response to neoadjuvant chemoradiotherapy. Int J Radiat Oncol Biol Phys 2012;83(2): 594–9.

87. Kim SH, Lee JM, Hong SH, et al. Locally advanced rectal cancer: added value of diffusion-weighted MR imaging in the evaluation of tumor response to neoadjuvant chemo- and radiation therapy. Radiology 2009;253(1):116–25.

88. Kim SH, Lee JY, Lee JM, et al. Apparent diffusion coefficient for evaluating tumour response to neoadjuvant chemoradiation therapy for locally advanced rectal cancer. Eur Radiol 2011;21(5):987–95.

89. Jung SH, Heo SH, Kim JW, et al. Predicting response to neoadjuvant chemoradiation therapy in locally advanced rectal cancer: diffusion-weighted 3 Tesla MR imaging. J Magn Reson Imaging 2012;35(1): 110–6.

90. Lambrecht M, Vandecaveye V, De Keyzer F, et al. Value of diffusion-weighted magnetic resonance imaging for prediction and early assessment of response to neoadjuvant radiochemotherapy in rectal cancer: preliminary results. Int J Radiat Oncol Biol Phys 2012;82(2):863–70.

91. Dzik-Jurasz A, Domenig C, George M, et al. Diffusion MRI for prediction of response of rectal cancer to chemoradiation. Lancet 2002;360(9329):307–8.

92. Curvo-Semedo L, Lambregts DM, Maas M, et al. Rectal cancer: assessment of complete response to preoperative combined radiation therapy with chemotherapy–conventional MR volumetry versus diffusion-weighted MR imaging. Radiology 2011; 260(3):734–43.

93. Carbone SF, Pirtoli L, Ricci V, et al. Assessment of response to chemoradiation therapy in rectal cancer using MR volumetry based on diffusion-weighted data sets: a preliminary report. Radiol Med 2012. [Epub ahead of print].

94. Mir N, Sohaib SA, Collins D, et al. Fusion of high b-value diffusion-weighted and T2-weighted MR images improves identification of lymph nodes in the pelvis. J Med Imaging Radiat Oncol 2010; 54(4):358–64.

95. Beer AJ, Eiber M, Souvatzoglou M, et al. Restricted water diffusibility as measured by diffusion-weighted MR imaging and choline uptake in (11) C-choline PET/CT are correlated in pelvic lymph nodes in patients with prostate cancer. Mol Imaging Biol 2011;13(2):352–61.

96. Budiharto T, Joniau S, Lerut E, et al. Prospective evaluation of 11C-choline positron emission tomography/computed tomography and diffusion-weighted magnetic resonance imaging for the nodal staging of prostate cancer with a high risk of lymph node metastases. Eur Urol 2011;60(1): 125–30.

97. Eiber M, Beer AJ, Holzapfel K, et al. Preliminary results for characterization of pelvic lymph nodes in patients with prostate cancer by diffusion-weighted MR-imaging. Invest Radiol 2010;45(1): 15–23.

98. Thoeny HC, Triantafyllou M, Birkhaeuser FD, et al. Combined ultrasmall superparamagnetic particles of iron oxide-enhanced and diffusion-weighted magnetic resonance imaging reliably detect pelvic lymph node metastases in normal-sized nodes of bladder and prostate cancer patients. Eur Urol 2009;55(4):761–9.

99. Pearce T, Philip S, Brown J, et al. Bone metastases from prostate, breast and multiple myeloma: differences in lesion conspicuity at short-tau inversion recovery and diffusion-weighted MRI. Br J Radiol 2012;85(1016):1102–6.

100. Gutzeit A, Doert A, Froehlich JM, et al. Comparison of diffusion-weighted whole body MRI and skeletal scintigraphy for the detection of bone metastases in patients with prostate or breast carcinoma. Skeletal Radiol 2010;39(4):333–43.

101. Lecouvet FE, El Mouedden J, Collette L, et al. Can whole-body magnetic resonance imaging with diffusion-weighted imaging replace Tc 99m bone scanning and computed tomography for single-step detection of metastases in patients with high-risk prostate cancer? Eur Urol 2012;62(1):68–75.

102. Luboldt W, Kufer R, Blumstein N, et al. Prostate carcinoma: diffusion-weighted imaging as potential alternative to conventional MR and 11C-choline PET/CT for detection of bone metastases. Radiology 2008;249(3):1017–25.

103. Xu X, Ma L, Zhang JS, et al. Feasibility of whole body diffusion weighted imaging in detecting bone metastasis on 3.0T MR scanner. Chin Med Sci J 2008;23(3):151–7.

104. Messiou C, Collins DJ, Giles S, et al. Assessing response in bone metastases in prostate cancer with diffusion weighted MRI. Eur Radiol 2011; 21(10):2169–77.

105. Reischauer C, Froehlich JM, Koh DM, et al. Bone metastases from prostate cancer: assessing treatment response by using diffusion-weighted imaging and functional diffusion maps–initial observations. Radiology 2010;257(2):523–31.

106. Kim CK, Park BK, Han JJ, et al. Diffusion-weighted imaging of the prostate at 3 T for differentiation of malignant and benign tissue in transition and peripheral zones: preliminary results. J Comput Assist Tomogr 2007;31(3):449–54.

107. Zelhof B, Pickles M, Liney G, et al. Correlation of diffusion-weighted magnetic resonance data with cellularity in prostate cancer. BJU Int 2009;103(7): 883–8.

108. Kim CK, Park BK, Kim B. High-b-value diffusion-weighted imaging at 3 T to detect prostate cancer: comparisons between b values of 1,000 and 2,000 s/mm2. AJR Am J Roentgenol 2010; 194(1):W33–7.

109. Reinsberg SA, Payne GS, Riches SF, et al. Combined use of diffusion-weighted MRI and 1H MR spectroscopy to increase accuracy in prostate cancer detection. AJR Am J Roentgenol 2007; 188(1):91–8.

110. Sato C, Naganawa S, Nakamura T, et al. Differentiation of noncancerous tissue and cancer lesions by apparent diffusion coefficient values in transition and peripheral zones of the prostate. J Magn Reson Imaging 2005;21(3):258–62.

Imaging of the Scrotum

Lejla Aganovic, MD*, Fiona Cassidy, MD

KEYWORDS

- Testis • Epididymis • Spermatic cord • Scrotal imaging • Testicular tumors • Torsion
- Epididymo-orchitis • Scrotal pseudotumors

KEY POINTS

- Most epididymal masses are benign.
- Most intratesticular masses are malignant.
- Scrotal pseudotumors such as hematoma, focal infection, segmental testicular infarction, fibrous pseudotumor, and polyorchidism can mimic tumors on imaging. There is a need for better understanding of these lesions to avoid unnecessary surgery.
- When scrotal ultrasonography is inconclusive, magnetic resonance imaging may provide important additional information.

INTRODUCTION

Ultrasonography is the first-line imaging technique for assessing acute and nonacute conditions of the scrotum and it is the only modality needed in most cases.[1] In certain cases in which clinical and ultrasound findings are inconclusive, magnetic resonance (MR) imaging may be useful because of its superior ability to characterize fat, blood products, fibrous tissue, and tissue perfusion.[2,3] This article describes the normal anatomy of the scrotum and reviews the ultrasound and MR imaging findings of a wide range of scrotal disorders that may be encountered. Several important imaging pitfalls are reviewed to minimize the risk of misdiagnosis that could lead to inappropriate patient treatment.

ANATOMY

The normal adult testis measures approximately 5 × 3 × 2 cm and is of homogeneous echotexture (Fig. 1). Each testis is enveloped by tunica albuginea, a fibrous capsule that is seen as a hyperechoic line (see Fig. 1). A fold of tunica albuginea projects into the testis and forms mediastinum testis, which is seen as a hyperechoic linear band. The tunica albuginea is covered by tunica vaginalis, which is a closed sac of peritoneum that consists of 2 layers: the visceral layer, which adheres to the testis, and the parietal layer, which lines the inside of the scrotal wall.[4] A potential space between the two layers of tunica vaginalis normally contains a few milliliters of fluid.[5] The testis is composed of multiple seminiferous tubules that coalesce toward the mediastinum to form a network of channels called the rete testis.[4] These channels pass through the mediastinum and tunica albuginea toward the epididymal head. The epididymis lies along the posterolateral aspect of the testis and is of similar echogenicity to the adjacent testis. It consists of head, body, and tail ducts, which then continue as the vas deferens in the spermatic cord. The spermatic cord contains vas deferens, testicular vessels, pampiniform venous plexus, and nerves.

IMAGING PROTOCOLS

The scrotum is examined by ultrasound with a patient in a supine position. The scanning is performed with high-frequency (5–12 MHz) linear array transducer. The testis and epididymis are

The authors have no financial disclosures.

Department of Radiology, VA Hospital, University of California San Diego, 3350 La Jolla Village Drive, San Diego, CA 92161, USA

* Corresponding author.

E-mail address: laganovic@ucsd.edu

Radiol Clin N Am 50 (2012) 1145–1165

http://dx.doi.org/10.1016/j.rcl.2012.08.003

0033-8389/12/$ – see front matter Published by Elsevier Inc.

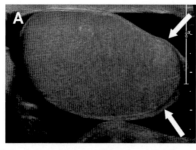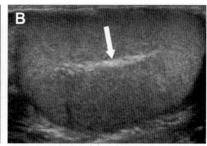

Fig. 1. Normal testis in a 26-year-old man. (*A*) Ultrasound appearance of a normal testis shows homogeneous echotexture. Tunica albuginea (*arrows*) is seen as an echogenic line surrounding the testis. The presence of hydrocele renders the tunica albuginea visible. (*B*) Mediastinum testis (*arrow*) is seen as an echogenic band oriented in craniocaudal direction.

examined in transverse and longitudinal planes. When there is a palpable abnormality, the patient places a finger over the lesion and targeted ultrasound evaluation of that area is performed. It is important to obtain one image that captures both testicles for comparison of echotexture and vascularity. This method is particularly valuable in the acute setting when torsion or infection is suspected. Color Doppler and pulsed color Doppler images are obtained to assess the vascularity of normal structures and for evaluation of focal masses. Color Doppler images need to be optimized to detect slow flow by using the lowest velocity scale and the lowest wall filter. Color gain setting is maximized for optimal sensitivity while limiting the excessive color noise. Because motion can mimic presence of blood flow on color Doppler images, imaging with pulsed color Doppler technique shows the presence of true blood flow and eliminates this potential pitfall. Evaluating the blood flow with power Doppler ultrasound is valuable when assessing perfusion in an acute setting such as torsion, scrotal trauma, and infection.

For MR imaging examinations, a 12.5-cm circular multipurpose surface coil is placed to cover the scrotum. Axial, coronal, and sagittal images are obtained with T1-weighted spin-echo sequences (recovery time [TR]/echo time [TE] 500–650/13–15) and T2-weighted fast spin-echo sequences (TR/TE 4000/100–120) with 3-mm to 4-mm slice thickness and a 0.5-mm gap. Axial precontrast T1 images are acquired with fat suppression, followed by postcontrast images in axial, coronal, and sagittal planes. All images are acquired with a small field of view (200 mm).

ACUTE SCROTUM

Epididymitis and Epididymo-orchitis

Epididymitis and epididymo-orchitis are the most common conditions that cause acute scrotal pain in adults. Infection most commonly affects the epididymis, although concomitant orchitis can occur in 20% of cases. The most common pathogens are *Escherichia coli*, *Pseudomonas* sp, and sexually transmitted *Chlamydia trachomatis* and *Neisseria gonorrhea*.[6] Isolated orchitis is rare and is most commonly caused by a virus.[7,8] Ultrasonographic findings in epididymitis include hypoechoic enlargement of the head and body with increased blood flow on Doppler images (**Fig. 2**). The entire epididymis or only focal areas may be involved. Scrotal wall thickening and hydrocele may also be present. When concurrent orchitis is present, the affected portions of the testis are hypoechoic and hypervascular (**Fig. 3**). Orchitis is most commonly diffuse, but may involve only a focal area. Abscess can occur as a complication of epididymo-orchitis. A focal, complex fluid collection with peripheral but no internal vascularity indicates an abscess (**Fig. 4**). Pus can collect between the layers of tunica vaginalis forming a pyocele, which often contains debris and septations (**Fig. 5**). Another complication of epididymitis is development of testicular ischemia, which occurs when epididymal edema compresses the testicular vessels, most commonly the draining veins.[9] This phenomenon can be observed on Doppler ultrasound or contrast-enhanced MR imaging (**Fig. 6**). Absent or decreased testicular blood flow can also be present in testicular torsion; however, in most cases, with torsion there is no hypervascularity of the epididymis, which is more typically seen with infection. The difference in epididymal vascularity therefore can help differentiate these two entities. Particularly if it is focal, orchitis can mimic an intratesticular tumor on imaging (**Fig. 7**). Follow-up imaging in these patients should be done to document resolution of infection and to exclude a neoplasm.

Testicular Torsion

Testicular torsion causes acute scrotal pain because of severe ischemia of the testis. The layers

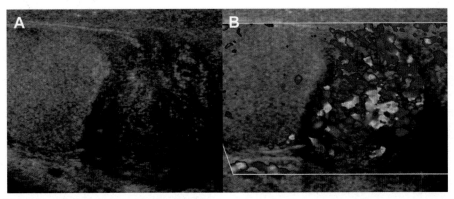

Fig. 2. Epididymitis. A 24-year-old man with scrotal pain. Gray-scale ultrasound images show enlarged, heterogeneous epididymal tail (*A*) that has increased vascularity on color Doppler images (*B*).

of tunica vaginalis normally fixate the testis posteriorly, preventing it from twisting. When an abnormally large tunica vaginalis is present, the posterior fixation is absent, allowing the testis to rotate freely within the scrotum. This abnormality is also known as bell-clapper deformity. Following the twist of the spermatic cord, obstruction of the testicular vessels occurs. Testicular torsion requires immediate surgery. If done within 6 hours, the success rate of the surgery is 100%, decreasing to 0% to 20% if it is more than 12 to 24 hours following the onset.[10] Torsion results in edema of the testis with decreased or absent blood flow. On gray-scale images, the testis is enlarged, heterogeneous, and hypoechoic. Later, as the hemorrhagic infarction occurs, hyperechoic areas in the affected testis can be seen. Color and power Doppler images have an advantage compared with the gray-scale images because of early detection of the absence of flow in the affected testis.

Depending on the duration and the degree of torsion, the amount of perfusion abnormality varies, initially affecting venous and then arterial flow. No detectable flow is eventually present on either color or power Doppler images (**Fig. 8**). After 6 hours from the onset of torsion, reactive hydrocele and skin thickening can be seen. After 24 hours, peritesticular tissues can become hyperemic because of reactive vascular response (**Fig. 9**).[11] The epididymis can become enlarged and, rarely, also hyperemic. The contralateral testis should always be imaged for comparison. When spontaneous detorsion occurs, increased blood flow may be detected caused by reactive hyperemia. This finding may represent a diagnostic challenge because epididymo-orchitis has similar imaging findings. The patient's symptoms can be helpful when differentiating these two entities. Patients with intermittent torsion or detorsion have resolution of acute symptoms with persistent

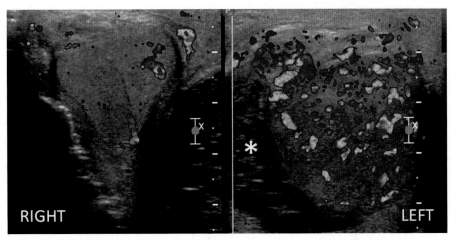

Fig. 3. Epididymo-orchitis. A 36-year-old man with left scrotal pain. Left testis and epididymis are enlarged and have increased vascularity on color Doppler images compared with the right side. Complex fluid is present surrounding the left testis, consistent with a pyocele (*asterisk*).

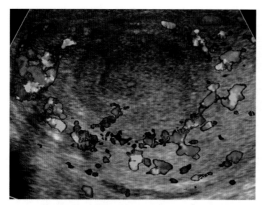

Fig. 4. Testicular abscess. A 26-year-old man with severe epididymo-orchitis. Color Doppler ultrasound image shows diffuse increase in vascularity of the testis. A central heterogeneous hypoechoic area is present with no flow. Surgery revealed abscess.

hypervascularity, whereas patients with infection have continued pain.

Ischemic testis with resulting hyperemic epididymis and peritesticular tissues can mimic epididymo-orchitis when, in a setting of infection, testicular ischemia occurs because of epididymal edema causing compression of the testicular vessels. When definite diagnosis cannot be made, surgical exploration may be warranted when an avascular or hypovascular testis is seen in conjunction with what appears to be a hyperemic epididymis, because torsion in those cases cannot be excluded.[12]

Segmental Testicular Infarction

Segmental testicular infarction is a rare entity that mainly affects men 20 to 40 years old. Predisposing

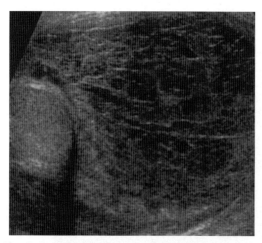

Fig. 5. Pyocele. Ultrasonography of the scrotum in a 39-year-old man with epididymo-orchitis shows a complex fluid collection with internal septations and loculations surrounding the testis.

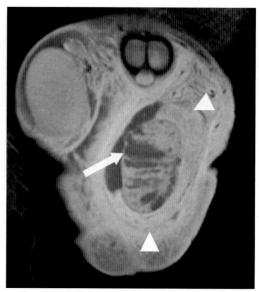

Fig. 6. Ischemia of the left testis caused by epididymo-orchitis. A 47-year-old man presents with a 4-day history of severe left scrotal pain. Postcontrast MR images of the scrotum show diffuse enlargement of the left epididymis (arrowheads) with thickening of the left scrotal wall. These structures also show increased enhancement compared with the contralateral side. Left testis has areas of decreased enhancement (arrow) that represent decreased perfusion and ischemia. This phenomenon is caused by compression of the testicular vessels in spermatic cord by edematous, inflamed epididymis.

factors include epididymo-orchitis and hematologic disorders such as sickle cell disease or vasculitis.[13] Patients may present with acute pain, although some patients may have chronic pain if the diagnosis was not made in the early phase. Ischemic process affects only one portion of the testis, which is typically oval or wedge shaped. Superior portions of the testis are more commonly involved because of lack of significant collateral vessels in that area.[13] On color Doppler images, the affected area shows no flow, whereas normal flow is preserved in the surrounding testicular tissue (Fig. 10).[14] This condition can be indistinguishable from a hypovascular tumor, especially if the tumor is of a smaller size, since small tumors can have diminished flow.[15] Because most testicular tumors have increased vascularity, absence of flow within a focal area in an appropriate clinical setting should prompt consideration of this entity. Diagnosis may be aided by MR imaging, which shows wedge-shaped abnormality with lack of internal enhancement. On postcontrast images, there can be intense rim enhancement surrounding the infracted area, which can be present in 90% of patients.[13] In a chronic setting, retraction of tunica

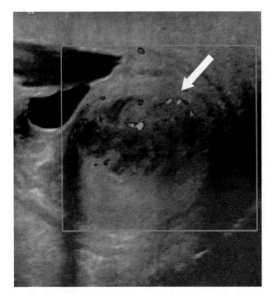

Fig. 7. Focal orchitis. A 34-year-old man with significant scrotal pain. Color Doppler ultrasound image shows heterogeneous area in the testis with some vascularity (*arrow*). No significant abnormality was noted in the rest of the testis. Based on the patient's presentation, focal orchitis was suspected. Patient was reimaged after a course of antibiotics to ensure that the abnormality was no longer present. Focal orchitis needs to be followed up to resolution to exclude a malignancy.

albuginea can be seen in the area containing the lesion caused by volume loss and fibrosis. Patients are managed conservatively so diagnosis of this entity on imaging can prevent unnecessary orchiectomy.

Trauma

Scrotal trauma is commonly associated with severe injuries to the scrotal contents including hematoma, fracture or rupture of the testicle, and peritesticular structures. Ultrasonography is valuable in diagnosing conditions, such as testicular rupture, that might require immediate surgery. Sensitivity of ultrasound for diagnosing testicular rupture reaches 100%.[16,17] Discontinuity of tunica albuginea, contour abnormality, and heterogeneous echotexture are signs of testicular rupture.[17,18] Abnormal contour of the testis is present because of extruded intratesticular parenchyma and is considered a secondary sign of tunica albuginea disruption (**Fig. 11**). Heterogeneous intratesticular lesions can be caused by rupture, although they can also be caused by hemorrhage or infarction. Isolated presence of a heterogeneous testis therefore should not be considered diagnostic of rupture, unless accompanied by tunica albuginea disruption or contour deformity. Color Doppler evaluation of the injured testis should always be performed because tunica albuginea injuries are commonly associated with focal or diffuse loss of vascularity. These avascular areas are commonly debrided. Hematocele is a collection of blood between the layers of tunica vaginalis. It can occur in an isolated form or can be associated with testicular rupture. Depending on the chronicity of the hematocele, it can present as hyperechoic collection in acute phase or can appear as anechoic fluid with septations in a more chronic setting. Presence of a large hematocele may obscure the evaluation of tunica albuginea and these patients may undergo surgery to assess the

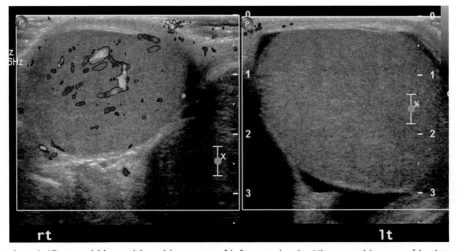

Fig. 8. Torsion. A 17-year-old boy with sudden onset of left scrotal pain. Ultrasound images of both testes were obtained for comparison. Left testis is enlarged compared with the right testis. Color Doppler images show absence of intratesticular blood flow in left testis and normal flow in the right testis. Torsion of the left testis was found at surgery.

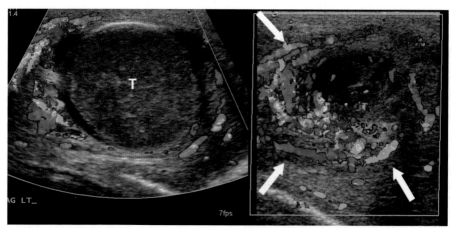

Fig. 9. Torsion. A 25-year-old man presents to the hospital 24 hours after the onset of sudden acute pain. Color Doppler ultrasound images show absence of flow in left testis (T), which is also diffusely hypoechoic. There is significant hyperemia of the surrounding paratesticular tissues (*arrows*). Surgery revealed a 720° testicular torsion.

continuity of the tunica. Hematomas can occur in testis, epididymis, and scrotal wall. Hematomas are round, avascular lesions on Doppler ultrasound and their appearance varies with age (**Fig. 12**). Acutely, they appear hyperechoic and with time they become more complex and hypoechoic. In a chronic setting, hematoma may mimic a neoplasm. In these cases, MR imaging can be helpful to exclude a neoplasm because hematomas are bright on T1-weighted images and have a dark hemosiderin rim on T2-weighted images (see **Fig. 12**). On postcontrast images, no enhancement is present, unlike tumors, which enhance avidly. Serial follow-up of intratesticular traumatic lesions should be done because up to 15% of tumors can be detected after an episode of trauma.[19] Traumatic lesions tend to resolve with time, unlike tumors, which continue to grow.[20,21]

Traumatic epididymitis occurs as sequela of contusion. Diffuse or focal enlargement of the epididymis is present with increase in vascularity. On imaging, this condition may mimic epididymitis; however, history is crucial in differentiating these 2 conditions.[20]

Fournier Gangrene

Fournier gangrene is a fulminant necrotizing fasciitis of the genitalia, scrotum, and perineum. Approximately 50% of patients have diabetes mellitus. Early diagnosis in Fournier gangrene is crucial because immediate surgical debridement and antibiotics can reduce the high mortality. Soft tissue

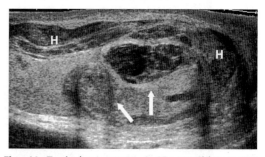

Fig. 11. Testicular rupture. A 25-year-old man sustained blunt trauma to the scrotum during a motorcycle accident. Ultrasound image shows a markedly abnormal testis with hypoechoic areas that represent intratesticular blood or infarcts (*arrows*). Testis has abnormal contour that indicates rupture. Complex fluid is present surrounding the testis, consistent with hematocele (H). At surgery, ruptured testis was found with extruded testicular contents through the tunica albuginea.

Fig. 10. Segmental testicular infarction. Acute scrotal pain in a 39-year-old man. Color Doppler ultrasound image shows an avascular hypoechoic oval area in the upper pole of the testis (*arrow*). The rest of the testicular parenchyma has normal vascularity.

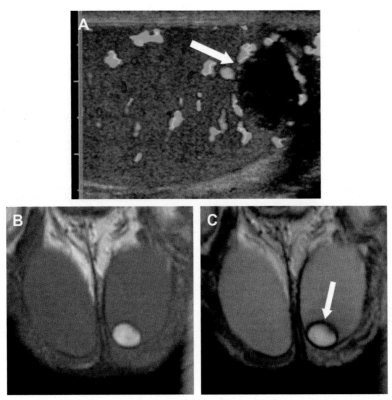

Fig. 12. Testicular hematoma. A 46-year-old man with history of scrotal trauma. (*A*) Sonographic image of left testis showed a well-defined hypoechoic mass in the lower pole with no vascularity (*arrow*). MR imaging was done to exclude a hypovascular tumor. The lesion is hyperintense on T1-weighted (*B*) and T2-weighted (*C*) images with a hypointense rim on T2-weighted images (*arrow*) caused by the presence of hemosiderin. Postcontrast images showed no enhancement of this lesion (not shown).

gas is a hallmark of this condition. Diagnosis is often made based on clinical examination; however, imaging may be required to confirm the diagnosis in questionable cases. Current imaging techniques include radiography, ultrasonography, and computed tomography (CT). On ultrasonographs, Fournier gangrene presents as scrotal wall thickening with echogenic foci that show dirty shadowing caused by the presence of gas (**Fig. 13**). The testis and epididymis often have a normal appearance.[22,23] CT has greater specificity for evaluating disease extent than radiography, ultrasonography, or physical examination.[22,23] CT can show asymmetric fascial thickening, any coexisting fluid collection or abscess, fat stranding around the involved structures, and subcutaneous emphysema secondary to gas-forming bacteria.[24]

NONACUTE SCROTUM

Nonacute conditions of the scrotum are divided into extratesticular and intratesticular. Extratesticular lesions are further categorized based on the site of origin into conditions affecting epididymis,

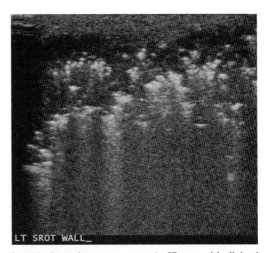

Fig. 13. Fournier gangrene. A 67-year-old diabetic with severe perineal and scrotal pain. Sonographic image shows left scrotal wall thickening. Multiple echogenic foci with dirty shadowing are present, representing gas in soft tissues.

spermatic cord, tunica vaginalis, or paratesticular area. Most (97%) solid extratesticular masses are benign, unlike intratesticular masses, which are predominantly malignant (95%).[25]

Extratesticular Lesions

Conditions of epididymis

Epididymal cysts Cystic masses in the epididymis include epididymal cysts and spermatoceles. Cystic appearance is caused by dilatation of tubules in the epididymis. They commonly present as palpable lesions. On ultrasonographs, these lesions are well-defined, anechoic structures with increased through-transmission. Epididymal cysts and spermatoceles cannot be reliably differentiated, although spermatoceles tend to be larger, contain internal echoes, and can be multilocular (**Fig. 14**).[26] Spermatoceles occur only in the epididymal head, whereas epididymal cysts can develop anywhere within the epididymis. No treatment of these cystic lesions is generally required, unless symptomatic. Patients who have undergone vasectomy have been reported to have increased incidence of epididymal cysts/spermatoceles, although some investigators report no such correlation.[27–29]

Adenomatoid tumor Adenomatoid tumor is the most common epididymal tumor. It is a benign neoplasm that most commonly originates in the tail of the epididymis.[30] Ultrasonography shows a round, well-defined hypoechoic epididymal lesion (**Fig. 15**). On MR imaging, this mass is slightly hypointense compared with the testicular parenchyma on T2-weighted images and, on post-contrast images, shows similar enhancement to the testis (**Fig. 16**).[31]

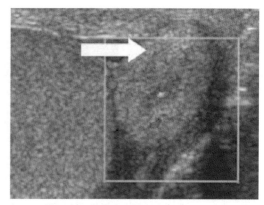

Fig. 15. Adenomatoid tumor in a 60-year-old man. Color Doppler ultrasound image shows a circumscribed homogeneous mass in the right epididymal tail (*arrow*) that is isoechoic to the testis and has internal vascularity.

Leiomyoma Leiomyomas are benign neoplasms that may arise from the smooth muscle anywhere in the body. Scrotal leiomyomas can arise from the epididymis, spermatic cord, tunica albuginea, and tunica dartos of the scrotal wall.[32] Leiomyoma is the second most common neoplasm of the epididymis. It appears as a nonspecific solid hypoechoic heterogeneous mass on ultrasonographs and may have cystic components and/or calcifications.[33] Following the appearance of leiomyomas elsewhere in the body, epididymal leiomyomas on T2-weighted MR imaging usually show low signal intensity similar to that of smooth muscle, which can be helpful in establishing this diagnosis (**Fig. 17**).

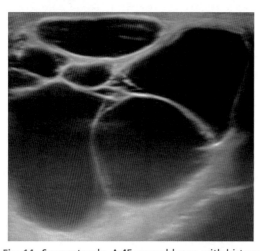

Fig. 14. Spermatocele. A 45-year-old man with history of vasectomy presents with a palpable mass. Ultrasonography of the left scrotum shows a large multilocular septated cystic lesion in the upper epididymis.

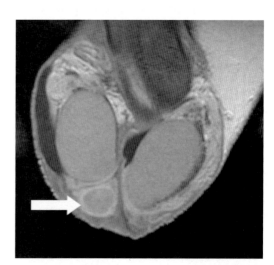

Fig. 16. Adenomatoid tumor in a 60-year-old man. Coronal postcontrast MR image shows a well-defined mass arising from the tail of the right epididymis (*arrow*) that shows similar enhancement to the normal testis.

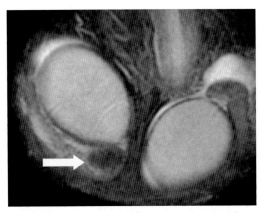

Fig. 17. Leiomyoma of epididymis. A 57-year-old man presented with a palpable mass in the scrotum. Coronal T2-weighted MR image shows a well-circumscribed mass in the tail of the epididymis (*arrow*). Because of the low T2 signal of the mass, diagnosis of leiomyoma was suspected, which was confirmed at surgery.

Sperm granuloma Sperm granulomas occur in almost 50% of patients following vasectomy. They represent a foreign body giant cell reaction to extravasated sperm and, although most of them are asymptomatic, they can present as painful nodules. On ultrasonographs, they present as a small (usually less than 1 cm) hypoechoic epididymal solid mass or masses (**Fig. 18**). These lesions can also occur at the cut ends of vas deferens in the superolateral portion of the scrotal sac.[34] To our knowledge, the MR imaging appearance of sperm granuloma has not yet been described.

Metastases Although uncommon, metastases should be considered when multifocal extratesticular lesions are seen, particularly in the setting of a known primary malignancy. Testicular involvement may also be present. The most frequent

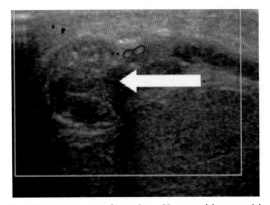

Fig. 18. Sperm granuloma in a 63-year-old man with history of vasectomy. Axial sonogram shows a small extratesticular hypoechoic mass (*arrow*) with minimal color Doppler flow.

primary tumors are lymphoma, leukemia, and prostate.[33]

Postvasectomy scrotum Vasectomy is one of the most effective methods of male contraception. It is performed by occluding and blocking the vas deferens. Chronic testicular pain can be present in 33% of patients after vasectomy.[35] Increased pressure in epididymal tubules caused by obstruction has been proposed as the mechanism of pain in these patients. On imaging, epididymal abnormalities are present in up to 50% of patients and these include diffuse enlargement, tubular ectasia of epididymis, spermatoceles, and sperm granulomas.[29] Presence of mobile echogenic material in epididymis has recently been described as a finding that can occur in 12% of patients.[27] In tubular ectasia of epididymis, multiple interfaces in enlarged epididymis are present (**Fig. 19**).[36] These changes are typically hypovascular and can be unilateral or bilateral. Although suggesting vasectomy, this sign can also be associated with other causes of vas obstruction, such as inguinal hernia repair or prostatitis. Tubular ectasia of rete testis can also be seen in patients after vasectomy.[37]

Conditions of tunica vaginalis

Fibrous pseudotumor Fibrous pseudotumor represents nodular reactive fibrous proliferation related to prior intrascrotal inflammation resulting in one or more fibrous masses most commonly arising from the tunica vaginalis. They can become mobile, resulting in a scrotolith or scrotal pearl. On ultrasonographs, the typical appearance is a hypoechoic mass or masses (sometimes with internal calcification) often associated with a hydrocele (in 50%) (**Fig. 20**A). On MR imaging they are of uniformly low intensity on T1-weighted and T2-weighted imaging because of the presence of fibrosis with delayed enhancement on postcontrast images (see **Fig. 20**B). It is important to recognize this benign condition and not mistake it for malignancy. If the diagnosis is made before surgery, treatment involves local excision rather than orchiectomy.[38]

Hydrocele Hydrocele is caused by collection of fluid between the layers of tunica vaginalis. It is a common cause of scrotal enlargement. Small hydroceles can be present in normal individuals and should not be interpreted as abnormal. There are many causes of hydrocele, including trauma, infection, tumors, torsion, and idiopathic and congenital causes.[39,40] A small hydrocele surrounds only a small fraction of testicular surface, whereas larger ones may surround the testis. In a setting of trauma or infection, hydroceles may contain blood or pus (see **Figs. 5**

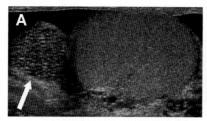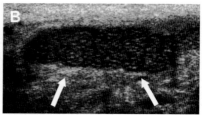

Fig. 19. Ductal ectasia of epididymis. A 53-year-old man with history of vasectomy 12 years ago. (*A, B*) Ultrasound images show diffuse thickening of epididymal head and body with dilatation of the tiny ducts (*arrows*) within the epididymis giving the speckled appearance characteristic of this condition.

and 11). If patient becomes symptomatic, hydrocelectomy can be performed.

Scrotal pearl Scrotal pearl is a calcified loose body lying between the membranes of the tunica vaginalis. The cause is unclear, although it may result from torsion of appendix testis or epididymis, hematoma, or may represent a dislodged fibrous pseudotumor of tunica vaginalis.[41] Repetitive microtrauma has also been described as a risk factor, with bikers having a high incidence of scrotal pearls (81%).[42] Scrotal pearls are usually round and solitary, although occasionally they are multiple, and measure up to 1 cm in diameter.[43] On ultrasonographs, they appear as a mobile hyperechoic focus with posterior acoustic shadowing (**Fig. 21**).

Conditions of the spermatic cord

Extratesticular lipoma Lipomas are the most common extratesticular tumors. They are typically well defined on ultrasonographs with homogeneous echotexture similar to that of subcutaneous fat and do not have internal color flow. However, the echogenicity of lipomas may be variable and they occasionally appear hypoechoic (**Fig. 22**).[44] In these cases, MR imaging may be helpful for confirmation. Lipomas are homogeneously bright

on T1 and T2 weighting, lose signal on fat-saturated images, and do not enhance.

Leiomyoma Scrotal leiomyomas can arise from the epididymis, spermatic cord, tunica albuginea, or scrotal wall. When they arise from the spermatic cord they are usually located in the scrotal part of spermatic cord; in contrast, leiomyosarcoma is usually located in the inguinal part of the spermatic cord. Imaging features of spermatic cord leiomyomas are similar to epididymal leiomyomas (discussed earlier).

Spermatic cord sarcomas The most common spermatic cord mass is a spermatic cord lipoma. However, if the diagnosis of lipoma is excluded, more than half of the spermatic cord masses are malignant, most commonly sarcomas.[25] Rhabdomyosarcoma (which mainly affects the pediatric population) is the most common, followed by liposarcoma and then leiomyosarcoma. The ultrasonographic appearance of spermatic cord sarcoma is typically a heterogeneous solid mass (because of hemorrhage and necrosis) with internal Doppler color flow (**Fig. 23**). On MR imaging, they appear as heterogeneous solid spermatic cord masses that generally enhance avidly but heterogeneously following administration of intravenous gadolinium. Liposarcomas may appear similar to lipomas but

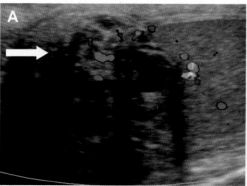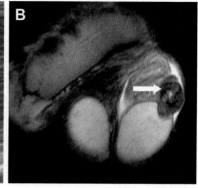

Fig. 20. Fibrous pseudotumor in a 39-year-old man. (*A*) Axial ultrasound image shows a heterogeneous hypervascular mass (*arrow*) that is not clearly definable as intratesticular or extratesticular. (*B*) Coronal T2-weighted MR image shows well-defined very-low-signal mass (*arrow*) that is likely arising from the tunica vaginalis and causing extrinsic impingement on the left testicle.

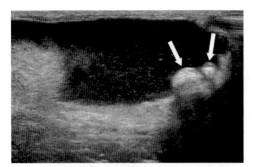

Fig. 21. Scrotoliths (scrotal pearls). Longitudinal ultrasound image shows 2 echogenic foci with posterior acoustic shadowing (*arrows*). Hydrocele is present.

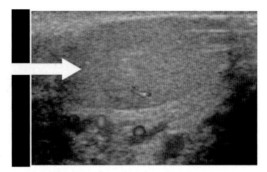

Fig. 22. Spermatic cord lipoma in a 58-year-old man. Ultrasound images of the right groin show a solid, homogeneous, slightly hypoechoic extratesticular mass (*arrow*) with no significant internal color flow.

usually show enhancing soft tissue septations or solid components and areas of calcification.[45] Macroscopic fat can be detected in approximately 80% of liposarcomas (see **Fig. 23**).[46,47]

Spermatic cord hematoma Spermatic cord hematoma occurs most commonly secondary to inguinal hernia repair but may be related to trauma, anticoagulation therapy, ruptured varicocele,[48] or

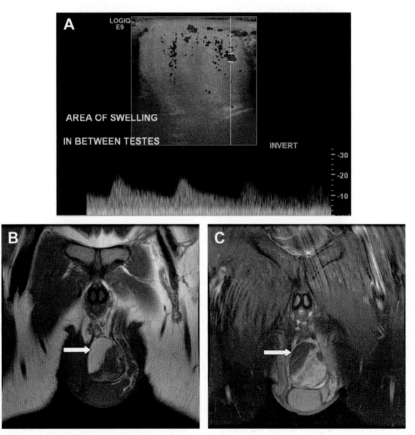

Fig. 23. Liposarcoma of the spermatic cord in a 68-year-old man. (*A*) Axial sonogram shows an echogenic solid extratesticular mass with internal vascularity shown by color Doppler. (*B, C*) Sagittal MR images show a suprates-ticular heterogeneous mass that is closely related to the left spermatic cord. Sagittal T1-weighted image (*B*) shows a large area of high signal intensity (*arrow*) within the mass that loses signal on postcontrast fat-saturated image (*C*) (*arrow*), confirming the presence of macroscopic fat. Avid heterogeneous enhancement of nonfatty portions of the mass is present.

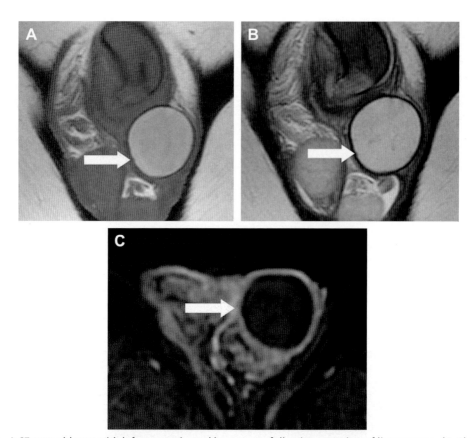

Fig. 24. A 67-year-old man with left spermatic cord hematoma following resection of liposarcoma. (*A, B*) Coronal T1-weighted and T2-weighted images show a well-defined high-signal-intensity mass (caused by methemoglobin) with a low-signal hemosiderin rim arising from the left spermatic cord (*arrows*). This lesion did not lose signal on fat-saturated images (not shown). (*C*) Axial postcontrast subtraction image (enhanced T1-weighted image minus unenhanced T1-weighted image) (*arrow*) shows no enhancement of the mass, confirming the diagnosis of a postsurgical hematoma.

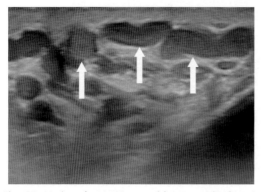

Fig. 25. Varicocele. A 45-year-old man with chronic dull scrotal pain. Gray-scale ultrasound image shows dilated vessels within pampiniform plexus (*arrows*). Internal echoes are present within the lumen caused by sluggish flow.

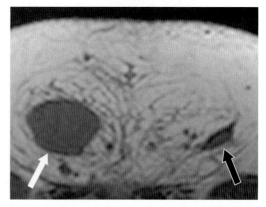

Fig. 26. Undescended testis. T1-weighted MR images through the pelvis show an undescended right testis in the right inguinal canal (*white arrow*). Normal left inguinal canal is present on the left side (*black arrow*).

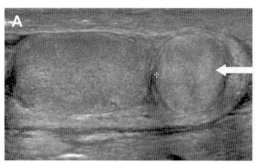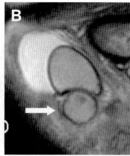

Fig. 27. Polyorchidism in a 46-year-old man. (*A*) Sagittal sonogram shows an extratesticular mass (*arrow*) that has similar echotexture to the testis. (*B*) Coronal T2-weighted MR image shows that the mass (*arrow*) is isointense to the testis and is surrounded by a hypointense rim corresponding with the tunica albuginea.

retroperitoneal hemorrhage. Ultrasonography shows a mixed-echogenicity inguinal or scrotal mass without internal color flow. MR typically shows a mass related to the spermatic cord that is hyperintense on T1 and T2 weighting (extracellular methemoglobin) with a low-signal rim on T2-weighted and T2*-weighted images (chronic hemosiderin)[38] without internal enhancement (**Fig. 24**). Peripheral enhancement may be seen because of the presence of granulation tissue.

Varicocele Varicoceles are abnormal dilatations of veins within the pampiniform plexus. Varicoceles are found in 20% to 40% of infertile men, and in only 15% of the general population.[49] Varicoceles can be diagnosed by physical examination, but sensitivity is only 70%, compared with ultrasonography which has sensitivity of 97%.[50] Scanning the patient in an upright position may improve detection. Varicoceles are more common on the left side because the left testicular vein is longer and enters the left renal vein at a 90° angle. Most varicoceles are caused by incompetent valves, but they are occasionally caused by a retroperitoneal mass that compresses or invades the renal vein or inferior vena cava. On ultrasonographs, varicoceles appear as serpiginous anechoic tubular structures with diameters larger than 2.5 mm.[51,52] Doppler images may show stasis, antegrade flow, or retrograde flow. Internal echoes are occasionally caused by sluggish flow

(**Fig. 25**). During Valsalva maneuver, varicoceles should increase in diameter and show reversal of blood flow. Isolated right varicoceles are rare and should prompt evaluation of retroperitoneum to exclude an underlying mass. Because varicoceles negatively affect spermiogenesis, removal of varicoceles often significantly improves the quality of sperm.

Other conditions of the paratesticular area

Undescended testicle Inguinal canal is the most common location for the undescended testis, although it may be present anywhere along the normal path of descent (**Fig. 26**).[53] Ultrasonography is helpful in depicting the undescended testis, which is generally atrophic and less echogenic than the normal testis. Undescended testis has increased risk of malignancy, typically seminoma.[54] The contralateral testis is also at increased risk for developing neoplasm and ultrasonography is a useful tool for surveilling these patients. Infertility can also be associated with this condition.

Polyorchidism Polyorchidism is thought to result from division of the genital ridge by peritoneal bands. It is commonly associated with cryptorchidism. The ultrasound appearance is of one or multiple paratesticular masses with identical echogenicity to normal testis. This diagnosis can be

Table 1 Extratesticular pseudotumors			
Epididymis	**Spermatic Cord**	**Tunica Vaginalis**	**Paratesticular Area**
Focal epididymitis	Hematoma	Fibrous pseudotumor	Hernia
Hematoma	—	Scrotal pearl	Polyorchidism
Sperm granuloma	—	—	Splenogonadal fusion
Sarcoidosis	—	—	—

confirmed by MR imaging because the masses have identical signal characteristics to the normal testis. In addition, the tunica albuginea is seen as a hypointense rim surrounding the supernumerary testes on T1-weighted and T2-weighted imaging (**Fig. 27**). Close clinical and imaging follow-up is recommended because the accessory testes have an increased risk of torsion and malignancy.[55]

Extratesticular lesions that can mimic tumors (pseudotumors) are summarized in **Table 1**.

Intratesticular Lesions

Testicular cysts

Testicular cysts include tunica albuginea cyst, simple cyst, and tubular ectasia of rete testis.

Tunica albuginea cysts occur at the periphery of the testis, originate from tunica albuginea, and are likely mesothelial in origin. On ultrasonographs they have appearance of simple cysts and are typically smaller than 5 mm (**Fig. 28**). These cysts commonly present as a palpable lump.

Simple intratesticular cysts are usually idiopathic, but may be posttraumatic or postinflammatory. They range from 2 mm to 2 cm and can be single or multiple. Unlike tunica albuginea cysts, simple cysts are usually not palpable even when large. Ultrasound examination reveals round anechoic lesions with increased through-transmission (see **Fig. 28**).[56] It is important to document absence of a perceptible wall, which can be seen in cystic teratomas.[57] Simple cysts in asymptomatic

patients require no follow-up, although some investigators suggest ultrasound surveillance.[58,59]

Tubular ectasia of rete testis is a benign condition that occurs because of obliteration of efferent ductules, which leads to cystic transformation. Up to 50% of patients have history of possible spermatic duct obstruction such as vasectomy or inguinal hernia repair.[37] This abnormality is often bilateral and is commonly associated with spermatoceles.[60] It is important to recognize this benign entity and not mistake it for a cystic neoplasm. On ultrasonographs, clusters of small cystic structures are present within the mediastinum testis. No solid areas are present between the cystic spaces (**Fig. 29**). Cystic components are usually only a few millimeters in size, but larger cysts can be present surrounding the tubular ectasia area.[37] In uncertain cases, MR imaging can be helpful to differentiate tubular ectasia and malignant tumors because tubular ectasia is isointense to hyperintense compared with testis on T2-weighted images, as opposed to malignant tumors, which are typically darker than testis on T2-weighted images.[60] Also, tubular ectasia, unlike the testicular tumors, does not enhance following administration of intravenous contrast.

Epidermoid cyst

Although rare (1%–2% of all resected testicular masses), testicular epidermoid cysts are the most common benign tumors originating in the testis. They are usually asymptomatic and found incidentally. The pathogenesis is uncertain but is thought to represent monodermal development of a teratoma or squamous metaplasia of the seminiferous epithelium or rete testis. The

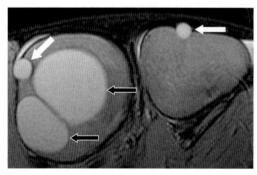

Fig. 28. Tunica albuginea cysts and intratesticular cysts. A 37-year-old man presents with bilateral palpable nodules. T2-weighted images of the scrotum show small cysts at the edge of both testes compatible with tunica albuginea cysts (*white arrows*). There are also 2 larger adjacent intraparenchymal cysts in the right testis (*black arrows*). The cysts appear simple and did not show abnormal enhancement on post-contrast images (not shown). Cystic tumors such as teratoma show thick walls with irregular enhancement and should be differentiated from simple cysts, which require no treatment.

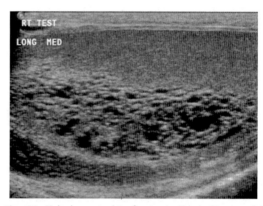

Fig. 29. Tubular ectasia of rete testis. A 46-year-old man with history of vasectomy. Longitudinal ultrasound image shows multiple tubular structures replacing the mediastinum. Doppler images did not show any flow within the rete testis. Tubular ectasia is a benign condition and should not be mistaken for a tumor.

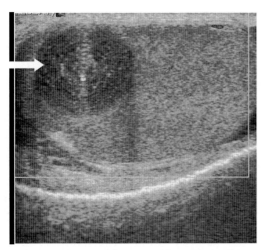

Fig. 30. A 42-year-old man with epidermoid cyst. Sagittal sonogram shows a well-defined hypoechoic intratesticular mass (*arrow*) with alternating hypoechoic and hyperechoic rings (onion appearance). Color Doppler showed no significant internal vascularity.

ultrasonographic appearance is typically a well-defined mixed-echogenicity intratesticular lesion with an onionskin or target appearance with no internal color flow (**Fig. 30**). It shows mixed signal on T2-weighted MR imaging with a low-signal rim and no significant postcontrast enhancement.[61]

Microlithiasis

Testicular microlithiasis is present in about 5% of the male population between 17 and 35 years of age.[62] This condition occurs because of development of intratubular calcifications 1 to 2 mm in size. On ultrasonographs, these calcifications appear as multiple, diffuse, small echogenic foci without acoustic shadowing (**Fig. 31**). Presence of 5 or more calcifications per transducer field is considered abnormal. Testicular microlithiasis is commonly associated with testicular abnormalities, such as infertility, cryptorchidism and neoplasms, and especially seminoma. Although microcalcifications exist in roughly 50% of germ cell tumors, most men with testicular microlithiasis do not develop testicular cancer.[63] The best management strategy for microlithiasis remains undecided and includes serial ultrasonographs, self-examinations, tumor marker screening, and testicular biopsy. However, recent investigators suggest that an intensive screening program for men with testicular microlithiasis might not be cost-effective and they recommend testicular self-examination, although symptomatic patients should be kept under closer surveillance.[63-65]

Intratesticular tumors

Most intratesticular solid masses represent malignant tumors, in contrast with extratesticular masses, which are nearly always benign. Intratesticular tumors include germ cell tumors, sex-cord and stromal tumors, and metastatic disease. Benign intratesticular lesions, lesions with malignant potential, and pseudotumors also occur in the testis (**Table 2**).

Germ cell tumors

Germ cell tumors represent 93% of intratesticular malignancy. Fifty percent of these are seminomas and 50% are nonseminomatous germ cell tumors (NSGCTs). NSGCTs include embryonal cell carcinoma, yolk-sac tumor, teratoma, choriocarcinoma, and mixed subtypes (the most common subtype). On ultrasonographs, seminomas are typically round, homogeneous tumors with increased vascularity (**Fig. 32**). In certain cases, seminoma can replace testicular parenchyma, which can make it difficult to differentiate from other infiltrative masses of the testis, such as leukemia and lymphoma (**Fig. 33**). The sonographic appearance

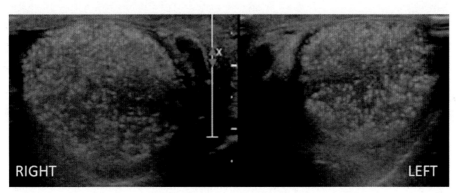

Fig. 31. Microlithiasis. Transverse ultrasound images of both testes show diffuse tiny nonshadowing foci throughout the testicular parenchyma that represent punctate calcifications.

Table 2
Intratesticular masses

Benign	Malignant Potential	Malignant	Pseudotumors
Leydig cell hyperplasia	Leydig cell tumor	Seminoma	Hematoma
Epidermoid cyst	Sertoli cell tumor	Nonseminomatous germ cell tumors: Yolk-sac tumor Embryonal cell carcinoma Teratocarcinoma Choriocarcinoma	Abscess
Lipoma	—	Lymphoma	Segmental infarction
Simple cyst	—	Metastases	Ectasia of rete testis

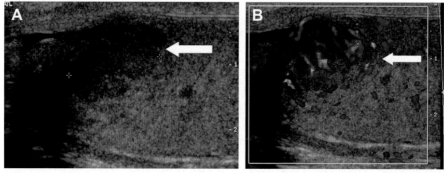

Fig. 32. A 34-year-old man with right testicular seminoma. (*A*) Sagittal sonogram shows a right intratesticular homogeneous hypoechoic mass (*arrow*). (*B*) Color Doppler image shows marked internal vascularity of the mass (*arrow*).

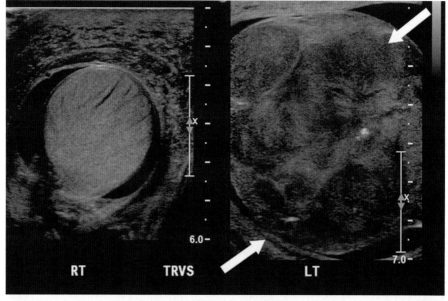

Fig. 33. Seminoma. A 24-year-old man presents with an enlarging left scrotal mass. Ultrasound images of both testes show markedly enlarged left testis that is completely replaced by a large hypoechoic mass (*arrows*). The tumor does not extend beyond the tunica albuginea. Surgery revealed seminoma.

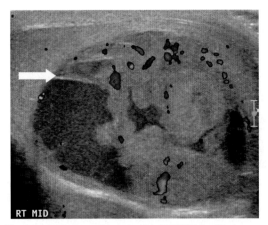

Fig. 34. A 28-year-old man with (NSGCT. Sagittal sonogram shows a markedly heterogeneous left intratesticular mass (*arrow*) with cystic and solid components. The solid components show marked color Doppler flow.

of NSGCT can be different from seminomas because these tumors tend to be more heterogeneous because of the presence of hemorrhage and necrosis (**Fig. 34**). MR imaging can be helpful in differentiating seminomas from NSGCT because seminomas tend to be homogeneous, whereas NSGCTs have heterogeneous signal and enhancement caused by necrosis and hemorrhage.[66] However, there may be overlap in the imaging characteristics of seminoma and NSGCT. Primary testicular tumors may, rarely, significantly involute in size after developing metastasis and may present as a small heterogeneous calcified area representing a burned-out tumor (**Fig. 35**).[67]

Sex-cord and stromal tumors

Leydig cell hyperplasia This rare benign condition is characterized by an increase in the number of Leydig cells in the testes and is often multifocal

and bilateral. It is usually an incidental finding in adults, although it can be hormone secreting in children and cause precocious puberty. On imaging, this entity manifests as an intratesticular nodule or nodules measuring 1 to 6 mm. Ultrasound and MR imaging features are nonspecific.[68]

Leydig cell tumors Leydig cell tumors comprise 1% to 2% of all testicular neoplasms. They are usually benign, but have malignant potential. In contrast with Leydig cell hyperplasia, these tumors are often hormonally active, leading to feminizing or virilizing syndromes. If this diagnosis is favored before surgery (because of the clinical presentation), tumor enucleation can be performed.[69] Imaging features are largely nonspecific, but marked homogeneous enhancement on MR imaging has been described (**Fig. 36**).[70]

Sertoli cell tumor Sertoli cell tumors account for less than 1% of testicular tumors. They are most common in younger patients (<40 years) and are mostly benign, although malignant subtypes exist. They do not usually secrete hormones. Twenty percent are bilateral. Reported ultrasound and MR imaging appearances are variable and nonspecific.[71,72]

Metastatic disease Metastatic disease comprises about 5% of intratesticular malignancy. The most common primary sites are lymphoma, leukemia, prostate, and kidney.

Testicular lymphomas (most commonly B cell subtype) comprise approximately 3% of all testicular neoplasms and are the most common testicular malignancy in men older than 60 years. Primary testicular lymphoma can occur but, more commonly, there is a known history of lymphoma elsewhere in the body. The imaging reflects lymphoma's infiltrative, nondestructive nature.[73]

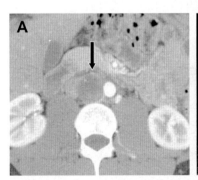
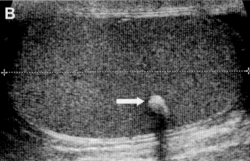

Fig. 35. Burned-out testicular tumor. (*A*) A 22-year-old man presented with an enlarged retroperitoneal lymph node (*black arrow*) and multiple lung metastases (not shown) on CT imaging. Biopsy of retroperitoneal lymph node revealed choriocarcinoma. (*B*) Ultrasound image of the right testis shows an echogenic focus with shadowing representing a calcified burned-out primary testicular choriocarcinoma that, on metastasizing, underwent regression (*white arrow*). No viable tumor was found in the orchiectomy specimen, consistent with a burned-out testicular tumor.

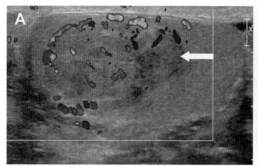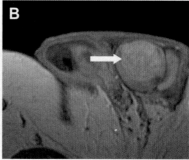

Fig. 36. Leydig tumor in a 51-year-old man. (*A*) Ultrasonography of the left testis shows a hypoechoic mass (*arrow*) with increased vascularity on color Doppler images. (*B*) Axial postcontrast T1-weighted MR imaging shows homogeneous hyperenhancement of the intratesticular mass (*arrow*) relative to the normal testicular tissue. The imaging characteristics of this tumor are not sufficient to make a diagnosis of a benign lesion.

Characteristic ultrasound findings are infiltration and enlargement of the testis by hypoechoic lymphoid tissue that may extend outside the testis, often into the epididymis. There is little mass effect and the shape of the testis is preserved (**Fig. 37**). MR imaging findings are similar; the testis is replaced by hypointense tissue on TI and T2 weighting, which shows mild enhancement on postcontrast images (less than the normal testicular parenchyma) (**Fig. 38**). Testicular lymphoma

occasionally presents as 1 or more focal masses. It may be bilateral in up to 20% of cases.

Other intratesticular tumors

Intratesticular lipoma Intratesticular lipomas are rare.[74] On ultrasonographs, they appear as echogenic, nonshadowing, nonvascular lesions and, on MR imaging, they follow the signal characteristics of fat and do not enhance. Testicular

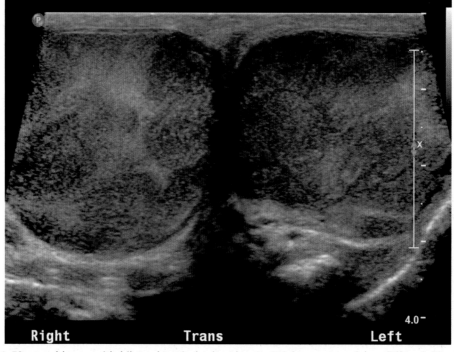

Fig. 37. A 59-year-old man with bilateral testicular lymphoma. Axial sonogram shows diffuse infiltration and enlargement of the testes by homogeneous hypoechoic tissue that is almost replacing both testes.

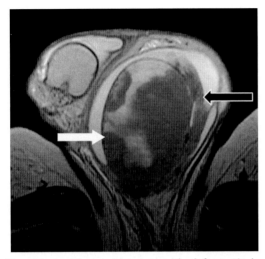

Fig. 38. A 68-year-old man with left testicular lymphoma. Axial T2-weighted MR image shows infiltrative hypointense tissue (*white arrow*) enlarging the left testis. The left epididymis (*black arrow*) showed heterogeneous signal and pathology confirmed epididymal involvement by lymphoma.

lipomatosis occurs exclusively in patients with Cowden disease (multiple hamartoma syndrome) in which multiple fat deposits are seen in the testes (**Fig. 39**).[75,76]

Adrenal rest tumors Adrenal rest tumors are benign testicular neoplasms derived from displaced cells of the primordial adrenal glands, and should be considered in a patient with increased levels of adrenocorticotropic hormone (particularly congenital adrenal hyperplasia) in whom ultrasonography shows multiple, bilateral hypoechoic nodules near the testicular hilum. The MR features are nonspecific.

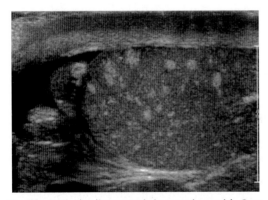

Fig. 39. Testicular lipomatosis in a patient with Cowden disease. Axial sonogram shows innumerable hyperechoic foci scattered throughout the right testis and epididymis with no acoustic shadowing and no Doppler color flow consistent with fat deposits.

SUMMARY

Radiologists play a pivotal role in characterizing scrotal lesions and knowledge of normal anatomy, imaging techniques, and imaging appearance of scrotal disorders is important for reaching the correct diagnosis. Ultrasonography continues to be the first-line imaging modality when evaluating the scrotum. Localizing the lesion correctly as intratesticular or extratesticular is crucial because most intratesticular masses are malignant, unlike extratesticular masses, which are overwhelmingly benign. Assessing the vascularity of the lesion is valuable in acute settings such as infection, trauma, and torsion. It is also essential in characterizing solid-appearing lesions because the absence of vascularity observed in hematoma, segmental testicular infarction, or abscess can suggest a benign rather than malignant lesion. When the correct diagnosis cannot be made by ultrasonography, MR imaging might be helpful. MR imaging has been found to add important information when diagnosing conditions such as hematoma, segmental testicular infarction, polyorchidism, lipoma, and fibrous pseudotumor. Familiarity with conditions that mimic tumors is important to avoid unnecessary surgery for lesions that could have been treated conservatively.

REFERENCES

1. Serra AD, Hricak H, Coakley FV, et al. Inconclusive clinical and ultrasound evaluation of the scrotum: impact of magnetic resonance imaging on patient management and cost. Urology 1998;51(6):1018–21.
2. Cassidy FH, Ishioka KM, McMahon CJ, et al. MR imaging of scrotal tumors and pseudotumors. Radiographics 2010;30(3):665–83.
3. Watanabe Y, Dohke M, Ohkubo K, et al. Scrotal disorders: evaluation of testicular enhancement patterns at dynamic contrast-enhanced subtraction MR imaging. Radiology 2000;217(1):219–27.
4. Dunnick NR, Sandier CM, Newhouse JH, et al. Anatomy and embryology. In: Dunnick NR, Sandier CM, Newhouse JH, et al, editors. Textbook of uroradiology. 3rd edition. Philadelphia: Lippincott Williams & Wilkins; 2001. p. 1–13.
5. Dogra VS, Gottlieb RH, Oka M, et al. Sonography of the scrotum. Radiology 2003;227(1):18–36.
6. Berger RE, Alexander ER, Harnisch JP, et al. Etiology, manifestations and therapy of acute epididymitis: prospective study of 50 cases. J Urol 1979; 121(6):750–4.
7. Freton RC, Berger RE. Prostatitis and epididymitis. Urol Clin North Am 1984;11:83–94.
8. Mittenmeyer BT, Lennox KW, Borski AA. Epididymitis: a review of 610 cases. J Urol 1966;95:390–2.

9. Eisner DJ, Goldman SM, Petronis J, et al. Bilateral testicular infarction caused by epididymitis. AJR Am J Roentgenol 1991;157(3):517–9.

10. Middleton WD, Middleton MA, Dierks M, et al. Sonographic prediction of viability in testicular torsion: preliminary observations. J Ultrasound Med 1997; 16(1):23–7 [quiz: 29–30].

11. Burks DD, Markey BJ, Burkhard TK, et al. Suspected testicular torsion and ischemia: evaluation with color Doppler sonography. Radiology 1990;175(3):815–21.

12. Nussbaum Blask AR, Rushton HG. Sonographic appearance of the epididymis in pediatric testicular torsion. AJR Am J Roentgenol 2006;187(6):1627–35.

13. Fernandez-Perez GC, Tardaguila FM, Velasco M, et al. Radiologic findings of segmental testicular infarction. AJR Am J Roentgenol 2005;184(5):1587–93.

14. Kramolowsky EV, Beauchamp RA, Milby WP 3rd. Color Doppler ultrasound for the diagnosis of segmental testicular infarction. J Urol 1993;150(3):972–3.

15. Flanagan JJ, Fowler RC. Testicular infarction mimicking tumour on scrotal ultrasound–a potential pitfall. Clin Radiol 1995;50(1):49–50.

16. Buckley JC, McAninch JW. Use of ultrasonography for the diagnosis of testicular injuries in blunt scrotal trauma. J Urol 2006;175(1):175–8.

17. Guichard G, El Ammari J, Del Coro C, et al. Accuracy of ultrasonography in diagnosis of testicular rupture after blunt scrotal trauma. Urology 2008; 71(1):52–6.

18. Micallef M, Ahmad I, Ramesh N, et al. Ultrasound features of blunt testicular injury. Injury 2001;32(1):23–6.

19. Wittenberg AF, Tobias T, Rzeszotarski M, et al. Sonography of the acute scrotum: the four T's of testicular imaging. Curr Probl Diagn Radiol 2006; 35(1):12–21.

20. Herbener TE. Ultrasound in the assessment of the acute scrotum. J Clin Ultrasound 1996;24(8):405–21.

21. Tumeh SS, Benson CB, Richie JP. Acute diseases of the scrotum. Semin Ultrasound CT MR 1991;12(2): 115–30.

22. Grant RW, Mitchell-Heggs P. Radiological features of Fournier gangrene. Radiology 1981;140(3):641–3.

23. Rajan DK, Scharer KA. Radiology of Fournier's gangrene. AJR Am J Roentgenol 1998;170(1):163–8.

24. Levenson RB, Singh AK, Novelline RA. Fournier gangrene: role of imaging. Radiographics 2008; 28(2):519–28.

25. Beccia DJ, Krane RJ, Olsson CA. Clinical management of non-testicular intrascrotal tumors. J Urol 1976;116(4):476–9.

26. Tessler FN, Tublin ME, Rifkin MD. Ultrasound assessment of testicular and paratesticular masses. J Clin Ultrasound 1996;24(8):423–36.

27. Frates MC, Benson CB, Stober SL. Mobile echogenicities on scrotal sonography: is the finding associated with vasectomy? J Ultrasound Med 2011; 30(10):1387–90.

28. Jarvis LJ, Dubbins PA. Changes in the epididymis after vasectomy: sonographic findings. AJR Am J Roentgenol 1989;152(3):531–4.

29. Reddy NM, Gerscovich EO, Jain KA, et al. Vasectomy-related changes on sonographic examination of the scrotum. J Clin Ultrasound 2004;32(8):394–8.

30. Leonhardt WC, Gooding GA. Sonography of intrascrotal adenomatoid tumor. Urology 1992;39(1):90–2.

31. Patel MD, Silva AC. MRI of an adenomatoid tumor of the tunica albuginea. AJR Am J Roentgenol 2004; 182(2):415–7.

32. Mak CW, Tzeng WS, Chou CK, et al. Leiomyoma arising from the tunica albuginea of the testis: sonographic findings. J Clin Ultrasound 2004; 32(6):309–11.

33. Akbar SA, Sayyed TA, Jafri SZ, et al. Multimodality imaging of paratesticular neoplasms and their rare mimics. Radiographics 2003;23(6):1461–76.

34. Noone TC, Semelka RC, Kubik-Huch RA, et al. Male pelvis. New York: John Wiley; 2002.

35. McMahon AJ, Buckley J, Taylor A, et al. Chronic testicular pain following vasectomy. Br J Urol 1992; 69(2):188–91.

36. Ishigami K, Abu-Yousef MM, El-Zein Y. Tubular ectasia of the epididymis: a sign of postvasectomy status. J Clin Ultrasound 2005;33(9):447–51.

37. Rouviere O, Bouvier R, Pangaud C, et al. Tubular ectasia of the rete testis: a potential pitfall in scrotal imaging. Eur Radiol 1999;9(9):1862–8.

38. Kim W, Rosen MA, Langer JE, et al. US MR imaging correlation in pathologic conditions of the scrotum. Radiographics 2007;27(5):1239–53.

39. Bree RL, Hoang DT. Scrotal ultrasound. Radiol Clin North Am 1996;34(6):1183–205.

40. Seigel MJ. The acute scrotum. Radiol Clin North Am 1997;35:959–75.

41. Linkowski GD, Avellone A, Gooding GA. Scrotal calculi: sonographic detection. Radiology 1985; 156(2):484.

42. Frauscher F, Klauser A, Stenzl A, et al. US findings in the scrotum of extreme mountain bikers. Radiology 2001;219(2):427–31.

43. Bushby LH, Miller FN, Rosairo S, et al. Scrotal calcification: ultrasound appearances, distribution and aetiology. Br J Radiol 2002;75(891):283–8.

44. Gooding GA. Sonography of the spermatic cord. AJR Am J Roentgenol 1988;151(4):721–4.

45. Bostwick DG. Spermatic cord and testicular adnexa. In: Bostwick DG, Eble JN, editors. Urologic surgical pathology. St Louis (MO): Mosby; 1997. p. 647–74.

46. Cramer BM, Schlegel EA, Thueroff JW. MR imaging in the differential diagnosis of scrotal and testicular disease. Radiographics 1991;11(1):9–21.

47. Cardenosa G, Papanicolaou N, Fung CY, et al. Spermatic cord sarcomas: sonographic and CT features. Urol Radiol 1990;12(3):163–7.

48. Gordon JN, Aldoroty RA, Stone NN. A spermatic cord hematoma secondary to varicocele rupture from blunt abdominal trauma: a case report and review. J Urol 1993;149(3):602–3.

49. Sakamoto H, Saito K, Shichizyo T, et al. Color Doppler ultrasonography as a routine clinical examination in male infertility. Int J Urol 2006;13(8):1073–8.

50. Trum JW, Gubler FM, Laan R, et al. The value of palpation, varicoscreen contact thermography and colour Doppler ultrasound in the diagnosis of varicocele. Hum Reprod 1996;11(6):1232–5.

51. Pilatz A, Altinkilic B, Kohler E, et al. Color Doppler ultrasound imaging in varicoceles: is the venous diameter sufficient for predicting clinical and subclinical varicocele? World J Urol 2011;29(5):645–50.

52. Wolverson MK, Houttuin E, Heiberg E, et al. High-resolution real-time sonography of scrotal varicocele. AJR Am J Roentgenol 1983;141(4):775–9.

53. Nguyen HT, Coakley F, Hricak H. Cryptorchidism: strategies in detection. Eur Radiol 1999;9(2):336–43.

54. Khatwa UA, Menon PS. Management of undescended testis. Indian J Pediatr 2000;67(6):449–54.

55. Baker LL, Hajek PC, Burkhard TK, et al. Polyorchidism: evaluation by MR. AJR Am J Roentgenol 1987; 148(2):305–6.

56. Gooding GA, Leonhardt W, Stein R. Testicular cysts: US findings. Radiology 1987;163(2):537–8.

57. Dambro TJ, Stewart RR, Barbara CA. The scrotum. In: Rumack CM, Charboneau JW, editors. Diagnostic ultrasound. 2nd edition. St Louis (MO): Mosby; 1998. p. 791–821.

58. Al-Jabri T, Misra S, Maan ZN, et al. Ultrasonography of simple intratesticular cysts: a 13 year experience in a single centre. Diagn Pathol 2011;6:24.

59. Shergill IS, Thwaini A, Kapasi F, et al. Management of simple intratesticular cysts: a single-institution 11-year experience. Urology 2006;67(6):1266–8.

60. Tartar VM, Trambert MA, Balsara ZN, et al. Tubular ectasia of the testicle: sonographic and MR imaging appearance. AJR Am J Roentgenol 1993;160(3):539–42.

61. Cho JH, Chang JC, Park BH, et al. Sonographic and MR imaging findings of testicular epidermoid cysts. AJR Am J Roentgenol 2002;178(3):743–8.

62. Peterson AC, Bauman JM, Light DE, et al. The prevalence of testicular microlithiasis in an asymptomatic population of men 18 to 35 years old. J Urol 2001; 166(6):2061–4.

63. Costabile RA. How worrisome is testicular microlithiasis? Curr Opin Urol 2007;17(6):419–23.

64. DeCastro BJ, Peterson AC, Costabile RA. A 5-year followup study of asymptomatic men with testicular microlithiasis. J Urol 2008;179(4):1420–3 [discussion: 1423].

65. Kosan M, Gonulalan U, Ugurlu O, et al. Testicular microlithiasis in patients with scrotal symptoms and its relationship to testicular tumors. Urology 2007; 70(6):1184–6.

66. Tsili AC, Tsampoulas C, Giannakopoulos X, et al. MRI in the histologic characterization of testicular neoplasms. AJR Am J Roentgenol 2007;189(6): W331–7.

67. Comiter CV, Renshaw AA, Benson CB, et al. Burned-out primary testicular cancer: sonographic and pathological characteristics. J Urol 1996;156(1):85–8.

68. Carucci LR, Tirkes AT, Pretorius ES, et al. Testicular Leydig's cell hyperplasia: MR imaging and sonographic findings. AJR Am J Roentgenol 2003; 180(2):501–3.

69. Henderson CG, Ahmed AA, Sesterhenn I, et al. Enucleation for prepubertal Leydig cell tumor. J Urol 2006;176(2):703–5.

70. Fernandez GC, Tardaguila F, Rivas C, et al. Case report: MRI in the diagnosis of testicular Leydig cell tumour. Br J Radiol 2004;77(918):521–4.

71. Liu P, Thorner P. Sonographic appearance of Sertoli cell tumour: with pathologic correlation. Pediatr Radiol 1993;23(2):127–8.

72. Drevelengas A, Kalaitzoglou I, Destouni E, et al. Bilateral Sertoli cell tumor of the testis: MRI and sonographic appearance. Eur Radiol 1999;9(9):1934.

73. Zicherman JM, Weissman D, Gribbin C, et al. Best cases from the AFIP: primary diffuse large B-cell lymphoma of the epididymis and testis. Radiographics 2005;25(1):243–8.

74. Harper M, Arya M, Peters JL, et al. Intratesticular lipoma. Scand J Urol Nephrol 2002;36(3):223–4.

75. Woodhouse JB, Delahunt B, English SF, et al. Testicular lipomatosis in Cowden's syndrome. Mod Pathol 2005;18(9):1151–6.

76. Woodhouse J, Ferguson MM. Multiple hyperechoic testicular lesions are a common finding on ultrasound in Cowden disease and represent lipomatosis of the testis. Br J Radiol 2006;79(946): 801–3.

Penile Imaging

Anuradha Shenoy-Bhangle, MD[a],*,
Rocio Perez-Johnston, MD[a], Ajay Singh, MD[b]

KEYWORDS

- Penile imaging • Peyronie • Penile fracture • Penile malignancy • Implants

KEY POINTS

- In Peyronie disease, magnetic resonance (MR) imaging is better than ultrasonography in detecting impalpable plaques and plaque dimensions, whereas calcified plaques are better visualized on ultrasonography.
- Ultrasonography with color Doppler technique is superior to MR imaging in evaluating vascular causes of erectile dysfunction.
- In penile fractures, MR imaging should be performed with the penis in the erect position to avoid kinking between the pendulous and fixed parts and thus enable better demonstration of the site of tunica albuginea disruption for surgical planning.
- MR imaging, with its superior soft tissue contrast and spatial resolution, is better than ultrasonography in both delineating primary penile malignancies and demonstrating lymph nodal involvement.
- Inflatable penile prostheses are MR imaging compatible, and hence the use of MR imaging to evaluate postsurgical changes is gaining widespread popularity.

INTRODUCTION

Various benign and malignant diseases of the penis are readily evaluated with cross-sectional imaging (ultrasonography [US], computed tomography [CT], and magnetic resonance [MR] imaging), which helps to confirm the clinical diagnosis, analyze extent of the disease, and guide appropriate treatment.

The imaging tools available in the evaluation of penile pathologies include high-resolution US complemented with color Doppler, MR imaging, CT, and retrograde urethrography (RGU).

Before imaging, a basic clinical evaluation that includes inspection and palpation should be performed by the radiologist; this not only serves in selecting the best imaging modality and examination technique but also eases interpretation of imaging findings.[1]

The aim of this article is to review normal anatomy as seen on US and MR imaging. The authors also review imaging appearance on MR imaging and discuss the imaging findings in a wide variety of benign and malignant conditions of the penis.

ANATOMY

The penile shaft is composed of 3 elongated tubular endothelium-lined cavernous structures (**Fig. 1**): the paired dorsolateral corpora cavernosa and the single midline ventral corpus spongiosum, which contains the urethra.

The 3 corpora combined are surrounded by 2 fascial layers: the superficial Colles fascia and the deeper Buck's fascia.

The tunica albuginea is the deepest fibrous layer and surrounds each corpus individually.

Anatomy with US and Color Doppler

Using high-frequency US linear probes, the ventral surface of the penis should be scanned in the longitudinal and transverse planes. The evaluation

[a] Department of Radiology, Division of Abdominal Imaging, Massachusetts General Hospital, White 280, 55 Fruit Street, Boston, MA 02115, USA; [b] Night Imaging Services, Department of Radiology, Division of Abdominal Imaging, Massachusetts General Hospital, White 280, 55 Fruit Street, Boston, MA 02115, USA
* Corresponding author.
E-mail address: ashenoy-bhangle@partners.org

Radiol Clin N Am 50 (2012) 1167–1181
http://dx.doi.org/10.1016/j.rcl.2012.08.009
0033-8389/12/$ – see front matter Published by Elsevier Inc.

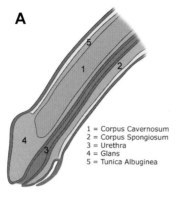

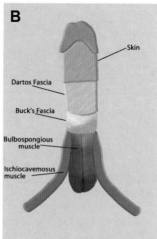

1 = Corpus Cavernosum
2 = Corpus Spongiosum
3 = Urethra
4 = Glans
5 = Tunica Albuginea

Skin
Dartos Fascia
Buck's Fascia
Bulbospongious muscle
Ischiocavemosus muscle

Fig. 1. (*A, B*) Penile anatomy: Sagittal cross section and undersurface view. (*A, From* Singh AK, Saokar A, Hahn PF, et al. Imaging of penile neoplasms. Radiographics 2005;25:1629–38; with permission and *B, From* Levenson RB, Singh AK, Novelline RA. Fournier gangrene: role of imaging. Radiographics 2008;28:519–28; with permission.)

is generally carried out in the flaccid state; however, while investigating erectile dysfunction and Peyronie disease, evaluation may be performed after intracavernosal injection of vasoactive drugs.

On transverse US images, the corpora cavernosa and corpus spongiosum demonstrate a homogeneous echotexture (**Fig. 2**). The surrounding tunica albuginea and Buck's fascia are inseparable

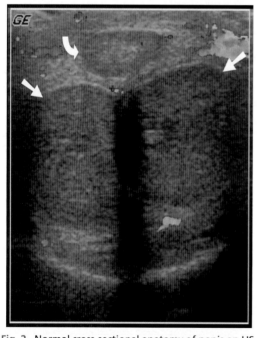

Fig. 2. Normal cross-sectional anatomy of penis on US. Transverse US images demonstrating homogeneous echotexture of the paired corpora cavernosa (*straight arrows*) and the midline corpus spongiosum (*curved arrow*).

and together appear as a thin echogenic line covering the 3 corpora. The outermost Colles fascia is typically not visualized. The urethra can be visualized as an anechoic structure after it is distended with fluid.

Vascular supply is from the cavernosal artery, the dorsal artery, and the urethral artery (from internal pudendal arteries).

Typically, one cavernosal artery (**Fig. 3**A) penetrates each corpus cavernosum and runs through it in a central position. The cavernosal artery branches into helicine arteries, which split into arterioles and connect with the corporeal sinusoidal spaces. The dorsal penile arteries (see **Fig. 3**B) and the urethral arteries supply the glans penis and corpus spongiosum. The dorsal penile arteries traverse the space between the tunica albuginea and the Buck's fascia. The penile skin is supplied by superficial arteries and veins lying above the Buck's fascia.

The venous drainage of the corpora cavernosa is through small emissary veins, which drain into the corpus spongiosum and the dorsal, cavernosal, and the crural veins.

On transverse US images, the cavernosal arteries appear as a pair of dots located medially within the corpora cavernosa. Likewise, the dorsal vessels are seen in the dorsal aspect of the penile shaft. The cavernosal arterial Doppler waveforms differ in the flaccid state and vary according to the phase of erection. The flaccid penis demonstrates monophasic waveforms with minimal diastolic flow (see **Fig. 3**). With the onset of erection, systolic and diastolic flows both increase; then, diastolic flow decreases to zero, ultimately undergoing flow reversal. The peak systolic velocities

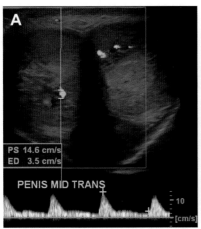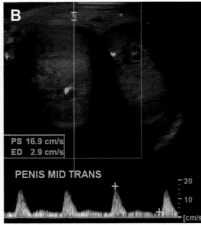

Fig. 3. Color Doppler US imaging of penis. (A) Doppler waveforms in the cavernosal artery demonstrate a peak systolic velocity of 14.6 cm/s in the flaccid state. (B) Doppler waveforms in the dorsal penile artery.

recorded in the normal cavernosal and dorsal arteries range between 11 and 20 cm/s. After intracavernous injection of prostaglandins, these can increase to greater than 35 cm/s.

MR IMAGING
Technique

With the patient in supine position, a towel is placed between the patient's legs to elevate the scrotum and penis. The penis is then dorsiflexed against the lower abdomen in the midline and taped in position to reduce the motion of the organ during the examination.

A surface coil (3 or 5 inches) for the penis is used for high-resolution images. A phased-array pelvic or body coil is used if the entire pelvis is to be imaged. Imaging protocols are customized to address the clinical question. MR appearance of the normal penis is described in (Table 1). A recent

small study by Scardino and colleagues[2] suggested that MR imaging of the erect penis after the injection of prostaglandin E1 into the corpora cavernosa has the potential to improve local staging. This technique, however, is not routinely used because of the risk of priapism in a minority of patients.

Additional points of importance on MR:

- Varying layering effects are a normal finding in the tumescent corpora cavernosa.
- The hypointense tunica albuginea is thinner around the corpus spongiosum.
- The most proximal part of the corpus spongiosum is the bulb surrounded by the low signal–intensity bulbospongiosus muscle, through which the urethra penetrates.
- The crura covered by the low signal–intensity ischiocavernosus muscle attaches the corpora cavernosa to the ischium.

Table 1
MR appearance

	T1-Weighted	T2-Weighted	Post Gadolinium
Corpora cavernosa and corpus spongiosum (Fig. 4)	Intermediate	High signal	Immediate enhancement of corpus spongiosum Gradual centrifugal enhancement of corpora cavernosa
Muscular walls of the urethra	Hypointense to corpus spongiosum	Hypointense to corpus spongiosum	No enhancement
Tunica albuginea and Buck fascia	Hypointense	Hypointense	No enhancement
Dartos fascia	Hypointense	Hypointense	No enhancement

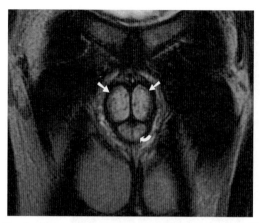

Fig. 4. MR anatomy of penis. Coronal T2-weighted MR image demonstrates high signal–intensity paired corpora cavernosa (*straight arrows*) and single corpus spongiosum (*curved arrow*), surrounded by a combined hypointense layer of the tunica albuginea and Buck's fascia.

BENIGN CONDITIONS
Peyronie Disease

Peyronie disease, an acquired condition of uncertain cause, is the most frequent cause of painful penile induration.[3,4] It is characterized by formation of fibrin plaques within the tunica albuginea, typically on the dorsal aspect, causing deformity and shortening of the penis.[5] These plaques may subsequently calcify.

The 2 clinical phases of this condition include the acute phase (usually lasts for 12–18 months) and the chronic phase.[6,7]

The role of imaging is to detect impalpable plaques and determine plaque dimensions. For these indications, MR is superior to US[8] because of superior contrast resolution. On MR imaging, the plaques appear as hypointense areas of thickening in the tunica albuginea on both T1-weighted and T2-weighted sequences (**Fig. 5**). On administration of gadolinium, some plaques may demonstrate enhancement. In a study conducted by Hauck and colleagues,[9] plaque enhancement was never associated with penile pain, which was considered an indicator of active disease.

On US, plaque calcification is better demonstrated than on MR imaging (**Fig. 6**). Penile calcification is not an uncommon incidental finding on CT of the pelvis (**Fig. 7**).

Erectile Dysfunction

The normally contracted state of the helicine arteries and the smooth muscle of the sinusoids maintain high vascular resistance in the flaccid penis. Stimulation causes the parasympathetic stimulation and dilatation of the helicine arteries and relaxes sinusoidal smooth muscles, increasing the flow of blood in the cavernosal arteries. This subsequently fills the cavernosal spaces, compressing the emissary veins against the tunica albuginea, decreasing venous outflow, and maintaining penile erection.

The vascular causes of erectile dysfunction includes arterial inflow disorder (**Fig. 8**A) and veno-occlusive disease. US is specific and sensitive in identifying vascular causes of erectile dysfunction.[10] Conventional angiography is also helpful and can be followed with angioplasty or stent placement to improve inflow. Cavernosometry with intracavernosal injection of prostaglandin E1 is the standard of reference.[11] Intracavernosal prostaglandin E1 (alprostadil) (**Fig. 8**B) is contraindicated in patients with a history of priapism, acute penile fracture, penile prosthesis, tumors invading the corpora, and clotting derangement.[12] There is an approximately 1% risk of priapism, which can be treated with evacuation of the corpora cavernosa or by pharmacologic means.[13]

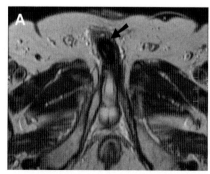
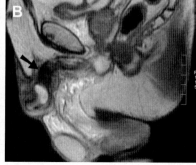

Fig. 5. Peyronie disease. (*A*) Axial T2-weighted image demonstrates a hypointense fibrous plaque (*arrow*). (*B*) Sagittal T2-weighted image in the same patient showing penile deformity and the hypointense penile plaque at the root of the penis (*arrow*).

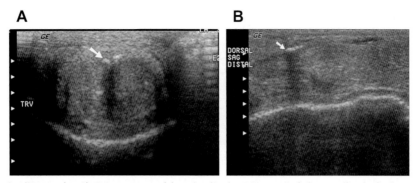

Fig. 6. Peyronie disease. (*A, B*) Transverse and longitudinal US images of the penile shaft demonstrate linear echogenic calcification (*arrows*) related to Peyronie disease.

MR imaging has a limited role in the evaluation of vascular causes, providing only noninvasive evaluation in cases of arteriogenic impotence.

Priapism

Priapism refers to prolonged painful erection, which can be of a low- or high-flow type (**Table 2**). Low-flow priapism is a medical emergency, leading to infarction and fibrosis if untreated. It is more common than high-flow priapism (**Fig. 9**).[15] The high-flow priapism is not an emergency and can be treated conservatively.

The diagnosis is based on clinical presentation, history, and measurement of oxygenation in aspirated corporeal blood.[16] Doppler US is usually not required but can be used to demonstrate patency of cavernosal arteries. Arteriolacunar fistula is seen as an area of turbulent high flow, occasionally with enlarged feeding vessels or draining veins. Cavernosal blood stasis appears as a fluid-fluid level, initially with tissue edema causing increased echogenicity of the corpora.

MR imaging can be used to delineate extent of infracted tissue in low-flow states, diagnose malignant infiltration of the corpora, and detect partial penile thrombosis.[17]

Arteriography can demonstrate a characteristic blush caused by an arteriolacunar fistula. Therapeutic embolization can be performed as part of the same procedure.

Inflammation

The causes include cavernous tissue ischemia (from maneuvers and prosthesis implantation), intracavernosal drug injections, improper catheterization, and endoscopic manipulation.

The role of US is in excluding abscess formation and involvement of the corpora cavernosa. Cellulitis appears as superficial soft tissue thickening and hyperemia without increase in vascularity of the underlying corpora. Increased echogenicity of the corpora as a result of edema and increased vascularity of the corpora is noted in cavernositis and spongiositis. Microabscesses are seen as small hypoechoic areas, whereas larger drainable abscesses appear as hypoechoic collections with internal echoes.[18]

The role of CT/MR imaging is in delineation of involvement of the perineum, abdominal wall, fascial planes, and buttocks. Abscesses demonstrate low signal intensity on T1-weighted sequences, high signal intensity on T2-weighted sequences, and

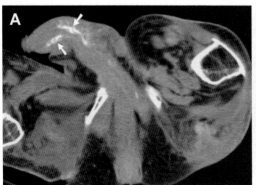
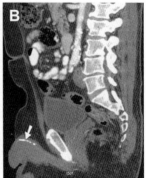

Fig. 7. Peyronie disease. Axial (*A*) and sagittal (*B*) CT images demonstrate tunica albuginea calcifications (*arrows*) related to Peyronie disease.

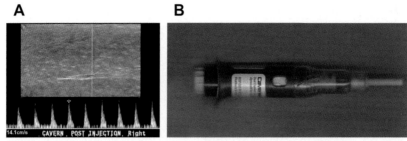

Fig. 8. US of erectile dysfunction in a 22-year-old man. (*A*) US after intracorporal injection of alprostadil shows no increase in the flow velocity (14.1 cm/s) in the cavernosal artery, indicating arterial inflow abnormality. Arterial flow of greater than 25 cm/s is considered normal during erection. (*B*) Alprostadil is injected intracorporally for evaluation of vascular causes of erectile dysfunction.

rim enhancement on postcontrast imaging. CT can demonstrate low-density fluid collections with rim enhancement.

Dorsal Vein Thrombosis

Clinically, dorsal vein thrombosis is seen as linear painful induration on the dorsum of the penile shaft. It can be caused by trauma and inflammation.[19] The roles of imaging are to confirm the diagnosis and to exclude underlying associated malignancy. Noncompressible hypoechoic dorsal and circumflex veins demonstrating the absence of color Doppler flow are diagnostic (**Fig. 10**).[20]

Corporal Thrombosis

Corporal thrombosis is characterized by induration and persistent pain in the proximal penile shaft. It can be idiopathic but it can also be post-traumatic (eg, post prolonged bicycling or vigorous intercourse). The role of Imaging is in differentiating corporal thrombosis from other causes. US shows predominantly hypoechoic areas within the corpora cavernosa with lack of vascularity. On MR imaging, varied signal intensity of the thrombus is noted, depending on the stage of degradation of hemoglobin with no enhancement on post gadolinium images.[21] Generally, it is hyperintense relative to the normal cavernosum

on T1-weighted images and hypointense on T2-weighted images.

Caciphylaxis is another vascular pathologic condition of the penis, characterized by ischemia caused by vascular occlusion related to extensive progressive vascular calcification. US can show occluded penile vessels and CT can demonstrate extensive arterial and tunica albuginea calcification. Usual disease progression to wet gangrene with superinfection warrants penile amputation.[22]

Penile Fibrosis

Penile fibrosis is associated with varied causes that can be related to erectile dysfunction.[23] It is commonly caused by Peyronie disease, trauma, untreated fracture, post removal of penile prosthesis, and intracavernosal agents for erectile dysfunction (especially papverine).

Imaging features on US include echogenic strands within the hypoechoic corpora cavernosa. On MR imaging, T2-weighted sequences demonstrate linear low signal–intensity areas within the high signal–intensity corpora.

Trauma

Painful swelling and deformity of the penile shaft are commonly seen after penile injury more commonly related to penile fractures (**Fig. 11**).

Table 2 Types of priapism		
	Low Flow	**High Flow**
Cause	Venous outflow blockage with many causes, including recreational and therapeutic drugs, leukemia, and sickle cell disease; 30%–50% are idiopathic[14]	Arteriolacunar fistula secondary to trauma or surgery
Oxygenation	Anoxic	Initially oxygenation maintained
Symptoms	Painful	Not as painful

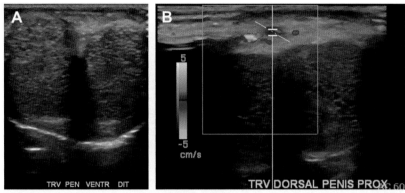

Fig. 9. A 17-year-old boy with a history of sickle cell anemia and acute priapism. (*A*) Transverse US image demonstrates edematous corpora cavernosa. (*B*) There is thrombosis of the dorsal veins related to sickle cell crisis causing low-flow type of priapism.

Penile fracture is a surgical emergency caused by traumatic rupture of the tunica albuginea. Trauma can also result in suspensory ligament rupture causing penile instability besides deformity.[24] Causes include sexual intercourse, falling on an erect penis, or, less commonly, masturbation.

The role of imaging is in demonstrating the presence and site of disruption of the tunica albuginea that requires surgical exploration.[25] It also can diagnose a coexisting urethral injury, which may be seen in 22% to 30% of acute fractures.[26]

MR imaging should be performed with the penis in the erect position to avoid kinking between the pendulous and the fixed parts. Disruption of the low signal–intensity tunica albuginea on both T1- and T2-weighted sequences is diagnostic. Rupture of the dorsal vein of the penis is a rare mimic of acute fracture.[27]

Gadolinium-enhanced T1-weighted sequence can be used to look for intracavernosal acute hematomas, which are isointense to the corpora on the unenhanced scans and thus may be better seen after contrast enhancement. Early focal enhancement at the site of rupture may be determined on dynamic contrast enhancement.[26] MR can also be used to diagnose suspensory ligament injures. If urethral injury is suspected in cases in which a fracture is clinically palpable, a retrograde urethrogram may be performed for diagnosis.

PENILE MALIGNANCIES

Penile neoplasms are rare, with an incidence of 0.1 to 7.9 per 100,000 male patients. In some areas such as Africa and South America, the incidence increases, representing up to 10% to 20% of all malignancies in men.[28] Neoplasms involving the penis can be classified as primary or secondary (**Fig. 12, Table 3**).[29,30]

The most frequent primary penile neoplasm is squamous cell carcinoma, which accounts for approximately 95% of cases.[31] It presents in the sixth decade, and multiple risk factors have been associated with this malignancy, such as poor hygiene, phimosis, chronic inflammatory conditions, and human papilloma virus infection, among others. However, it rarely presents in circumcised patients, likely because of the lack of accumulation of smegma that is produced from desquamated epithelial cell.[30]

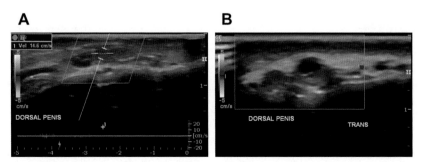

Fig. 10. Dorsal vein thrombosis in a 45-year-old man. (*A, B*) US with Doppler demonstrates linear serpigenous veins on the dorsum of the penile shaft with lack of flow consistent with dorsal vein thrombosis.

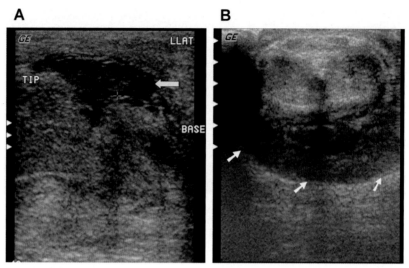

Fig. 11. Penile trauma. (*A*) Sagittal US image of the penile shaft demonstrates discontinuity of the tunica albuginea and on the dorsal aspect of corpora cavernosa by hematoma (*arrow*) in a patient with penile fracture. (*B*) Cross-sectional image of the penile shaft demonstrates hematoma (*arrows*) encircling the penile shaft by approximately 270°.

The glans is the most frequently involved location, occurring in 48% of cases (**Fig. 13**), followed by the prepuce (21%), coronal sulcus (6%), and penile shaft (2%).[28,30] The Buck's fascia acts as a barrier to cavernosal invasion and hematogenous spread. Thus, penile carcinoma spreads frequently via lymphatic vessels. The location of lymphatic spread depends on the location of the primary lesion (**Table 4**).

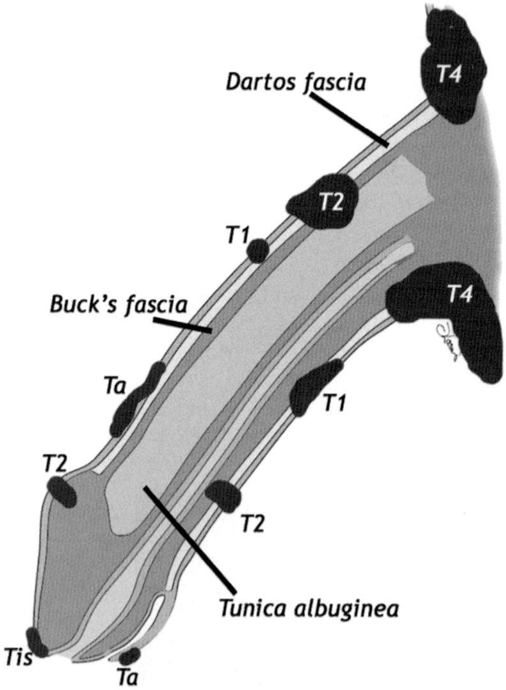

The main prognostic factors for penile carcinoma are the degree of invasion by the primary tumor and involvement of draining lymph nodes.[32] Physical examination can predict the tumor size and the extent of cavernosal involvement with high positive predictive value and has traditionally assessed nodal involvement in the inguinal region, however, MR imaging is a more sensitive method to assess the extent of the involvement (**Fig. 14**).[33]

Fig. 12. Staging of primary penile malignancies. (*From* Singh AK, Saokar A, Hahn PF, et al. Imaging of penile neoplasms. Radiographics 2005;25:1629–38; with permission.)

Labels in figure: Dartos fascia, T4, T2, T1, Buck's fascia, T4, Ta, T1, T2, T2, Tunica albuginea, Tis, Ta

Table 3 Histologic types of neoplasm involving the penis	
Primary	Squamous cell carcinoma Sarcoma: epitheloid sarcoma, Kaposi sarcoma, leiomyosarcoma, rhabdomyosarcoma Others: melanoma, basal cell carcinoma, lymphoma
Secondary	Prostate, bladder, colon, rectum, stomach, lung, thyroid

Data from Grimm MO, Spiegelhalder P, Heep H, et al. Penile metastasis secondary to follicular thyroid carcinoma. Scand J Urol Nephrol 2004;38:253–5; and Perdomo JA, Hizuta A, Iwagaki H, et al. Penile metastasis secondary to cecum carcinoma: a case report. Hepatogastroenterology 1998; 45:1589–92.

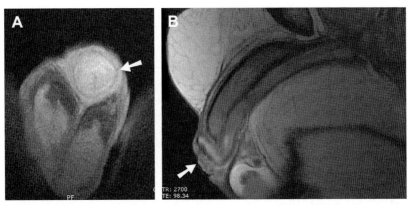

Fig. 13. Penile carcinoma of the glans. (*A*) Coronal gadolinium-enhanced image demonstrates a heterogeneously enhancing mass (*arrow*) involving the glans. (*B*) Sagittal T2-weighted image demonstrates contour abnormality of the glans (*arrow*).

Staging

The Jackson classification and TNM classification are the 2 staging systems used for penile cancer (**Table 5**). The presence and degree of lymph node involvement represent the most important prognostic factors. Nodal disease occurs in 20% of T1 lesions and in 47% to 66% of T2 to T4 lesions.[34] Other factors that determine the lymphatic spread are the histologic grade, the vertical growth, and the presence of vascular or lymphatic invasion.[35]

Imaging

Imaging is useful in assessing the local invasion, regional lymph nodes, and distant metastases. US has been the primary modality for cross-sectional imaging because of its widespread availability and low cost. Squamous cell carcinoma usually presents as a hypoechoic heterogeneous lesion, which may present as small hyperechoic spots, resulting from ulceration and small foci of entrapped gas. Infiltration of the tunica albuginea is seen as interruption of the thin echogenic line of the tunica albuginea.

CT plays a limited role in the primary tumor evaluation and local invasion; however, it is considered the modality of choice for distant metastasis evaluation (**Fig. 15**). The most common sites of metastases are the lungs, liver, and retroperitoneum.

MR imaging has superior soft-tissue contrast and spatial resolution compared with US and is useful for staging purposes. Squamous cell carcinomas are usually hypointense relative to the

Table 4 Lymphatic spread according to the location of the primary lesion	
Location	Lymphatic involvement
Skin penis and prepuce	Superficial inguinal nodes
Glans	Deep inguinal and external iliac nodes
Corpora cavernosa, corpus spongiosum, urethra	Internal iliac nodes

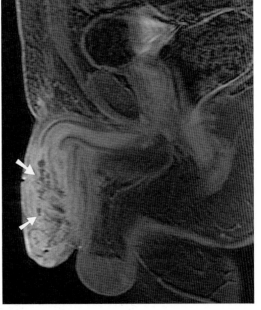

Fig. 14. Penile carcinoma. Sagittal contrast-enhanced image demonstrates enhancing tumor with extensive infiltration of the corpora cavernosa (*arrows*) and tunica albuginea, extending up to the skin.

Table 5
Staging systems used for penile cancer

Classification	Stage	Involvement
Jackson	1	Confined to the penile gland
	2	Invasion of the shaft or corpora
	3	Metastatic inguinal lymph nodes—surgical
	4	Invasion of adjacent structures, inoperable metastatic inguinal lymph nodes
TNM	T-	
	Tx	Primary tumor cannot be assessed
	T0	No evidence of primary tumor
	Tis	Carcinoma in situ
	T1	Invasion of subepithelial connective tissue
	T2	Invasion of one or more corpora
	T3	Invasion of urethra or prostate
	T4	Invasion of other adjacent structures
	N-	
	Nx	Regional lymph nodes cannot be assessed
	N0	No regional metastatic lymph nodes
	N1	Single superficial inguinal lymph node metastasis
	N2	Metastases in multiple or bilateral superficial inguinal lymph nodes
	N3	Unilateral or bilateral metastatic deep inguinal or pelvic lymph nodes
	M-	
	Mx	Distant metastasis cannot be assessed
	M0	No evidence of distant metastases
	M1	Distant metastasis, including common iliac lymph nodes

corpora on both T1- and T2-weighted images. On contrast-enhanced images, the lesion remains hypointense compared with the corpora.

MR imaging also plays an important role in the determination of lymph node involvement, especially in detecting pelvic and retroperitoneal lymph nodes. However, the suspicion of metastases to the lymph nodes based on size criteria (short axis >10 mm) alone has limitations because the node size does not allow differentiation between nodal metastases and nodal hyperplasia. The sensitivity of MR imaging for detection of nodal

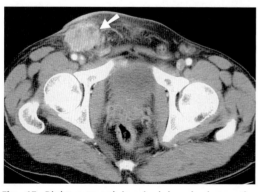

Fig. 15. Right external inguinal lymphadenopathy. Contrast-enhanced CT shows enlarged right eternal inguinal lymph node (*arrow*) in a patient with penile squamous cell cancer.

involvement ranges from 24% to 75% for urogenital malignancies.[36] To overcome the limitations of anatomic lymph node assessment, functional MR imaging using diffusion-weighted images and ultrasmall superparamagnetic iron oxide, also known as ferumoxtran-10 is under investigation for clinical use.

Normal lymph nodes engulf ultrasmall superparamagnetic iron oxide nanoparticles, whereas malignant lymph nodes affected by metastatic disease do not take up the contrast material (**Fig. 16**). Promising results have been found in patients with testicular, bladder, and penile cancer, but further investigation is needed for clinical validation.[37,38]

Primary nonsquamous and secondary malignancies such sarcomas, melanoma, basal-cell carcinoma, and lymphoma of the penis are very rare. Kaposi sarcoma has increased in frequency with the onset of acquired immunodeficiency syndrome.[39]

Penile lymphoma presents as a well-vascularized lesion that presents as a mass, plaque, or skin ulcer. Infiltration of the corpora cavernosum is common.[40] Kaposi sarcoma presents as a well-defined mass or variable echogenicity often limited to the glans.[39]

Carcinoma of the male urethra usually occurs in the bulbous and membranous portions of the urethra. The type of epithelium lining changes

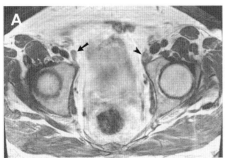
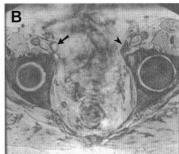

Fig. 16. MR imaging of lymph nodes with ultrasmall superparamagnetic iron oxide (USPIO). Normal-sized right external iliac lymph nodes (A, arrow) demonstrate no uptake on USPIO imaging (B, arrow) consistent with malignant infiltration of these nodes. Left external iliac lymph node (arrowheads) shows normal USPIO uptake.

according to the location: transitional cells are present in the prostatic and membranous segments, stratified and pseudostratified columnar epithelium is in the bulbous portion, and squamous cells are in the fossa navicularis and urethral meatus. Thus, squamous cell carcinoma and then transitional cell carcinoma are the most common neoplasms of the anterior urethra.[41]

Most penile metastases (Fig. 17) are secondary to direct invasion from other pelvic tumors. Spread from distant organs has been reported, representing less that 30% of secondary penile involvement.[42] Penile metastases present as multiple palpable nodules and may be associated with pain, hematuria, or urinary outflow obstruction.

Imaging

Metastatic extension from adjacent organs presents as diffuse infiltration of the penile shaft and multiple nodules. Interruption of the tunica albuginea at the base of the penis represents direct infiltration from the primary tumor.

When diffuse secondary involvement of the shaft is present, the lesions may be difficult to assess with US, observing mild alteration of the penile echogenicity. In these patients, tumor nodules can be identified with contrast-enhanced US.[43]

MR imaging features of epitheloid sarcomas are nonspecific and may be isointense on T1- and T2-weighted images, hypointense compared with the corpora, and hypointense to the corpora on contrast-enhanced images.[44] Rhabdomyosarcomas are isointense relative to the skeletal muscle on T1-weighted images, hyperintense on T2-weighted images, and heterogeneous after contrast administration.[45] Urethral carcinomas and metastatic nodules are usually hypointense relative to the corpora both on T1 and T2-weighted images.[46]

Prosthesis Implantation

Penile implants remain a mainstay for the treatment of erectile dysfunction unresponsive to other, less-invasive methods. Most implants are inserted in a patient with organic causes of impotence, such as diabetes, neuropathy, or atherosclerosis or post pelvic surgery.[47] The 3 types of devices include 3-piece hydraulic, 2-piece hydraulic, and semirigid types.

1. The 3-piece hydraulic is the most popular device, accounting for 70% of all devices used (AMS 700 series, Alpha 1, and Titan; Mentor).
2. The 2-piece hydraulic devices constitute 20% and include Ambicor (AMS) and Mark 2 (Mentor).

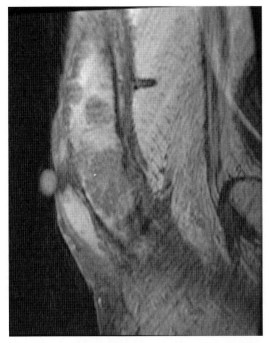

Fig. 17. Penile metastases. Sagittal T2-weighted sequence demonstrates multiple hypointense rounded metastases in the corpora cavernosa from prostate cancer.

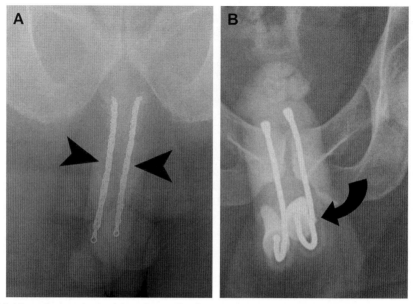

Fig. 18. Semirigid penile prosthesis. (*A*) Radiograph of pelvis demonstrates the first-generation semirigid penile prosthesis (*arrowheads*). (*B*) Radiograph of pelvis demonstrates semirigid penile prosthesis with fracture of the left metallic wire, secondary to blunt trauma. The magnified view better shows the fracture and resulting step-off (*curved arrow*).

3. Semirigid devices are the least popular and constitutes 10%. AMS 600/650 is the typical semirigid device (**Fig. 18**). Their advantages include low cost and low rate of mechanical failure. The disadvantages include constant erection, increased chronic pain, and erosion.[48]

Mechanism

The AMS 700TM series (**Figs. 19–22**) consists of a 3-piece inflatable penile implant that includes a reservoir, a pump, and a pair of cylinders. Fluid movement from reservoir to the cylinders produces erection. Ambicor prostheses consist of

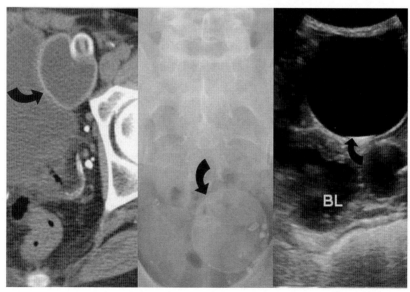

Fig. 19. AMS 700TM Series: 3-Piece Inflatable Penile Implant. Axial CT, plain film, and US images demonstrate the reservoir (*curved arrow*) of the inflatable penile prosthesis. The reservoir stores hydraulic fluid.

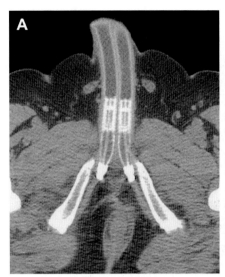

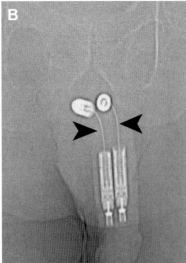

Fig. 20. Penile prosthesis. (*A*) Axial CT shows a 1-piece inflatable penile prosthesis, which offers a compromise between the multicomponent inflatable and the semirigid device. It does not become as erect as the rigid one, and it does not deflate as much as the multicomponent inflatable prosthesis. (*B*) Scout film shows Ambicor penile prosthesis, consisting of paired tension wires (*arrowheads*).

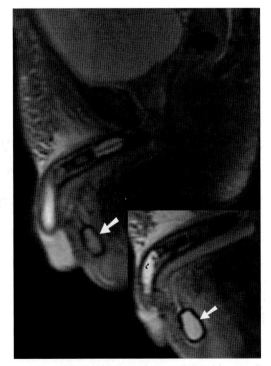

Fig. 21. AMS Ambicor: 2-piece inflatable penile implant. Sagittal T2-weighted MR image demonstrates the penile and the scrotal component of the prosthesis. The prosthesis consists of a pair of cylinders implanted in the penis and a single pump bulb (*straight arrows*) implanted in the scrotum.

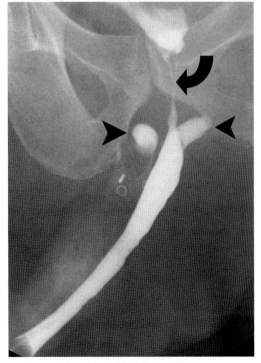

Fig. 22. Penile prosthesis and urethral stricture. A patient with a 1-piece inflatable prosthesis (*arrowheads*) demonstrating stricture in the prostatic and bulbar urethra (*curved arrow*).

a pair of cylinders and a pump in the scrotum. The Omniphase prosthesis is a self-contained inflatable prosthesis, in which a distal inflation pump transfers fluid from the posterior to the central reservoir.

US provides adequate visualization of the corporeal cylinders, the scrotal pump, and some portions of the tubing. The abdominal reservoir may or not be visualized, depending on the patient's body habitus and the depth of placement in the pelvis. The reservoir may easily be mistaken for a fluid collection or a bladder diverticulum.[47]

Inflatable prostheses are MR imaging compatible, and the use of MR imaging to evaluate postsurgical changes is becoming more widely popular. The hydraulic cylinders are hyperintense on T2-weighted images. Ideally, inflatable devices should be imaged in both "inflation" and "deflation" sequences. The silicone in semirigid devices is hypointense on T2-weighted images.[8]

The complications associated with prostheses include fluid leak, pump retraction, kinking of the tubing, tissue erosion, infection (3% risk), aneurysmal dilatation of the corporeal cylinders, and infection. Prosthetic tear can usually be identified as fluid extravasation and deformity of the cylinder.[49]

REFERENCES

1. Bertolotto M, Pavlica P, Serafini G, et al. Painful penile induration: imaging findings and management. Radiographics 2009;29:477–93.
2. Scardino E, Villa G, Bonomo G, et al. Magnetic resonance imaging combined with artificial erection for local staging of penile cancer. Urology 2004;63:1158–62.
3. Hakim LS. Peyronie's disease: an update-the role of diagnostics. Int J Impot Res 2002;14:321–3.
4. Pryor JP, Ralph DJ. Clinical presentations of Peyronie's disease. Int J Impot Res 2002;14:414–7.
5. El-Sakka AI, Hassoba HM, Pillarisetty RJ, et al. Peyronie's disease is associated with an increase in transforming growth factor-beta protein expression. J Urol 1997;158:1391–4.
6. Schwarzer U, Sommer F, Klotz T, et al. The prevalence of Peyronie's disease: results of a large survey. BJU Int 2001;88(7):727–30.
7. Kadioglu A, Akman T, Sanli O, et al. Surgical treatment of Peyronie's disease: a critical analysis. Eur Urol 2006;50(2):235–48.
8. Kirkham AP, Illing RO, Minhas S. MR imaging of non malignant penile lesions. Radiographics 2008;28: 837–53.
9. Hauck EW, Hackstein N, Vosshenrich R, et al. Diagnostic value of magnetic resonance imaging in Peyronie's disease: a comparison both with palpation and ultrasound in the evaluation of plaque formation. Eur Urol 2003;43(3):293–300.
10. Golijanin D, Singer E, Davis R, et al. Doppler evaluation of erectile dysfunction. I. Int J Impot Res 2007; 19(1):37–42.
11. Golijanin D, Singer E, Davis R, et al. Doppler evaluation of erectile dysfunction. II. Int J Impot Res 2007; 19(1):43–8.
12. Hatzimouratidis K, Hatzichristou DG. A comparative review of the options for treatment of erectile dysfunction: which treatment for which patient? Drugs 2005; 65(12):1621–50.
13. Linet OI, Ogrinc FG. Efficacy and safety of intracavernosal alprostadil in men with erectile dysfunction. The Alprostadil study group. N Engl J Med 1996; 334(14):873–7.
14. El-Bahnasawy MS, Dawood A, Farouk A. Low flow priapism: risk factors for erectile dysfunction. BJU Int 2002;89(3):285–90.
15. Pryor J, Akkus E, Alter G, et al. Priapism. J Sex Med 2004;1(1):116–20.
16. Berger R, Billups K, Brock G, et al. Report of the American Foundation for Urologic Disease 9AFUD) Thought Leader Panel for evaluation and treatment of priapism. Int J Impot Res 2001;13(Suppl 5):S39–43.
17. Pretorius ES, Siegelman ES, Ramchandani P, et al. MR imaging of the penis. Radiographics 2001;21: S283–99 (Spec no).
18. Serafini G, Bertolotto M, Lacelli F, et al. Penile inflammation. In: Bertolotto M, editor. Color Doppler US of the penis. Berlin (Germany): Springer-Verlag; 2008. p. 147–51.
19. Schmidt BA, Schwarz T, Schellong SM. Spontaneous thrombosis of the deep dorsal penile vein in a patient with thrombophilia. J Urol 2000;164:1649.
20. Shapiro RS. Superficial dorsal penile vein thrombosis (penile Mondor's phlebitis): ultrasound diagnosis. J Clin Ultrasound 1996;24:272–4.
21. Zandrino F, Musante F, Mariani N, et al. Partial unilateral intracavernosal hematoma in a long distance mountain biker: a case report. Acta Radiolo 2004; 45:580–3.
22. Guvel S, Yaycioglu O, Kilinc F, et al. Penile necrosis in end-stage renal disease. J Androl 2004;25:25–9.
23. Gonzalez- Cadavid NF. Mechanisms of penile fibrosis. J Sex Med 2009;6(Suppl 3):353–62.
24. Li CY, Agarwal V, Minhas S, et al. The penile suspensory ligament: abnormalities and repair. BJU Int 2007;99(1):117–20.
25. Abolyosr A, Moneim AE, Abdrlatif AM, et al. The management of penile fracture based on clinical and magnetic resonance imaging findings. BJU Int 2005;96(3):373–7.
26. Uder M, Gohl D, Takahashi M, et al. MRI of penile fracture: diagnosis and therapeutic follow-up. Eur Radiol 2002;12(1):113–20.
27. Nehru- Babu M, Hendry D, Ai-Saffar N. Rupture of the dorsal vein mimicking fracture of the penis. BJU Int 1999;84(1):179–80.

28. Algaba F, Horenblas S, Pizzocaro G, et al. EAU guidelines on penile cancer. Eur Urol 2002;42:199–203.

29. Pow-Sang MR, Benavente V, Pow-Sang JE, et al. Cancer of the penis. Cancer Control 2002;9:305–14.

30. Burgers JK, Badalament RA, Drago JR. Penile cancer. Clinical presentation, diagnosis, and staging. Urol Clin North Am 1992;19:247–56.

31. Lucia MS, Miller GJ. Histopathology of malignant lesions of the penis. Urol Clin North Am 1992;19: 227–46.

32. Mosconi AM, Roila F, Gatta G, et al. Cancer of the penis. Crit Rev Oncol Hematol 2005;53:165–77.

33. Lont AP, Besnard AP, Gallee MP, et al. A comparison of physical examination and imaging in determining the extent of primary penile carcinoma. BJU Int 2003;91(6):493–5.

34. Ornellas AA, Seixas AL, Marota A, et al. Surgical treatment of invasive squamous cell carcinoma of the penis: retrospective analysis of 350 cases. J Urol 1994;151:1244–9.

35. Slaton JW, Morgenstern N, Levy DA, et al. Tumor stage, vascular invasion and the percentage of poorly differentiated cancer: independent prognostic factors for inguinal lymph node metastasis in penile squamous cancer. J Urol 2001;165:1138–42.

36. Paño B, Sebastia C, Buñesch L, et al. Pathway of lymphatic spread in male urogenital Pelvic maligngncies. Radiographics 2011;31:135–60.

37. Mouli SK, Zhao LC, Omary RA, et al. Lymphotropic nanoparticle enhanced MRI for the staging of genitourinary tumors. Nat Rev Urol 2010;7(2):84–93.

38. Harisinghani MG, Saksena M, Ross RW, et al. A pilot study of lymphotrophic nanoparticle-enhanced magnetic resonance imaging technique in early stage testicular cancer: a new method for noninva–sive lymph node evaluation. Urology 2005;66(5):1066–71.

39. Guiterrez HJ, Vegas GA, Moyano SA, et al. Kaposi's sarcoma of the penis: our experience and review of the literature. Arch Esp Urol 1995;48:153–8.

40. Villalba LB, Castelló XB, Puig RV, et al. Lymphoma of the penis. Sonographic findings. J Ultrasound Med 2001;20:929–31.

41. Mostofi FK, Davis CJ, Sesterhenn IA. Carcinoma of the male and female urethra. Urol Clin North Am 1992;19:347–57.

42. Belville WD, Cohen JA. Secondary penile malignancies: the spectrum of presentation. J Surg Oncol 1992;51:134–7.

43. Bertolotto M, Serafini G, Dogliotti L, et al. Primary and secondary malignancies of the penis: ultrasound features. Abdom Imaging 2005;30:108–12.

44. Oto A, Meyer J. MR appearance of penile epithelioid sarcoma. AJR Am J Roentgenol 1999;172:555–6.

45. Agrons GA, Wagner BJ, Lonergan GJ, et al. From the archives of the AFIP: genitourinary rhabdomyosarcoma in children— radiologic-pathologic correlation. RadioGraphics 1997;17:919–37.

46. Demuren OA, Koriech O. Isolated penile metastasis from bladder carcinoma. Eur Radiol 1999;9: 1596–8.

47. Bertolotto M, Serafini G, Savoca G, et al. Colo Doppler US of the postoperative penis: Anatomy and surgical complications. Radiographics 2005; 25:731–48.

48. Zermann DH, Kutzenberger J, Sauerwein D, et al. Penile prosthetic surgery in neurologically impaired patients: long-term followup. J Urol 2006;175: 1041–4.

49. Carson CC, Mulcahy JJ, Govier FE. Efficacy, safety and patient satisfaction outcomes of the AMS 700CX inflatable penile prosthesis: results of a long-term multicenter study. J Urol 2000;164:376–80.

Imaging in Male Infertility

Syed Arsalan Raza, MBBS, FRCR[a,b], Kartik S. Jhaveri, MD[a,b,*]

KEYWORDS

• Male infertility • Male subfertility • Ultrasound • Male reproduction • Cryptorchidism • Varicocele

KEY POINTS

- Male infertility is a common problem, with 7% of all men confronted with infertility problems. Male factors are present in up to 50% of involuntarily childless couples.
- Male infertility is often correctable. It may be a presenting symptom of an occult underlying condition.
- The primary role of imaging is to identify an anatomically correctable cause of infertility.
- Imaging is critically important in the detection of testicular position and its abnormalities, as well as in the assessment of causes of obstructive azoospermia.

INTRODUCTION

Infertility is defined as the "failure to conceive after regular unprotected sexual intercourse in the absence of known reproductive pathology," over a period of 1 or 2 years.[1] Male infertility or subfertility causes and/or contributes to approximately 50% of involuntarily childless couples. Male factors are identifiable in approximately 1 in 13 couples attempting to conceive, and approximately 7% of all men are confronted with infertility problems.[2–6] Although in the majority of the patients no cause can be found and such are labeled as having idiopathic infertility, approximately 30% of patients have a physical cause to explain infertility.

BASIC SCIENCE CONCEPTS IN MALE REPRODUCTION

Male reproduction requires integrated functionality of the hypothalamic-pituitary-gonadal hormonal axis, male ductal system, prostate, bladder neck, and penis. Sound knowledge of embryology, anatomy, and physiology is helpful in the comprehension and recognition of imaging-detectable anatomic and pathologic features of male infertility.

Embryology

There are 3 excretory organs involved in the formation of reproductive tract: the pronephros, mesonephros, and metanephros. The pronephros develops in the third fetal week and evolves into of Wolffian ducts. The mesonephros develops as the pronephros degenerates and temporarily acts as the functioning kidneys. The ureters and the permanent kidneys are developed from the ureteric buds (branching and eventually detaching from the Wolffian duct at 5 weeks) and metanephric blastema, respectively. The Wolffian duct persists, maturing into the male internal genital tract. The Mullerian ducts start developing at 5 weeks under the induction stimulus from Wolffian ducts and involute after forming the prostatic utricle and appendix of the testis. The urogenital sinus arises from the cloaca and develops into the bladder and urethra. The urethra gives rise to the prostate gland.[7]

Dr. Raza is now with the Department of Diagnostic Imaging, Cape Breton Regional Hospital, 1482 George Street, Sydney, Nova Scotia B1P 1P3, Canada. Funding sources: None.
Conflicts of interest: None.
[a] Department of Medical Imaging, University of Toronto, 150 College Street, Room 112, Toronto, Ontario M5S 3E2, Canada; [b] Abdominal Imaging, University Health Network, Mt. Sinai and Women's College Hospital, 610 University Avenue, 3-957, Toronto, Ontario M5G 2M9, Canada
* Corresponding author. Abdominal Imaging, University Health Network, Mt. Sinai and Women's College Hospital, 610 University Avenue, 3-957, Toronto, Ontario M5G 2M9, Canada.
E-mail address: kartik.jhaveri@uhn.ca

radiologic.theclinics.com

Anatomy and Physiology

The testis is responsible for spermatogenesis. It is compartmentalized into approximately 400 seminiferous lobules, each containing 1 to 3 tubules that contain developing germ cells and Sertoli cells. Sertoli cells play a critical role in supporting spermatogenesis. The interstitial spaces contain Leydig cells, which produce testosterone. These U-shaped seminiferous tubules connect and drain into the rete testis within the mediastinum of the testis. The tubules of the rete testis drains into 10 to 12 efferent ducts, which exit the superior pole of testis posteriorly and form a single, highly convoluted epididymal tubule, approximately 3 to 5 m in length and constituting the major portion of the epididymis. The epididymis performs 3 functions: sperm maturation, sperm storage, and sperm transit. Arising from the tail of the epididymis, the vas deferens is a thick muscular tube 2 to 2.5 mm in outer diameter but with a 300- to 500-μm intraluminal diameter, which travels within the spermatic cord through the inguinal canal. As vas deferens enters the deep inguinal ring, it diverges from the testicular vessels and travels within the retroperitoneum toward the prostate gland. It terminates behind the bladder base where its ampulla is joined with seminal vesicles, forming the ejaculatory duct. The paired seminal vesicles lie posterosuperiorly to the prostate gland, storing and producing the bulk of the fluid that makes up semen. Seminal vesicle abnormalities result in diminished semen volume, low pH, and low fructose levels. The ejaculatory ducts open into the prosthetic urethra at the level of verumontanum, through which the semen is propelled into the urethra during ejaculation.

The process of sperm production derives its blood supply from 3 sources: the testicular artery, the deferential artery, and the cremesteric artery. The testicular artery is the main blood supply, surrounded by an intricate network of anastomotic veins known as the pampiniform plexus. This plexus provides a countercurrent heat-exchange mechanism maintaining testicular temperature 2° to 4°C below the body temperature. The plexus forms a single vein in the region of the inguinal canal, which than ascends to drain into the inferior vena cava on the right and the renal vein on the left.

An intact hypothalamic-pituitary-gonadal hormonal axis is essential for sperm production, and can be pharmacologically manipulated. The hypothalamic hormones regulate the pituitary hormones. The 2 pituitary hormones are luteinizing hormone–releasing hormone (LHRH), which stimulates testicular Leydig cells to release testosterone, and follicle-stimulating hormone (FSH), which stimulates Sertoli cells to maintain spermatogenesis.[8]

Penile anatomy is important in the diagnostic evaluation of erectile dysfunction with Doppler sonography. There are paired dorsolaterally located corpora cavernosa, surrounded by the thick fibrous sheath of tunica albuginea. These structures consist of multiple smooth muscle and endothelial-lined sinusoids, capable of considerable volume expansion. The single, ventrally located corpus spongiosum (enveloped by a thinner layer of tunica albuginea) surrounds the penile urethra. The 3 corpora are surrounded by the more superficial Buck fascia. The penis is supplied by branches of the internal pudendal artery, which continues as the penile artery. After giving off the bulbar artery (supplying the proximal shaft), the penile artery further divides into the dorsal and cavernosal arteries, both of which are end arteries. Variant anatomy is recognized in penile arterial supply.[9,10] Complex neurochemical events lead to relaxation of the smooth muscle of the sinusoids and the cavernosal arteries, with significant elevation in cavernosal artery flow causing engorgement of the cavernosal sinusoids, resulting in penile lengthening and tumescence.

DIFFERENTIAL DIAGNOSIS AND CLINICAL EVALUATION

The causative factors for impaired sperm production and function can be related to different congenital or acquired etiology acting at pretesticular, testicular, or posttesticular level (Table 1). Increasingly, genetic factors can be identified in each etiologic category, and some of these are now used in the diagnostic workup of selected groups of patients.[11]

A detailed clinical history and thorough physical examination of the couple is essential. Together with the semen analysis, this helps in establishing the etiology of infertility or the need for adjunctive laboratory or imaging evaluation in most cases.

Normal semen parameters are described in Table 2, and multiple associated abnormal conditions are explained in Table 3. Semen analysis identifies azoospermia in 5% to 10% of infertile males.[12] Azoospermia may be secondary to defective spermatogenesis (nonobstructive) or obstruction of the male ductal system (obstructive). Nonobstructive azoospermia is associated with small testes,[13] and patients are likely to require reproduction-assisted techniques such as intracytoplasmic sperm injection (ICSI). By comparison, obstructive azoospermia may be amenable to surgical treatment. Fewer than 3% of cases are attributable to a hormonal cause. Nevertheless, hormonal analysis remains important in establishing whether infertility is a result of hypothalamic/pituitary deficiency or

Table 1
Differential diagnosis of male infertility

Categories	Subcategories	Causes
Idiopathic		Unknown etiology (about 50%)
Pretesticular causes	Hypogonadotropic hypogonadism	Idiopathic Prader-Willi syndrome Laurence-Moon-Biedl syndrome CNS tumors Drugs (eg, dopamine agonists)
	Pituitary failure	Tumor Infarction Radiation Granulomatous disease Prolactinomas Isolated LH/FSH deficiency Thalassemia Cushing disease
	Estrogen excess	Sertoli cell tumors Leydig tumors Liver failure Obesity
	Cortisol excess/deficiency	Adrenal hyperplasia Adrenal adenoma or carcinoma Congenital adrenal hyperplasia Lung tumors Adrenal hyperplasia Adrenal adenoma or carcinoma Congenital adrenal hyperplasia
Testicular	Chromosomal	Klinefelter syndrome Noonan syndrome Anorchia Testicular dysgenesis Germ cell aplasia Myotonic dystrophy
	Nonchromosomal	Varicocele Cryptorchidism Tumor Trauma Radiation Heat Drugs/chemotherapy Orchitis Granulomatous disease Sickle cell disease
Posttesticular	Congenital blockage	Congenital bilateral absence of vas deferens Utricle cysts Mullerian cysts Wolffian cysts
	Acquired blockage	Inflammatory or traumatic stenosis of ejaculatory ducts Functional ejaculatory duct obstruction (diabetes or APKD) Epididymal obstruction secondary to infection
	Ejaculatory or sexual dysfunction	

Abbreviations: APKD, autosomal dominant polycystic kidney disease; FSH, follicle-stimulating hormone; LH, luteinizing hormone.

Table 2
Normal human semen characteristics

2010 WHO Parameters	Percentile (95% CI)
Semen volume	1.5 mL (1.4–1.7)
Total sperm number	39 million (33–46)
Sperm concentration	15 million/mL (12–16)
Vitality	58% live (55–63)
Progressive motility	32% (31–34)
Total (progressive + nonprogressive) motility	40% (38–42)
Morphologically normal forms	4.0% (3.0–4.0)

Abbreviations: CI, confidence interval; WHO, World Health Organization.

Data from Cooper TG, Noonan E, von Eckardstein S, et al. World Health Organization reference values for human semen characteristics. Hum Reprod Update 2010;16(3): 231–45.

primary testicular failure. A simplified approach to the diagnostic assessment of azoospermia is shown in **Fig. 1**. Detailed clinical algorithms according to different physical and biochemical parameters have been described in literature.[14]

The primary role of imaging is to identify an anatomically correctable cause of infertility.[15] A thorough imaging evaluation is required for the most appropriate and cost-effective therapy to be delivered.

IMAGING TECHNIQUES
Scrotal Ultrasonography

The superficial nature of the scrotal sac allows ultrasonography to be used as the first-line imaging modality in diagnostic evaluation. It is performed using a high-frequency duplex echo transducer probe (7.5 MHz and higher). The probe length should allow accurate long-axis measurements of the testis, with the patient examined in the supine recumbent position. Multiple parameters are assessed including testicular size, anatomic variants, and abnormalities of the testes, epididymides, and proximal genital tract. Color flow and Doppler assessment should be performed as an integral part of examination to assess vasculature in the testis and spermatic cord.

The normal adult testis has a volume of 15 to 20 mL. Testicular volumes appear to correlate with semen profiles.[16] Sakamoto and colleagues[17] investigated the accuracy of orchidometry and ultrasonography for measuring testicular volume, and found Lambert's formula to be the most accurate:

$$\text{Volume (mL)} = \text{Length} \times \text{Width} \times \text{Anteroposterior depth (cm)} \times 0.71$$

The prevalence of scrotal abnormalities in infertile men has been reported as between 38% and 65%.[17,18] In these respective studies, 67% and 58% of these abnormalities had not been detected clinically. Reduced testicular tumors have been reported in 0.5% of infertile men, a higher prevalence than in the general population.[18]

Table 3
Nomenclature related to pathologic semen quality

Nomenclature	Definition
Oligozoospermia	Sperm concentration $<15 \times 10^6$/mL; total sperm number $<39 \times 10^6$/mL
Asthenozoospermia	$<32\%$ progressively motile spermatozoa
Teratozoospermia	$<4\%$ morphologically normal spermatozoa
Oligo-astheno-teratozoospermia	Disturbance of all 3 parameters
Azoospermia	No spermatozoa in the ejaculate
Cryptozoospermia	Spermatozoa absent from fresh preparation but observed in a centrifuged pellet
Aspermia	No ejaculate
Leukospermia(leukocytospermia)	$>1 \times 10^6$ mL leukocytes in the ejaculate

Data from World Health Organization. WHO laboratory manual for the examination and processing of human semen. 5th edition. Geneva (Switzerland): World Health Organization; 2010.

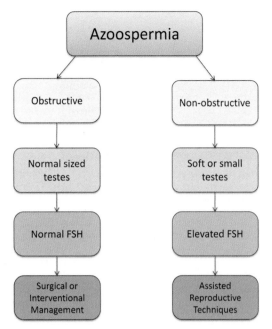

Fig. 1. Simplified algorithm showing the types and management of azoospermia. FSH, follicle-stimulating hormone. (*Modified from* Jhaveri KS, Mazrani W, Chawla TP, et al. The role of crosssectional imaging in male infertility: a pictorial review. Can Assoc Radiol J 2010;61(3):144–55; with permission.)

Transrectal Ultrasonography

Transrectal ultrasonography (TRUS) is used in the evaluation of azoospermia to exclude obstruction and to determine the absence of hypoplasia of the seminal vesicles and ejaculatory ducts. A high-frequency (6.5–7.5 MHz) endorectal probe is used with the bladder partially filled (to provide an acoustic window), with the patient lying in a lateral decubitus position. A preprocedure digital examination may help to assess the rectal cavity and exclude any rectal lesion. The prostate gland, seminal vesicles, vasa deferentia, and ejaculatory ducts are systemically evaluated in axial and sagittal planes.

ULTRASONOGRAPHIC APPEARANCE OF NORMAL MALE GENITAL ORGANS

The normal prostate gland (**Fig. 2**) is a symmetric, triangular, and ellipsoid structure surrounded by a thin echogenic capsule. It measures approximately 4 cm in transverse, 3 cm in anteroposterior, and 4 cm in craniocaudal dimensions, with a normal volume of 20 to 25 mL and a weight of approximately 20 g.

The seminal vesicles (**Figs. 3** and **4**) are hypoechoic, paired elongated structures, with a few fine internal echoes and a network of tubules

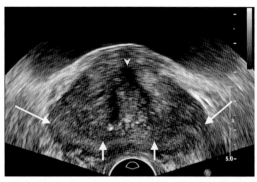

Fig. 2. Transrectal ultrasonography (TRUS) transverse image of a normal prostate gland showing the urethra (*arrowhead*), transitional zone (*short arrows*), and peripheral zone (*long arrows*). Note the foci of calcification in the transitional zone commonly seen in benign prostatic hyperplasia.

with septations. These vesicles lie cephalad to the prostate and posterior to the urinary bladder in a bow-tie configuration. Typically they are less than 3 cm in length, 1.5 cm in width, and 1.5 cm in anteroposterior diameter, with a mean volume of around 14 mL.

The vasa deferentia (see **Fig. 4**) are seen axially as a pair of oval, convoluted, tubular structures located medial to the seminal vesicles and just cephalad to the prostate, with an echotexture similar to the seminal vesicles.

The ejaculatory duct (**Fig. 5**) is formed by the convergence and confluence of the seminal vesicle and the terminal portion of the vas deferens. The duct appears as a small, hypoechoic (paired) structure with a caliber of 2 mm, crossing the prostate gland obliquely to terminate in the prostatic urethra, lateral and proximal to the verumontanum.

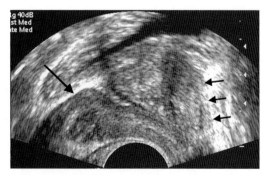

Fig. 3. Sagittal TRUS image showing the normal left seminal vesicle (*long arrow*) and fibromuscular stroma of the prostate gland (*short arrows*). (*From* Jhaveri KS, Mazrani W, Chawla TP, et al. The role of cross-sectional imaging in male infertility: a pictorial review. Can Assoc Radiol J 2010;61(3):144–55; with permission.)

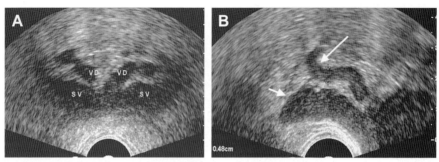

Fig. 4. (A) Transverse TRUS image showing the normal vas deferens (VD) and seminal vesicles (SV). (B) Sagittal TRUS image showing the normal right vas deferens (*long arrow*) and right seminal vesicle (*short arrow*). (*From* Jhaveri KS, Mazrani W, Chawla TP, et al. The role of cross-sectional imaging in male infertility: a pictorial review. Can Assoc Radiol J 2010;61(3):144–55; with permission.)

The entire course, from the seminal vesicle to the urethra, can be visualized on the sagittal plane.

Color Doppler Ultrasonography of the Penis

Dynamic assessment of the penile vasculature can be performed using stimulated color Doppler ultrasonography to assess for erectile dysfunction. A high-frequency linear-array probe with a small footprint is used. The penis, held in anatomic position by the patient, is assessed with high-resolution gray-scale imaging to assess for fibrotic plaque disease, focal cavernosal fibrosis or calcification, and disruption of tunica albuginea. Baseline imaging allows identification of optimum injection sites, and location of the cavernosal arteries as anatomic variants is common. Vasculature is then assessed with intracavernosal injection of 10 to 20 μg of prostaglandin E_1 (PGE_1) after assessing for contraindications and obtaining informed consent (especially alerting as regards the risk of priapism). The cavernosal artery is sampled for accurate velocity measurements. The peak systolic and end-diastolic velocities are assessed every 5 minutes after the administration of PGE_1 for up to 30 minutes.[19,20]

Magnetic Resonance Imaging

Magnetic resonance (MR) imaging can provide a noninvasive alternative to traditional vasography, which is invasive and carries risks, including strictures of the vas deferens. High-resolution, multiplanar images provide detailed anatomy of the reproductive tract. MR imaging assessment of the pelvis is ideally performed on 1.5-T or 3-T field-strength systems using phased-array or endorectal coils if available (**Figs. 6** and **7**). An antiperistaltic agent administered intravenously (usually 20 mg hyoscine butylbromide or 1 mg glucagon after screening for contraindications) is recommended to reduce bowel-motion artifacts.

PRETESTICULAR ABNORMALITIES

The main causes of pretesticular infertility are endocrinopathies (see **Table 1**). Endocrinopathies are investigated by biochemical profile assessment and, increasingly, with genetic testing.[11] There is a very limited role for pelvic imaging in these cases, but MR imaging is frequently used to evaluate the brain for suspected pituitary masses. Prolactin-producing adenomas are the most

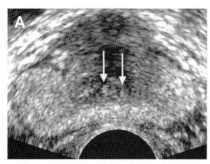
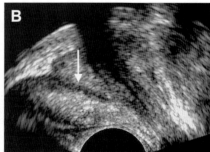

Fig. 5. (A, B) TRUS images in axial (A) and sagittal (B) planes demonstrating ejaculatory ducts (*arrows*). (*From* Jhaveri KS, Mazrani W, Chawla TP, et al. The role of cross-sectional imaging in male infertility: a pictorial review. Can Assoc Radiol J 2010;61(3):144–55; with permission.)

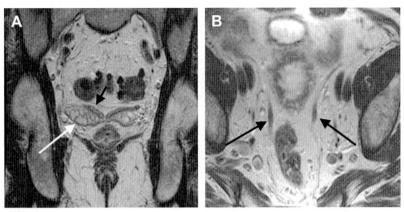

Fig. 6. (*A, B*) Coronal (*A*) and axial (*B*) T2-weighted (T2W) MR images showing normal seminal vesicle (*white arrow*) and vas deferens (*black arrows*). (*From* Jhaveri KS, Mazrani W, Chawla TP, et al. The role of cross-sectional imaging in male infertility: a pictorial review. Can Assoc Radiol J 2010;61(3):144–55; with permission.)

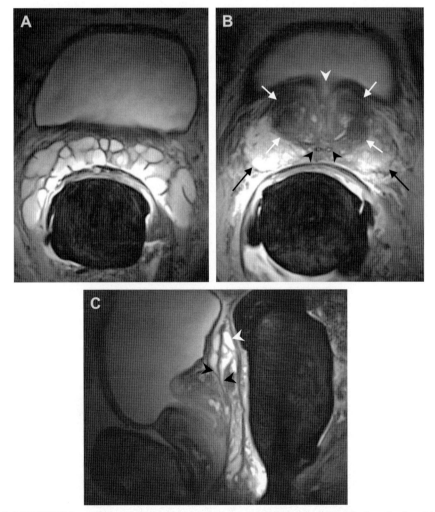

Fig. 7. (*A*) Axial T2W MR image performed with endorectal coil (*A*) showing fluid-filled seminal vesicles. (*B*) Axial T2W image at lower level shows T2 hyperintense peripheral zone (*black arrows*) and T2 hypointense transitional zone (*white arrows*), which define the prostate gland. Both ejaculatory ducts (*black arrowheads*) and urethra (*white arrowhead*) are seen in midline. (*C*) Sagittal T2 image in the same patient showing seminal vesicles (*white arrowhead*) and formation of ejaculatory ducts (*black arrowheads*) draining into urethra in the region of verumontanum.

common pituitary tumors, which exert a negative effect on testicular function through suppression of gonadotropin hormones.

TESTICULAR ABNORMALITIES

Primary testicular causes of infertility include congenital and acquired causes. Imaging has a limited role in congenital causes, where the diagnosis is often made clinically. In such congenital cases, imaging may demonstrate testicular atrophy.

Varicocele

Varicocele is defined as abnormal dilatation of the pampiniform venous plexus. Varicocele is a common finding, present in 12% to 20% of the adult male population, and is usually asymptomatic. However, varicocele is the most common abnormality identified in men with primary male factor infertility, present in up to 25% to 50%. The effect of varicocele is not established as a causative factor in the context of infertility. A meta-analysis showed no significant overall benefit from treatment of varicocele in terms of improved fertility.[21] However, one of the largest multicenter trials did show a clinically significant effect.[22] Varicoceles are correctable, and semen parameters can be improved in up to 44% of patients after repair.[23] The proposed effect of varicocele is mediated through semen abnormalities, decreased testicular volume, and decline in Leydig cell function, and therefore it can be considered as a cofactor of impaired sperm production.[24]

Diagnosis is confirmed on scrotal ultrasonography when veins within the pampiniform plexus measure greater than 3 mm in diameter and dilate further during the Valsalva maneuver (**Figs. 8** and **9**). Varicoceles are usually left sided. If right-sided varicoceles are detected, retroperitoneal abnormality should be excluded. Tubular ectasia

of the rete testis may cause confusion with varicoceles and should be assessed carefully (**Fig. 10**). Color flow Doppler allows identification of reversal of flow in incompetent pampiniform veins, and improves diagnostic accuracy. A Valsalva maneuver should be performed during the Doppler examination. The degree of venous reflux during Valsalva may be graded as static (grade I), intermittent (grade II), or continuous (grade III). Grade III reflux is considered significant, grade II is indeterminate, and grade I is of doubtful significance.[25,26]

The current guidelines of the American Urological Association advise treatment for in men with varicoceles, impaired semen quality, and documented subfertility who have a female partner with normal fertility or correctable infertility.[27] The current trend is to perform artery-sparing, lymphatic-sparing, inguinal or subinguinal microsurgical varicocelectomy, which has been reported to be associated with lower recurrence and complication rates, with greater improvements in semen quality in comparison with radiographic embolization or nonmicrosurgical approaches.[28]

Cryptorchidism

Cryptorchidism is the most frequent congenital birth defect in male children, and may occur as an isolated disorder or in association with other congenital anomalies (syndromic cryptorchidism).[29] The incidence of cryptorchidism varies between 2% and 9% at birth (related to geographic variations) and reduces to 1% to 2% by 3 months of age, owing to delayed spontaneous descent.[30–32] It can also occur as an acquired disorder diagnosed during infancy and childhood.[32,33] This so-called acquired cryptorchidism is defined as the ascent of the testis into a cryptorchid position after normal scrotal position at birth, and its cumulative incidence by age

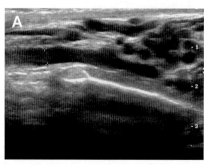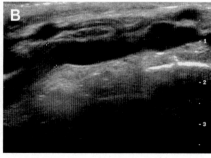

Fig. 8. (*A, B*) Gray-scale ultrasound images demonstrating dilated spermatic vein (*A*), which increases in size after Valsalva maneuver (*B*). (*From* Jhaveri KS, Mazrani W, Chawla TP, et al. The role of cross-sectional imaging in male infertility: a pictorial review. Can Assoc Radiol J 2010;61(3):144–55; with permission.)

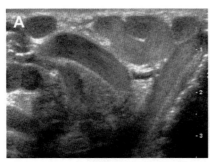
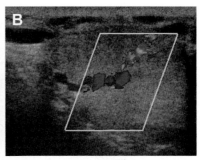

Fig. 9. (A) Gray-scale ultrasound image through the pampiniform plexus shows dilated vascular channels. (B) Doppler ultrasound image through left testis shows intratesticular component of varicocele. (From Jhaveri KS, Mazrani W, Chawla TP, et al. The role of cross-sectional imaging in male infertility: a pictorial review. Can Assoc Radiol J 2010;61(3):144–55; with permission.)

24 months can be even higher than that observed at birth.[34]

Cryptorchidism is present in 2% to 9% of infertile men.[35] Fertility is considerably reduced in patients with bilateral cryptorchidism, where azoospermia is found in up to 42% of patients and paternity is achieved in only 35% to 53%.[36] The anatomic location of the testis outside the scrotum results in impaired spermatogenesis, and can be a cause of subfertility. The interaction of genetic and environmental factors in the pathogenesis of cryptorchidism and its effects has been recently described.[11]

With regard to the testes' abnormal position, 72% are located in the inguinal canal (Fig. 11) and are commonly seen as an oval mass, 20% are prescrotal, and 8% are abdominal in location.[37] In the absence of an intrascrotal testis at ultrasonography, an undescended testis should be sought by scanning along the path of testicular descent, through the pelvis, and along the inguinal canal. MR imaging may be useful for the imaging of pelvic testes (Fig. 12). Absent or ectopic testes are relatively uncommon, reported in only 3% to 5% of cases of presumed cryptorchidism.[38]

Another role for imaging in cryptorchidism is tumor surveillance. Approximately 5% to 10% of patients with testicular carcinoma have undescended testes, and 2% to 8% of patients with undescended testes have carcinoma in situ, 50% of whom develop a testicular carcinoma (Fig. 13). Testicular biopsy is therefore required before sperm retrieval.

Testicular Atrophy

Several testicular insults can result in testicular atrophy and subsequent oligozoospermia or azoospermia. Examples include testicular torsion, trauma, orchitis, sickle cell disease, tumor, chemotherapy, and radiation therapy (Figs. 14–16). In addition to global reduction in the volume of testis, decrease in both the testicular reflectivity and vascularity are common findings. The epididymis usually appears normal.

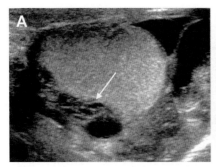
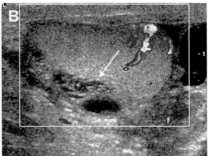

Fig. 10. (A, B) Gray-scale ultrasound image of right testis (A) showing cystic dilatation of the rete testis (arrow). Doppler assessment (B) shows absence of flow within the dilated channels excluding intratesticular varicocele (arrow). (From Jhaveri KS, Mazrani W, Chawla TP, et al. The role of cross-sectional imaging in male infertility: a pictorial review. Can Assoc Radiol J 2010;61(3):144–55; with permission.)

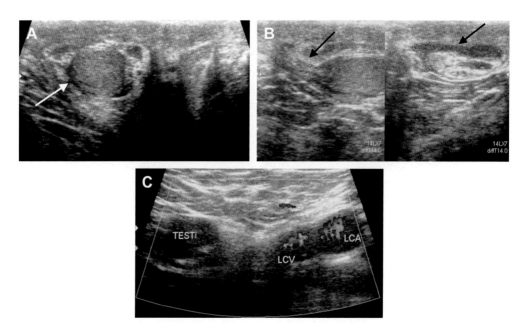

Fig. 11. (*A–C*) Gray-scale ultrasound images through the left inguinal region show undescended testis (*white arrow in A*). The left epididymis is clearly visualized in orthogonal planes (*black arrows in B*). Left inguinal vessels are seen in the vicinity (LCA and LCV in *C*).

Orchitis and Epididymo-Orchitis

Infective disorders of the testis and epididymis are common causes of acute scrotal pain; if chronic, they may cause spermatogenic arrest and result in testicular atrophy.

Pure orchitis is uncommon and is most often results from mumps virus.[39] The testis and epididymis may appear enlarged, hypoechoic, and hyperemic on ultrasonography during an acute episode, resulting in marked testicular atrophy in 30% of cases.

Epididymo-orchitis results from a range of organisms including *Neisseria gonorrhoeae* and *Chlamydia trachomatis*; rarer causes, such as mumps and sarcoidosis, tend to cause bilateral changes.[40] Gray-scale ultrasound findings include testicular enlargement and heterogeneity of echotexture associated with an enlarged hypoechoic or hyperechoic epididymis. Color Doppler ultrasonography shows hyperemia in both testis and epididymis (see **Fig. 14**).[41] Epididymitis can result in postinflammatory obstruction of the epididymis.

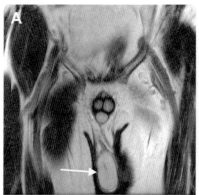
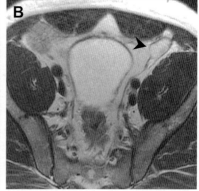

Fig. 12. (*A*) Coronal T2W MR image shows a single right testis within the scrotal sac (*white arrow*). (*B*) Axial T2W image through the lower pelvis shows undescended testis (*black arrowhead*) in the left anterior pelvis. (*From Jhaveri KS, Mazrani W, Chawla TP, et al. The role of cross-sectional imaging in male infertility: a pictorial review. Can Assoc Radiol J 2010;61(3):144–55; with permission.*)

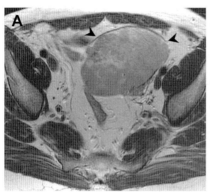
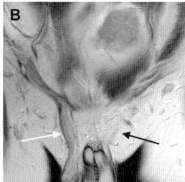

Fig. 13. (A) Axial T2W MR image through the lower pelvis shows a large heterogeneous intermediate T2 signal mass (*black arrowheads*) confirmed pathologically as tumor complicating left undescended testis. (B) Coronal T2W MR image showing absence of left spermatic cord (*black arrow*) and normal right-sided structures (*white arrow*). (*From* Jhaveri KS, Mazrani W, Chawla TP, et al. The role of cross-sectional imaging in male infertility: a pictorial review. Can Assoc Radiol J 2010;61(3):144–55; with permission.)

The goal of diagnostic evaluation and antimicrobial therapy is to avoid transmission of infection to the female partner and to eliminate the adverse effects of infection on semen quality and sperm function, thereby reducing the risk of subsequent infertility.

Testicular Microlithiasis

Testicular microlithiasis is a condition of unknown etiology whereby multiple small punctate calcifications are present within the seminiferous tubules of the testes (at least 5 echogenic foci in a single transducer field). A higher than expected frequency of testicular microlithiasis is reported in infertile men,[42] and it is associated with an increased risk of testicular cancer.[43] However, following up patients with isolated testicular microlithiasis using ultrasonography is controversial,

and should be dictated by other concurrent risk factors.

POSTTESTICULAR ABNORMALITIES/ OBSTRUCTIVE AZOOSPERMIA

Obstruction of the ductal system accounts for up to 40% of azoospermia,[44] and should be suspected when the physical examination and serum hormone profile are normal. Obstructive disorders causing azoospermia are divided into congenital and acquired causes and can occur anywhere along the excretory ductal system including the epididymis, vas deferens, seminal vesicle, ejaculatory duct, and urethra (Fig. 17). The 2 main treatment strategies are surgical correction of the obstruction and sperm retrieval followed by ICSI.

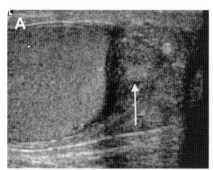
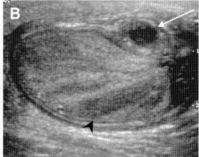

Fig. 14. (A) Sagittal gray-scale ultrasound image of right hemiscrotum shows an enlarged, hypoechoic right epididymis (*white arrow*), which was found to be hyperemic (Doppler image not shown). (B) Sagittal gray-scale image through the left hemiscrotum shows hypoechoic and heterogeneous appearance of left testis (*black arrowhead*), which reflects associated orchitis. The left epididymis is also enlarged and containing a focal hypoechoic area (*white arrow*), suggesting early abscess formation. Appearances are consistent with bilateral epididymo-orchitis. (*From* Jhaveri KS, Mazrani W, Chawla TP, et al. The role of cross-sectional imaging in male infertility: a pictorial review. Can Assoc Radiol J 2010;61(3):144–55; with permission.)

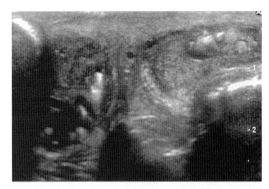

Fig. 15. Gray-scale ultrasound image showing bilateral chronic epididymitis with calcification (causative etiology was tuberculosis in this case). (*From* Jhaveri KS, Mazrani W, Chawla TP, et al. The role of cross-sectional imaging in male infertility: a pictorial review. Can Assoc Radiol J 2010;61(3):144–55; with permission.)

Congenital Bilateral Absence of the Vas Deferens

Congenital bilateral absence of the vas deferens (CBAVD) (**Fig. 18**) is the most common cause of congenital vas deferens obstruction, seen in approximately 2% of patients under investigation for infertility and accounting for 4% to 17% of cases of azoospermia.[8] CBAVD is found in nearly all patients with cystic fibrosis, and up to 82% of patients with CBAVD have at least one mutation in the cystic fibrosis gene.[45] Identification is therefore important, as it may prompt genetic counseling and management. The genetic associations of CBAVD also manifest as concurrent Wolffian duct abnormalities.[46,47] Abnormalities of the seminal vesicle are observed in 90% of cases of CBAVD, with complete absence of seminal vesicles in about 40% of cases. Renal abnormalities such as renal agenesis, crossed fused ectopia, or ectopic pelvic kidney may also be associated with CBAVD.

TRUS shows absence of ampulla of the vas deferens and may reveal associated seminal vesicle abnormalities such as absence, hypoplasia (**Fig. 19**), cysts, calcification, and hyperechoic appearance.[48] Scrotal ultrasonography shows dilatation of the efferent ducts. The head of the epididymis stops abruptly at the junction of the body and tail where the agenesis begins. Renal sonography should be performed to exclude unilateral renal agenesis (see **Fig. 19**). Sperm retrieval with ICSI is the treatment of choice, as surgical reconstruction is not possible.[8]

Congenital Cystic Lesions of the Ductal Tract

Seminal vesicle cysts
Congenital seminal vesicle cysts are rare (see **Figs. 17** and **18**). These cysts are frequently associated with an ectopic ureter draining into the seminal vesicle from a dysplastic kidney or unilateral renal agenesis (see **Fig. 18**), explained by a common embryologic mesonephric origin.[49] The seminal vesicle is the second most common site of ureteric ectopy after the prostatic urethra.

Prostatic cysts
Midline cysts (**Figs. 20** and **21**) can be classified according to their sperm content. Cysts of utricular and Mullerian origin do not contain sperm, whereas the Wolffian cysts that arise in the ejaculatory ducts (**Fig. 22**) do contain sperm.

Utricle cysts are confined to the prostate and are strictly midline. These cysts are usually smaller (no more than 15 mm in long axis), do not communicate with the urethra, and are commonly associated with other congenital anomalies, such as intersex disorders, cryptorchidism, and hypospadias. Mullerian duct cysts result from failure of complete regression of the Mullerian duct in utero.

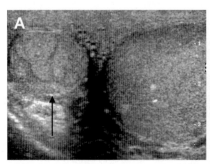
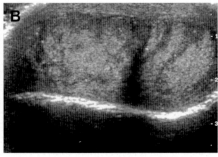

Fig. 16. Combined view of both testes (*A*) and sagittal view of right hemiscrotum (*B*) shows atrophic heterogeneous appearance of right testis containing scattered foci of calcification (*arrow*). The patient had previous orchitis. (*From* Jhaveri KS, Mazrani W, Chawla TP, et al. The role of cross-sectional imaging in male infertility: a pictorial review. Can Assoc Radiol J 2010;61(3):144–55; with permission.)

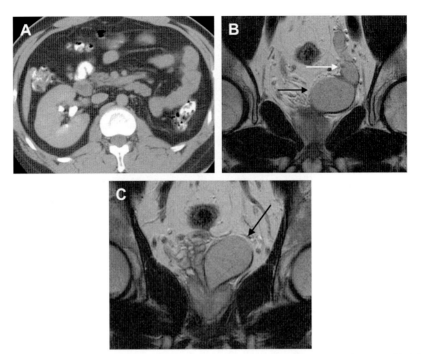

Fig. 17. (A) Axial computed tomography (CT) image through upper abdomen shows absence of left kidney. (B, C) Coronal T2W MR images show ectopic insertion of left ureteric remnant (*white arrow in B*) into the left seminal vesicle (*black arrows in B and C*). Abnormal insertion of the ureter has resulted in cystic dilatation of left seminal vesicle. (*From* Jhaveri KS, Mazrani W, Chawla TP, et al. The role of cross-sectional imaging in male infertility: a pictorial review. Can Assoc Radiol J 2010;61(3):144–55; with permission.)

These cysts can be much larger, may extend above the prostate gland, and are prone to hemorrhage. On TRUS, they appear as spherical hypoechoic foci in the prostate with posterior acoustic enhancement.[46] In the absence of an extraprostatic component, the appearances of Mullerian and utricular cysts are indistinguishable on TRUS. MR imaging can be useful in delineation of the origin of the abnormality. MR imaging may also allow differentiation from posterior bladder diverticula and vas deferens cysts, which can have similar appearances on TRUS. Wolffian duct cysts

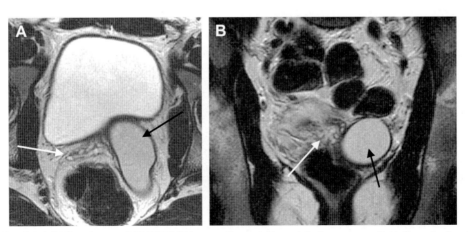

Fig. 18. (A, B) Axial (A) and coronal (B) T2W MR images through the pelvis show congenital left seminal vesicle cyst (*black arrow*) and hypoplastic right seminal vesicle (*white arrow*). (*From* Jhaveri KS, Mazrani W, Chawla TP, et al. The role of cross-sectional imaging in male infertility: a pictorial review. Can Assoc Radiol J 2010;61(3):144–55; with permission.)

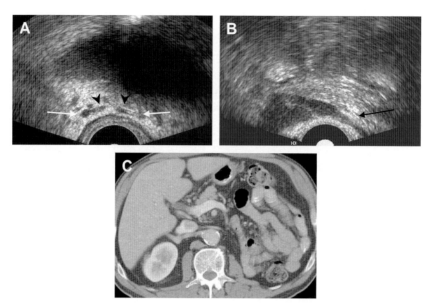

Fig. 19. (*A*) Transverse TRUS image showing atretic seminal vesicles (*white arrows*) and vas deferens (*black arrowheads*). (*B, C*) In another patient, transverse TRUS image (*B*) shows normal-appearing right seminal vesicle with absence of left seminal vesicle (*black arrow in B*). Axial CT image (*C*) through the upper abdomen shows absence of left kidney. (*From* Jhaveri KS, Mazrani W, Chawla TP, et al. The role of cross-sectional imaging in male infertility: a pictorial review. Can Assoc Radiol J 2010;61(3):144–55; with permission.)

are usually midline and can also become very large, extending beyond the prostate.[50] Paramedian or lateral intraprostatic cysts of Wolffian duct origin are rarely seen in clinical practice.

Large cysts can be aspirated transrectally under ultrasound guidance, but the results are often short lived.[50] Patients with midline cysts tend to have the most favorable outcomes following transurethral resection.[51]

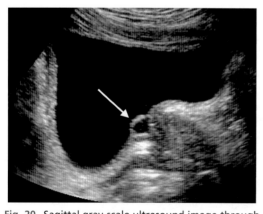

Fig. 20. Sagittal gray-scale ultrasound image through urinary bladder and prostate shows a midline Mullerian cyst (*arrow*), which extends above the prostatic base. (*From* Jhaveri KS, Mazrani W, Chawla TP, et al. The role of cross-sectional imaging in male infertility: a pictorial review. Can Assoc Radiol J 2010;61(3): 144–55; with permission.)

Acquired Causes of Obstruction of the Ductal Tract

Seminal vesicles

Acquired seminal vesicle cysts are secondary to obstruction. Etiology includes benign prostatic enlargement, prostatic malignancy, and prostatic surgery. Adult polycystic kidney disease has been associated with marked dilatation of the seminal vesicles (megavesicles) (**Fig. 23**). This phenomenon has been attributed to atonicity, a functional rather than mechanical obstruction.[52]

Ejaculatory ducts

Obstruction of the ejaculatory duct is an uncommon but potentially correctable cause of male factor infertility. The causes can be divided into congenital (including compression by median cysts) and acquired, including distal inflammatory and traumatic stenoses of ejaculatory ducts (see **Fig. 22**; **Fig. 24**). The presence of calculi in the distal ejaculatory ducts at the level of the ampulla is a relatively common occurrence, and may be associated with dilatation of the proximal duct and evidence of obstruction.[46] Obstruction of the ejaculatory duct can be iatrogenic, a potential complication of bladder neck repairs,[47] or result from prolonged catheterization at the level of the ejaculatory duct.

Vas deferens

Obstruction of the vas deferens can occur as a complication of inguinal hernia repair or scrotal surgery as well as deliberate closure in elective

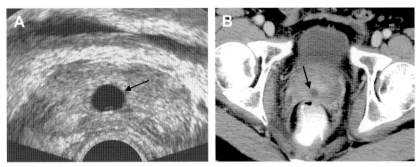

Fig. 21. (A, B) Transverse TRUS (A) and axial CT (B) images showing a small midline utricle cyst (arrows) within the prostate gland. (From Jhaveri KS, Mazrani W, Chawla TP, et al. The role of cross-sectional imaging in male infertility: a pictorial review. Can Assoc Radiol J 2010;61(3):144–55; with permission.)

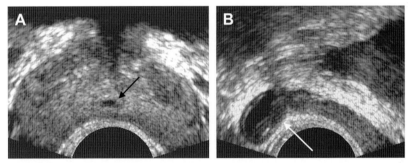

Fig. 22. (A, B) Transverse TRUS images show right ejaculatory duct cyst (black arrow in A) causing right seminal vesicle obstruction and cyst formation (white arrow in B). (From Jhaveri KS, Mazrani W, Chawla TP, et al. The role of cross-sectional imaging in male infertility: a pictorial review. Can Assoc Radiol J 2010;61(3):144–55; with permission.)

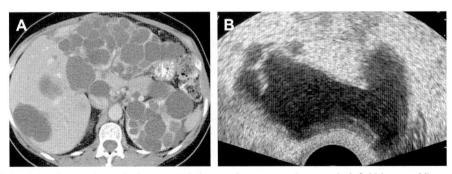

Fig. 23. (A) Axial CT image through the upper abdomen shows extensive cysts in left kidney and liver, consistent with polycystic disease. (B) Transverse TRUS image shows cystic dilatation of both seminal vesicles. (From Jhaveri KS, Mazrani W, Chawla TP, et al. The role of cross-sectional imaging in male infertility: a pictorial review. Can Assoc Radiol J 2010;61(3):144–55; with permission.)

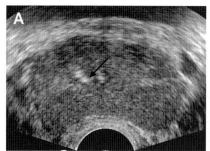
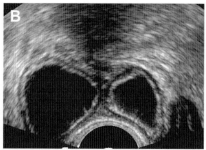

Fig. 24. (*A, B*) TRUS images showing ejaculatory duct calcifications (*black arrow in A*) and resultant obstruction, causing cystic dilatation of seminal vesicles (*B*). (*From* Jhaveri KS, Mazrani W, Chawla TP, et al. The role of cross-sectional imaging in male infertility: a pictorial review. Can Assoc Radiol J 2010;61(3):144–55; with permission.)

vasectomy. Testicular fibrosis–related impairment of germ cell function can occur with prolonged obstruction secondary to vasectomy, which can reduce fertility following potential reversal.[53]

Epididymis

Epididymal obstruction (**Fig. 25**) should be suspected in patients with oligozoospermia or azoospermia and a normal ejaculate volume. Epididymal obstruction can occur as a sequel of acute (gonococcal) or subacute (chlamydial) infections, iatrogenic factors (surgical removal of an epididymal cyst), or trauma. Scrotal ultrasonography may demonstrate epididymal enlargement and a hypoechoic appearance caused by prior epididymitis. There may be dilatation of the rete testis, although marked postinfectious sclerosis may mask this finding. Postvasectomy appearances of epididymis are characteristic. There is epididymal dilatation, with an inhomogeneous appearance on ultrasonography described as ectasia of the epididymis. In addition, epididymal cysts can develop.[54]

Erectile Dysfunction

Erectile dysfunction (ED) has been defined as the consistent inability to attain or maintain penile erections of sufficient quality to allow satisfactory sexual activity.[19,55] Approximately 52% of men aged 40 to 70 years experience ED, with up to 10% suffering from severe ED.[56] The physical causes can be divided into problems with arterial inflow, problems with the venous occlusion mechanism, or structural penile abnormalities.

Peak systolic velocity between 25 and 35 cm/s is used for diagnosing arterial insufficiency in cavernosal artery.[56] Doppler sonography can also allow visualization of stenoses. Ancillary findings include high-velocity jets and damped waveforms as a result of proximal stenoses.[20] An abnormal Doppler study prompts further evaluation by arteriography to allow surgical planning if appropriate. The diagnosis of venogenic ED secondary to venous incompetence or leakage is suggested by the presence of normal arterial flow and end-diastolic velocities of greater than 5 cm/s.[56–58] Cavernosography is the gold-standard imaging technique for demonstration of venous leak, and therefore should be performed to define the anatomy for surgical planning.[20] False-positive results for venous leak may occur in young patients with suboptimal response to PGE$_1$ caused by high anxiety and increased sympathetic drive.[59] Pyronie disease is a benign, localized connective-tissue

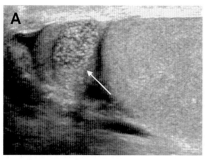
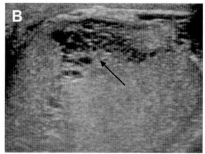

Fig. 25. (*A, B*) Gray-scale ultrasound images of left hemiscrotum demonstrating proximal epididymal obstruction (*white arrow in A*) and dilatation of the rete testis (*black arrow in B*). (*From* Jhaveri KS, Mazrani W, Chawla TP, et al. The role of cross-sectional imaging in male infertility: a pictorial review. Can Assoc Radiol J 2010;61(3):144–55; with permission.)

disorder of unknown etiology that causes fibrous thickening of the penile tunica albuginea. Pyronie disease could be associated with both arterial incompetence and venous leakage, leading to ED in a proportion of affected patients (range, 4%–80%).[60] Standard gray-scale ultrasonography may delineate the plaques as hyperechoic, irregular thickening of the tunica albuginea with or without calcification.[61]

SUMMARY

Knowledge of normal male reproductive anatomy, familiarity with diagnostic imaging options, and awareness of potential causes and treatment options are critical for radiologists involved in multidisciplinary management of male infertility. The underlying causative factor of male infertility is often correctable, and may be associated with occult health-threatening conditions. This article presents the important embryologic, anatomic, and physiologic concepts underpinning male reproduction, explains common and uncommon abnormalities resulting in male infertility, and discusses management strategies.

REFERENCES

1. Rowe PJ, World Health Organization. WHO manual for the standardized investigation, diagnosis, and management of the infertile male. Cambridge (United Kingdom); New York: Published on behalf of the World Health Organization by Cambridge University Press; 2000.
2. Hull MG, Glazener CM, Kelly NJ, et al. Population study of causes, treatment, and outcome of infertility. Br Med J (Clin Res Ed) 1985;291(6510):1693–7.
3. Greenhall E, Vessey M. The prevalence of subfertility: a review of the current confusion and a report of two new studies. Fertil Steril 1990;54(6):978–83.
4. Thonneau P, Marchand S, Tallec A, et al. Incidence and main causes of infertility in a resident population (1,850,000) of three French regions (1988-1989). Hum Reprod 1991;6(6):811–6.
5. Mosher WD, Pratt WF. Fecundity and infertility in the United States: incidence and trends. Fertil Steril 1991;56(2):192–3.
6. Forti G, Krausz C. Clinical review 100: evaluation and treatment of the infertile couple. J Clin Endocrinol Metab 1998;83(12):4177–88.
7. Sadler TW, Langman J. Langman's medical embryology. 12th edition. Philadelphia: Wolters Kluwer Health/Lippincott Williams & Wilkins; 2012.
8. Stahl PJ, Stember DS, Goldstein M. Contemporary management of male infertility. Annu Rev Med 2012;63(1):525–40.
9. Bahren W, Gall H, Scherb W, et al. Arterial anatomy and arteriographic diagnosis of arteriogenic impotence. Cardiovasc Intervent Radiol 1988;11(4):195–210.
10. Quam JP, King BF, James EM, et al. Duplex and color Doppler sonographic evaluation of vasculogenic impotence. AJR Am J Roentgenol 1989;153(6):1141–7.
11. Krausz C. Male infertility: pathogenesis and clinical diagnosis. Best Pract Res Clin Endocrinol Metab 2011;25(2):271–85.
12. Papadimas J, Papadopoulou F, Ioannidis S, et al. Azoospermia: clinical, hormonal, and biochemical investigation. Arch Androl 1996;37(2):97–102.
13. Moon MH, Kim SH, Cho JY, et al. Scrotal US for evaluation of infertile men with azoospermia. Radiology 2006;239(1):168–73.
14. Turek PJ. Practical approaches to the diagnosis and management of male infertility. Nat Clin Pract Urol 2005;2(5):226–38.
15. Jhaveri KS, Mazrani W, Chawla TP, et al. The role of cross-sectional imaging in male infertility: a pictorial review. Can Assoc Radiol J 2010;61(3):144–55.
16. Arai T, Kitahara S, Horiuchi S, et al. Relationship of testicular volume to semen profiles and serum hormone concentrations in infertile Japanese males. Int J Fertil Womens Med 1998;43(1):40–7.
17. Sakamoto H, Saito K, Oohta M, et al. Testicular volume measurement: comparison of ultrasonography, orchidometry, and water displacement. Urology 2007;69(1):152–7.
18. Pierik FH, Dohle GR, van Muiswinkel JM, et al. Is routine scrotal ultrasound advantageous in infertile men? J Urol 1999;162(5):1618–20.
19. Halls J, Bydawell G, Patel U. Erectile dysfunction: the role of penile Doppler ultrasound in diagnosis. Abdom Imaging 2009;34(6):712–25.
20. Wilkins CJ, Sriprasad S, Sidhu PS. Colour Doppler ultrasound of the penis. Clin Radiol 2003;58(7):514–23.
21. Ficarra V, Cerruto MA, Liguori G, et al. Treatment of varicocele in subfertile men: the Cochrane review—a contrary opinion. Eur Urol 2006;49(2):258–63.
22. Madgar I, Weissenberg R, Lunenfeld B, et al. Controlled trial of high spermatic vein ligation for varicocele in infertile men. Fertil Steril 1995;63(1):120–4.
23. Dohle GR, Colpi GM, Hargreave TB, et al. EAU guidelines on male infertility. Eur Urol 2005;48(5):703–11.
24. The influence of varicocele on parameters of fertility in a large group of men presenting to infertility clinics. World Health Organization. Fertil Steril 1992;57(6):1289–93.
25. Beddy P, Geoghegan T, Browne RF, et al. Testicular varicoceles. Clin Radiol 2005;60(12):1248–55.
26. Kocakoc E, Serhatlioglu S, Kiris A, et al. Color Doppler sonographic evaluation of inter-relations between diameter, reflux and flow volume of testicular veins in varicocele. Eur J Radiol 2003;47(3):251–6.

27. Report on varicocele and infertility. Fertil Steril 2004; 82:142–5.

28. Al-Kandari AM, Shabaan H, Ibrahim HM, et al. Comparison of outcomes of different varicocelectomy techniques: open inguinal, laparoscopic, and subinguinal microscopic varicocelectomy: a randomized clinical trial. Urology 2007;69(3):417–20.

29. Main KM, Skakkebæk NE, Virtanen HE, et al. Genital anomalies in boys and the environment. Best Pract Res Clin Endocrinol Metab 2010;24(2):279–89.

30. Virtanen HE, Toppari J. Epidemiology and pathogenesis of cryptorchidism. Hum Reprod Update 2008;14(1):49–58.

31. Boisen KA, Kaleva M, Main KM, et al. Difference in prevalence of congenital cryptorchidism in infants between two Nordic countries. Lancet 2004; 363(9417):1264–9.

32. Wohlfahrt-Veje C, Boisen KA, Boas M, et al. Acquired cryptorchidism is frequent in infancy and childhood. Int J Androl 2009;32(4):423–8.

33. Villumsen AL, Zachau-Christiansen B. Spontaneous alterations in position of the testes. Arch Dis Child 1966;41(216):198–200.

34. Acerini CL, Miles HL, Dunger DB, et al. The descriptive epidemiology of congenital and acquired cryptorchidism in a UK infant cohort. Arch Dis Child 2009; 94(11):868–72.

35. Hadziselimovic F, Cryptorchidism. Its impact on male fertility. Eur Urol 2002;41(2):121–3.

36. Lee PA, Coughlin MT. Fertility after bilateral cryptorchidism. Evaluation by paternity, hormone, and semen data. Horm Res 2001;55(1):28–32.

37. Edey AJ, Sidhu PS. Male infertility: role of imaging in the diagnosis and management. Imaging 2008; 20(2):139–46.

38. Nguyen HT, Coakley F, Hricak H. Cryptorchidism: strategies in detection. Eur Radiol 1999;9(2): 336–43.

39. Subramanyam B, Horii S, Hilton S. Diffuse testicular disease: sonographic features and significance. Am J Roentgenol 1985;145(6):1221–4.

40. Stewart VR, Sidhu PS. The testis: the unusual, the rare and the bizarre. Clin Radiol 2007;62(4):289–302.

41. Dogra VS, Gottlieb RH, Oka M, et al. Sonography of the scrotum. Radiology 2003;227(1):18–36.

42. Aizenstein RI, DiDomenico D, Wilbur AC, et al. Testicular microlithiasis: association with male infertility. J Clin Ultrasound 1998;26(4):195–8.

43. Bach AM, Hann LE, Hadar O, et al. Testicular microlithiasis: what is its association with testicular cancer? Radiology 2001;220(1):70–5.

44. Jarow JP, Espeland MA, Lipshultz LI. Evaluation of the azoospermic patient. J Urol 1989;142(1):62–5.

45. Donat R, McNeill AS, FitzPatrick DR, et al. The incidence of cystic fibrosis gene mutations in patients with congenital bilateral absence of the vas deferens in Scotland. Br J Urol 1997;79(1):74–7.

46. Kuligowska E, Fenlon HM. Transrectal US in male infertility: spectrum of findings and role in patient care. Radiology 1998;207(1):173–81.

47. Hendry WF. Disorders of ejaculation: congenital, acquired and functional. Br J Urol 1998;82(3):331–41.

48. Cornud F, Amar E, Hamida K, et al. Imaging in male hypofertility and impotence. BJU Int 2000; 86(Suppl 1):153–63.

49. Patel B, Gujral S, Jefferson K, et al. Seminal vesicle cysts and associated anomalies. BJU Int 2002; 90(3):265–71.

50. Meacham RB, Townsend RR, Drose JA. Ejaculatory duct obstruction: diagnosis and treatment with transrectal sonography. Am J Roentgenol 1995; 165(6):1463–6.

51. Schroeder-Printzen I, Ludwig M, Kohn F, et al. Surgical therapy in infertile men with ejaculatory duct obstruction: technique and outcome of a standardized surgical approach. Hum Reprod 2000; 15(6):1364–8.

52. Hendry WF, Rickards D, Pryor JP, et al. Seminal megavesicles with adult polycystic kidney disease. Hum Reprod 1998;13(6):1567–9.

53. Raleigh D, O'Donnell L, Southwick GJ, et al. Stereological analysis of the human testis after vasectomy indicates impairment of spermatogenic efficiency with increasing obstructive interval. Fertil Steril 2004;81(6):1595–603.

54. Jarvis L, Dubbins P. Changes in the epididymis after vasectomy: sonographic findings. Am J Roentgenol 1989;152(3):531–4.

55. Schwartz AN, Wang KY, Mack LA, et al. Evaluation of normal erectile function with color flow Doppler sonography. AJR Am J Roentgenol 1989;153(6):1155–60.

56. Benson CB, Aruny JE, Vickers MA. Correlation of duplex sonography with arteriography in patients with erectile dysfunction. Am J Roentgenol 1993; 160(1):71–3.

57. Fitzgerald SW, Erickson SJ, Foley WD, et al. Color Doppler sonography in the evaluation of erectile dysfunction: patterns of temporal response to papaverine. AJR Am J Roentgenol 1991;157(2):331–6.

58. Fitzgerald SW, Erickson SJ, Foley WD, et al. Color Doppler sonography in the evaluation of erectile dysfunction. Radiographics 1992;12(1):3–17 [discussion: 18–9].

59. Gontero P, Sriprasad S, Wilkins CJ, et al. Phentolamine re-dosing during penile dynamic colour Doppler ultrasound: a practical method to abolish a false diagnosis of venous leakage in patients with erectile dysfunction. Br J Radiol 2004;77(923):922–6.

60. Lopez JA, Jarow JP. Penile vascular evaluation of men with Peyronie's disease. J Urol 1993;149(1): 53–5.

61. Golijanin D, Singer E, Davis R, et al. Doppler evaluation of erectile dysfunction—part 2. Int J Impot Res 2007;19(1):43–8.

Imaging of Male Pelvic Trauma

Laura L. Avery, MD[a],*, Meir H. Scheinfeld, MD, PhD[b]

KEYWORDS

- Bladder trauma • Testicular trauma • Testicular rupture • Penile trauma • Penile fracture

KEY POINTS

- Prompt imaging plays an important role in the evaluation of male pelvic soft tissue trauma, particularly in the evaluation of bladder, scrotal, and penile/urethral injuries. Using appropriate imaging modalities, with optimization of contrast administration when appropriate, is essential for accurate diagnosis.
- Traumatic bladder rupture, either extraperitoneal or intraperitoneal, is diagnosed with high accuracy using computed tomography cystography, thus allowing for either conservative or surgical repair, respectively.
- Suspicion of urethral injury warrants evaluation with retrograde urethrography to evaluate for the presence of injury and injury location (anterior versus posterior).
- Early identification of laceration of the testicular tunica albuginea, usually with ultrasound but occasionally with magnetic resonance imaging, is essential given the need for emergent surgical repair.
- Penile injuries require surgical exploration and repair when the tunica albuginea of the corpus cavernosum is ruptured. Understanding both normal penile anatomy and the imaging appearance of corpus rupture (as opposed to a hematoma) is imperative for proper diagnosis and management.

INTRODUCTION

Male pelvic trauma, including bladder, urethral, penile, and scrotal injuries, are uncommon, but when they occur, prompt diagnosis and treatment are required. Many of these injuries occur in the context of multitraumatized patients in whom other injuries and potential hemodynamic instability may lead to clinical distraction from these injuries. Various imaging modalities have been developed to diagnose these injuries with a high diagnostic accuracy in a timely manner. Rapid recognition of pathologic conditions is essential for timely and appropriate intervention, with delay having the potential for development of complications and/or loss of function. Imaging and clinical aspects of bony and vascular pelvic injuries have been covered elsewhere.[1–5] This article will focus on the soft tissue organs with a review of the proper imaging techniques, regional anatomy, and common injury patterns encountered in the evaluation of the traumatized male pelvis.

BLADDER TRAUMA

Bladder injuries can be caused by either blunt or penetrating trauma. The bladder's position deep within the bony pelvis provides moderate protection from injury. Bladder injury may be seen in multitraumatized patients, and in general, the probability of bladder injury increases with the degree of bladder distention.[6] In one study, there was a 22% mortality rate in trauma patients whose presentations include a ruptured bladder, with patient death usually related to the polytrauma.[7]

[a] Division of Emergency Radiology, Department of Radiology, Harvard Medical School, Massachusetts General Hospital, 55 Fruit Street, FHD-210, Boston, MA 02114, USA; [b] Division of Emergency Radiology, Montefiore Medical Center, Albert Einstein College of Medicine, 111 East 210 Street, Bronx, NY 10467, USA
* Corresponding author.
E-mail address: lavery@partners.org

Radiol Clin N Am 50 (2012) 1201–1217
http://dx.doi.org/10.1016/j.rcl.2012.08.010
0033-8389/12/$ – see front matter © 2012 Elsevier Inc. All rights reserved.

Blunt traumatic injury of the bladder frequently occurs with deceleration injuries such as occurs in motor vehicle collisions; 83% to 97% of patients with bladder rupture have associated pelvic fractures.[7,8] Conversely, only approximately 10% of patients with pelvic fractures sustain bladder injuries.[9,10] Traumatic bladder ruptures may be either extraperitoneal or intraperitoneal. Extraperitoneal rupture occurs in 54% to 56% of cases, whereas intraperitoneal rupture accounts for 38% to 40% of injuries.[11] Combined injuries are uncommon and range from 5% to 8% of cases.[11]

One analysis concluded that radiographic investigation of the bladder is necessary when both pelvic fracture and gross hematuria are present.[10] If only one is present, then other clinical factors should influence the decision of whether dedicated bladder imaging should be performed. This was confirmed in a recent consensus statement.[11]

Because of its high accuracy, computed tomography (CT) cystography is the test of choice to investigate bladder wall integrity.[12,13] After the trauma team determines urethral continuity based on clinical examination or retrograde urethrography (RUG), bladder catheterization is performed. CT cystography requires adequate distention of the bladder with retrograde filling using a minimum of 300 mL of iodinated contrast material (Box 1). Gadolinium-based contrast has also been used in patients with a known life-threatening reaction to iodinated contrast.[14] Although in the past, conventional cystography was performed,[15] CT cystography has a demonstrated accuracy approaching 100% and provides efficient and timely evaluation, particularly in the multitrauma patient in whom CT cystography can be performed following standard abdominal and pelvic trauma

CT imaging.[12,16] Although CT cystography may expose the patient to a larger quantity of radiation than fluoroscopic imaging, CT imaging has the advantage of rapid acquisition, no need to transfer the patient to a different imaging room, and the potential to diagnose additional injuries.

Extraperitoneal bladder rupture is nearly always associated with pelvic fractures.[11] Classically, this was presumed to be caused by bony pelvic fragments directly lacerating the bladder wall. Currently, however, it is thought that injury is usually caused by a burst or shearing mechanism that results in rupture of the anterolateral aspect of the bladder during traumatic deformation of the bony pelvis.[11,17]

The classic CT finding of extraperitoneal bladder rupture is contrast extravasation around the base of the bladder, confined to the perivesicular and prevesicular space (of Retzius) (Fig. 1). On axial CT scans, the presence of irregular extraperitoneal areas of contrast extravasation anterior and lateral to the bladder is commonly described as having a "molar tooth" appearance (with the crown of the tooth anterior to the bladder and the roots of the tooth on either side of the bladder).[6] On coronal images, the contrast opacified bladder may assume a "teardrop"- or "pear"-shaped configuration, similar to its classic appearance using conventional cystography.[18] This shape is caused by a combination of compression by pelvic hematoma and extravasated urine.

In simple extraperitoneal ruptures, contrast extravasation is limited to the perivesical space. In complex ruptures, contrast may dissect into adjacent fascial planes and extraperitoneal spaces, including the thigh, penis, and anterior abdominal wall. Contrast may reach the scrotum if the urogenital diaphragm or it superior fascia is disrupted (Fig. 2).[19]

Historically, extraperitoneal bladder rupture was managed with good results with either urethral or suprapubic catheter drainage and follow-up cystography after 10 days.[20] Some series have described common complications using this approach.[21] Currently, catheter drainage is favored for low-grade injuries; however, in more complex injuries and in ones that involve the bladder neck, operative treatment is favored.[22] When the patient is going to surgery for operative orthopedic repair of the bony pelvis, bladder repair is commonly performed simultaneously.[23]

Intraperitoneal bladder rupture usually occurs when a full, already thinned, bladder sustains an abdominal and pelvic impact, causing a sudden large increase in intravesical pressure. In the adult, the bladder dome is covered by a thin layer of peritoneum, and it is the part of the bladder that is

---

Box 1
CT cystogram

1. Retrograde bladder catheterization is usually performed by the trauma team before imaging.

2. Trauma protocol CT of the abdomen and pelvis is performed to exclude vascular contrast extravasation.

3. Drain the bladder to eliminate urine and blood.

4. The bladder is filled retrograde using a minimum of 300 mL of sterile dilute contrast (20 mL Iothalamate Meglumine 60% (Conray) in 500 mL of saline) under gravity drip 40 cm above the patient.

5. Repeat CT of the pelvis, with multiplanar reconstructions.

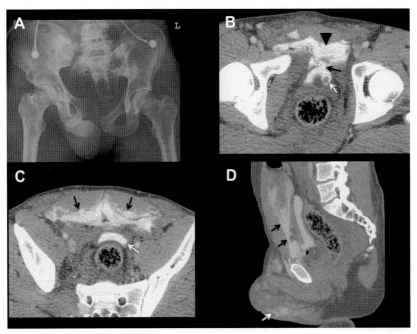

Fig. 1. Extraperitoneal bladder rupture. (A) Frontal pelvic portable radiograph from a trauma series demonstrates a displaced vertical shear fracture with elevation of the right hemipelvis and marked diastasis at the pubic symphysis. (B) Axial CT cystogram image demonstrates extravasation of contrast from the anterior base of the bladder (black arrow). Contrast extends into the prevesicular space (black arrow head). A Foley catheter is identified in the bladder lumen (white arrow). (C) Axial CT cystogram image more superior than in B demonstrates extraperitoneal contrast accumulation along the anterior pelvic wall (black arrows). Contrast material is identified in the bladder lumen (white arrow). (D) Sagittal CT scan demonstrates the extent of extraperitoneal contrast extravasation into the anterior abdominal/pelvic wall (black arrows). Contrast also extends inferiorly into the scrotum (white arrow), consistent with disruption of the urogenital diaphragm.

poorly protected from sudden increases in pressure. The bladder only fully descends into the pelvis by 20 years of age. Therefore, in children, more of the bladder is intraperitoneal and intraperitoneal rupture is more prevalent in children.[24] An enlarged prostate gland in an older man may increase the risk of intraperitoneal rupture as a result of the bladder being more distended at baseline in this population.

On CT cystography, contrast extravasation will be visualized as contrast entering into the peritoneal cavity (Fig. 3). Contrast is seen surrounding loops of bowel, separating leaves of mesentery and layering in the paracolic gutters.[6] Even when this is seen, an extraperitoneal component to rupture should be searched for to exclude a combined intraperitoneal-extraperitoneal injury.

Nearly all intraperitoneal bladder ruptures require surgical exploration and repair.[22,25] These injuries are usually large and do not heal with prolonged catheterization alone. Urine continues to leak into the abdominal cavity, leading to urinary ascites, abdominal distention, electrolyte disturbances,

and possible chemical peritonitis.[22] With injury limited to the bladder such that laparotomy is not necessary, laparoscopic repair has been successfully performed in humans and cystoscopic repair has been performed in an animal model.[26]

BLADDER HERNIA

Bladder hernia is an uncommon complication of pelvic trauma and occurs secondary to a traumatic abdominal wall hernia or pelvic ring disruption. Bladder hernia may be seen is the setting of pubic symphysis diastasis, such that the bladder is trapped between the pubic bones (Fig. 4). When this is discovered, it must be relayed promptly to the orthopedic team to prevent bladder entrapment or injury that may occur during pelvic reduction or surgery.[27–29] Rupture of the rectus abdominis muscle or avulsion of its tendon from the pubis may occur after a blunt or penetrating anteroposterior force to the pelvis. This defect may be an additional site of bladder herniation and entrapment (see Fig. 4).

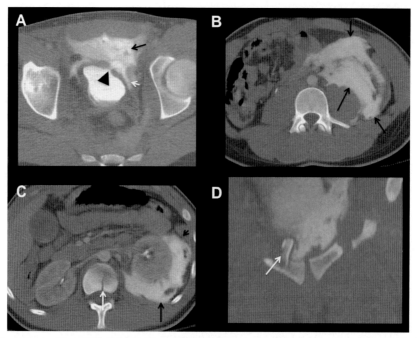

Fig. 2. Complex extraperitoneal bladder rupture. (*A*) Axial CT scan through the base of the bladder demonstrates extravasation of contrast into the prevesicular (*black arrow*) and perivesical spaces (*white arrow*). The location of bladder perforation is indicated (*black arrowhead*). (*B* and *C*) Axial CT scans at progressively more superior levels demonstrate contrast material dissecting through fascial planes in the left retroperitoneum and extending into the perirenal and posterior pararenal spaces (*black arrows*). Note the sagittal lumbar spine fracture (*white arrow in image C*). (*D*) Coronal CT scan of the pelvis demonstrates a displaced fracture fragment of the right pubic rami (*white arrow*) as a possible source for bladder perforation seen in *A*.

URETHRAL INJURIES

A brief anatomic overview of the urethra is presented, as evaluation of urethral trauma requires understanding of male urethral anatomy (**Fig. 5**). The urethra is approximately 22 cm in length[30] and extends from the base of the bladder to the external urethral meatus. The posterior urethra is made up of the prostatic and membranous segments, with the membranous segment being the narrowest urethral segment.[31] The anterior urethra consists of the bulbous and penile (or pendulous) segments. The portion of the urethra within the glans penis is mildly dilated relative to the remainder of the penile urethra and is termed the fossa navicularis. The urogenital diaphragm separates the anterior and posterior segments. The membranous urethra and prostate are anchored to the anterior pubic arch by the puboprostatic ligaments.[32]

Male urethral injuries are rare, with less than one-tenth of a percent of noniatrogenic trauma cases resulting in urethral injuries.[33] Iatrogenic injury is believed to be more common.[34–36] Noniatrogenic urethral injuries are seen in the setting of significant pelvic trauma (eg, motor vehicle accidents and falls from a height) or straddle-type injuries. Classically, it was thought that the posterior urethra at the level of the membranous urethra was the most commonly injured portion of the urethra occurring in conjunction with pelvic fractures. Now it is thought that it is actually the proximalmost portion of the bulbous urethra, just distal to the urogenital diaphragm, that is injured.[33,37] Anterior urethral injuries are more common with straddle-type injuries caused by a crush mechanism. This occurs when the relatively immobile bulbous urethra is compressed against the inferior aspect of the pubis.[38]

Proper and prompt diagnosis is imperative to decrease the morbidity associated with urethral injuries. For example, in the acute setting, misdirection of a bladder catheter through an injured urethra may upgrade a partial injury into a complete injury. Additionally, unrecognized and incompletely treated lacerations may result in chronic urethral strictures because of the formation of fibrous scar tissue.

Clinical signs may be present that suggest urethral injury and warrant RUG before bladder catheter placement. These signs include blood at the urethral meatus, swelling or hematoma of the

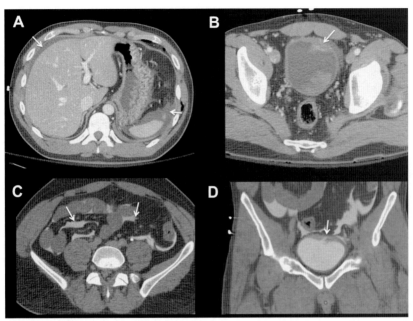

Fig. 3. Intraperitoneal bladder rupture. (*A*) Axial intravenous contrast-enhanced portal venous phase CT scan demonstrates low- to mixed-density fluid around the liver and spleen (*white arrows*). (*B*) Axial intravenous contrast-enhanced portal venous phase CT scan through the bladder demonstrates high-attenuation clot layering dependently in the bladder with thickening along the left anterolateral bladder wall (*white arrow*). (*C*) CT cystogram image demonstrates free contrast in the peritoneal cavity interdigitated among bowel loops and leaves of mesentery (*arrows*). (*D*) Coronal image demonstrates focal interuption of the dome of the bladder with extravasation of contrast into the peritoneal cavity (*arrow*).

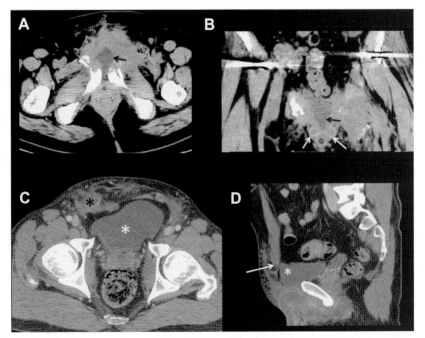

Fig. 4. Bladder hernia. (*A*) Axial contrast-enhanced CT scan from a patient who sustained an open-book fracture of the pelvis demonstrates bladder herniation though the pubic symphysis (*black arrow*) following orthopedic reduction. (*B*) Coronal image demonstrates the bladder (*black arrow*) to be resting on the dorsum of the penis (*white arrows*). (*C* and *D*) Axial and sagittal CT scans from a different patient who also sustained an open-book pelvic fracture demonstrates herniation of the bladder (*white asterisk*) over the pubis secondary to avulsion of the inferior rectus abdominis tendon (*white arrow*) with adjacent hematoma (*black asterisk*).

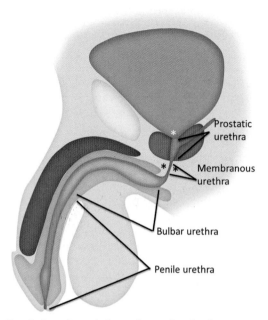

Fig. 5. Drawing of the male urethra in the sagittal plane. The various segments of the urethra including prostatic, membranous, bulbar, and penile portions are illustrated. The bladder neck (*white asterisk*) and level of the urogenital diaphragm (*black asterisks*) are key anatomic landmarks for the classification of urethral injuries when performing urethrography.

perineum or penis, inability to void, and a "high-riding" prostate gland on digital rectal examination.[33] Imaging of the male urethra is best performed using RUG (**Box 2, Fig. 6**). Retrograde contrast opacification of the urethra is performed via instillation of contrast material through a small catheter with its balloon inflated in the fossa navicularis. When the patient is stable, the examination is ideally performed under fluoroscopic visualization with real-time imaging. In an unstable patient, images can be obtained portably in the trauma bay after the injection of contrast. At the authors' institution, when urethral evaluation is essential, a more concentrated dilute contrast (40 mL Iothalamate Meglumine 60% (Conray) in 500 mL saline as opposed to 20 mL Iothalamate Meglumine 60% (Conray) in 500 mL saline for cystography) is injected into the urethra and a pelvic CT scan is performed (termed a CT-RUG) following standard CT. The increased density of the concentrated contrast helps distinguish the contrast from vascular or excreted bladder contrast.

Although the portable-RUG and CT-RUG techniques are generally able to determine only the presence or absences of urethral injury, with only limited information about the exact location of the injury, they are important time-saving screening examinations to be considered in specific

---

Box 2
Retrograde urethrogram
1. A 16-F or 18-F Foley catheter or a hysterosalpingogram catheter is flushed with radiopaque contrast to avoid air bubbles.
2. The glans penis and urethral meatus are cleaned with antiseptic.
3. The catheter is inserted into the penis and the balloon is partially inflated (1–2 mL) in the fossa navicularis.
4. The penis is then pulled laterally to straighten the urethra under moderate traction.
5. A precontrast "scout" image is obtained, because prostatic calcifications may be confused for extravasated contrast.
6. Under fluoroscopic visualization, 20–30 mL of contrast is injected with the goal of filling the entire urethra.
7. If spasm of the external sphincter prevents posterior urethral filling, slow, gentle pressure may allow opacification.
8. Static images are obtained to demonstrate the identified pathologic condition.

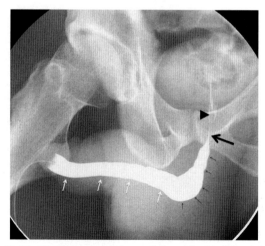

Fig. 6. Normal retrograde urethrogram with filling of the entire urethra. The prostatic urethra demonstrates the normal impression of the verumontanum (*black arrowhead*). The membranous urethra is the narrowest portion of the urethra on the normal urethrogram (*large black arrow*). Small black arrows denote the bulbar portion of the anterior urethra. The white arrows denote the penile portion of the anterior urethra.

situations. For example, in an unstable patient, this information may be sufficient to proceed to suprapubic catheter placement or cystoscopically guided Foley catheter placement.

Urethral injuries have been traditionally classified anatomically as either anterior or posterior. Additional classification systems have been proposed, with the Goldman classification based on anatomic location of injury being the most frequently used system (Table 1).[31,39] This system defines 5 types of urethral injuries. In type I injuries, the puboprostatic ligaments are ruptured, resulting in stretching of the prostatic urethra without urethral urothelial discontinuity (Fig. 7). In type II injuries, the membranous urethra is torn above an intact urogenital diaphragm; this causes contrast extravasation about the prostate but prevents contrast from extravasating inferiorly into the perineum (Fig. 8). Type III urethral injury is characterized by contrast material extravasation into the pelvic extraperitoneal space and also into the perineum as a result of interruption of the urogenital diaphragm (Fig. 9). Type IV injuries occur at the bladder base and are particularly concerning because of involvement of the internal sphincter, which is important for urinary continence (Fig. 10). Type V injuries are injuries that involve only the anterior urethra (Fig. 11).

Regarding treatment, all penetrating injuries are generally explored and debrided immediately.[40] In general, when retrograde drainage of the bladder via urethral catheterization is not possible, a suprapubic catheter is placed. Once urinary drainage is secure, reconstruction of blunt urethral injury may be delayed for weeks to months, thereby allowing time for other injuries to be managed and pelvic hematoma and inflammation to decrease. If there is another indication for immediate surgical exploration, such as penile fracture, bladder neck injury, or rectal tear, the urethra may be repaired concurrently.[36]

Although complete anterior urethral injuries are treated with suprapubic drainage and delayed repair, there are multiple opinions as to the optimal treatment of posterior urethral injuries, including primary realignment, immediate repair, and delayed repair.[22] Primary realignment of posterior urethral injuries, commonly endoscopically, has become increasingly popular[41,42]; however, other data suggest that this may lead to a higher rate of late complications.[36,43] Even in cases of incomplete injury, recent data indicate that stricture-free healing is more likely with suprapubic catheter placement alone.[44] The initially placed or a postrepair urethral catheter may still be in place when the patient presents for follow-up fluoroscopy, which is done to assess for persistent extravasation or possible stricture formation.

SCROTAL TRAUMA

Scrotal trauma is relatively uncommon and accounts for less than 1% of all cases of trauma annually.[45] Frequently blunt testicular trauma is isolated to the scrotum instead of being associated with multitraumatic injuries. Scrotal injuries frequently are sports related and caused by projectiles such as baseballs or by a direct kick to the groin. As a result, younger men are most often injured with a peak age range between 10

Table 1
Goldman system for classification of urethral injuries at urethrography

Injury Type	Injury Description	Urethrographic Appearance
I	Stretching or elongation of an intact posterior urethra resulting from ligament rupture	Intact but stretched urethra
II	Membranous urethral disruption above an intact urogenital diaphragm	Contrast extravasation above the urogenital diaphragm, no inferior contrast extravasation into the perineum
III	Disruption of the membranous urethra with injury of the urogenital diaphragm	Contrast extravasation above the urogenital diaphragm and below the urogenital diaphragm into the perineum
IV	Bladder neck injury extending into the proximal urethra	Extraperitoneal contrast extravasation around the bladder base
V	Isolated anterior urethral injury as from a straddle-type injury	Contrast extravasation below the urogenital diaphragm, confined to the anterior urethra

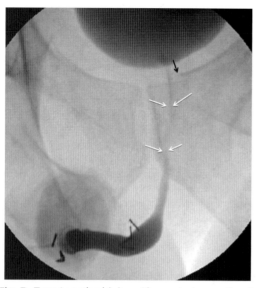

Fig. 7. Type I urethral injury. The posterior urethra is stretched (*white arrows*) but intact. Note the left superior pubic ramus fracture (*black arrow*).

and 30 years. A blunt force to the scrotum may result in testicular contusion, hematoma, or fracture/rupture. A testicular rupture is defined as a rupture of the tunica albuginea with extrusion of the seminiferous tubules. Approximately 50 kg of force is required to rupture a normal tunica albuginea.[46] The right testis is more prone to injury than the left testis, likely because of its superior location and greater propensity to be trapped against the pubis or inner thigh.[47] Testicular fracture/rupture is a surgical emergency, with immediate repair

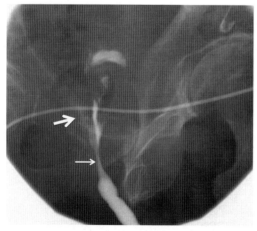

Fig. 8. Type II urethral injury. Contrast extravasation is seen adjacent to the prostatic urethra (*large white arrow*). Contrast does not extend below the intact urogenital diaphragm, indicated by the membranous urethra (*small white arrow*).

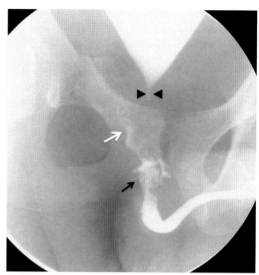

Fig. 9. Type III urethral injury. In this patient there is posterior urethral injury extending through the urogenital diaphragm to involve the bulbous urethra. Retrograde urethrogram reveals contrast material extravasation at and below the membranous urethra (*black arrow*) and a component above the urogenital diaphragm (*white arrow*). Complete disruption of the membranous urethra was diagnosed. Urethral transection results in dislocation of the bladder superiorly, which in this case is filled with excreted contrast from a prior contrast-enhanced CT scan. Note the narrowed and elevated bladder base (*arrowheads*) because of pelvic hematoma.

improving the preservation of fertility and hormonal function.

The normal adult testis measures approximately 5 cm in length and 2 to 3 cm in the transverse dimensions.[48] Many layers cover and protect the testis. Of these layers, the tunica vaginalis and tunica albuginea are import anatomic structures to be aware of when evaluating for traumatic injury. The tunica vaginalis is a double-layered serous membrane derived from the processus vaginalis of the peritoneum.[49] The tunica's inner visceral layer covers most of the testis and epididymis, and the outer parietal layer lines the internal spermatic fascia of the scrotal wall. Within the potential space between the layers, hydroceles or hematoceles may accumulate. The small physiologic volume of fluid normally found in this space allows mobility and provides cushioning to the testis, thus offering mild protection from injury.

The visceral layer of the tunica vaginalis is closely attached to the tunica albuginea of the testis. The tunica albuginea is a fibrous capsule that covers the testis and appears on ultrasound as an echogenic rim surrounding the testis (**Fig. 12**). Additionally, the fibrous nature of the

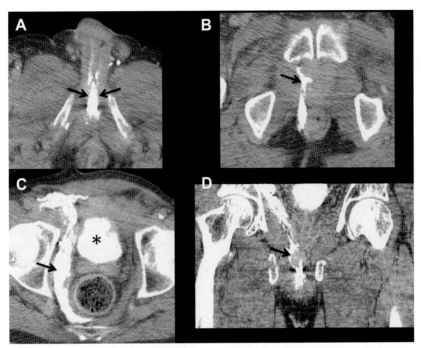

Fig. 10. Type IV urethral injury. A CT retrograde urethrogram was performed (*arrows*). (*A*) Axial CT scan at the level of the penis demonstrates contrast opacification of the bulbar urethra. (*B*) More superiorly, there is contrast extravasation above the urogenital diaphragm (*arrow*). (*C*) More superiorly, at the level of the superiorly displaced urinary bladder, excreted contrast from prior CT (*asterisk*) is seen within the bladder. Extraperitoneal contrast is noted along the right pelvic sidewall (*arrow*). (*D*) Coronal CT scan demonstrates urethral injury extending into the bladder base with extravasation of contrast and clot (*arrow*). This was confirmed at cystoscopy.

tunica gives it low signal on T1- and T2-weighted magnetic resonance (MR) images.[50] In cases of testicular fracture/rupture, the tunica albuginea is lacerated.

Ultrasonography is the most frequent modality used to evaluate the injured scrotum. Ultrasound has a high sensitivity for diagnosing testicular injury.[47,51] The sonographic features of an injured testis include focal areas of altered testicular echogenicity corresponding to areas of contusion or infarction, discrete intraparenchymal fracture plane, discontinuity of the tunica albuginea with irregular contour, and hematocele formation (**Figs. 13 and 14**).[45,47,51,52] The ultrasound findings of a heterogeneous testicular echotexture with a loss of normal testicular contour without directly demonstrating tunica albuginea discontinuity is sufficient to diagnose testicular rupture with a sensitivity of 100% and a specificity of 65% to 93.5% (**Fig. 15**).[51–53] Identifying the discontinuity

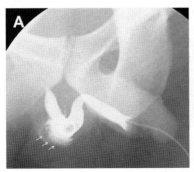

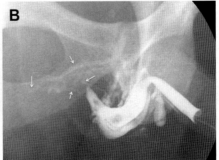

Fig. 11. Type V urethral injury, caused by straddle-type injury. Retrograde urethrogram demonstrates disruption of the bulbous urethra with extravasation inferior to the urethra. (*B*) Extensive venous intravasation of contrast is seen on later images (*arrows*).

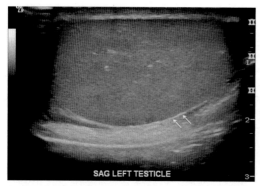

Fig. 12. Normal testicular ultrasound. The normal testicle has homogeneous intermediate echotexture. Arrows define the thin echogenic tunica albuginea, which surrounds the testicle.

within the tunica albuginea may increase confidence for the diagnosis of testicular rupture. The identification of testicular rupture is an indication for surgical exploration and repair.[53] Surgical exploration may also be warranted when a hematocele is present without other evidence of rupture.[53,54] Evolving treatment algorithms have favored exploration only in cases of large (>5 cm) or expanding scrotal hematomas. Thus, close follow-up with serial ultrasound measurements of the hematocele/hematoma may be needed in conservatively managed patients.

At times, MR imaging may be helpful to better define the pattern of testicular injury (Fig. 16). On T1-weighted images, the normal testes have homogeneous intermediate signal, whereas on T2-weighted images, the testes have homogeneous high signal.[50] High T2-weighted signal is expected given that the testes are composed of

the fluid containing seminiferous tubules.[55] Heterogeneous low T2-weighted signal in the context of trauma should raise the possibility of testicular hematoma. Still interruption of the low signal tunica albuginea is diagnostic of rupture.[56,57] The relatively long acquisition time and limited availability for MR examinations make this modality imperfect for initial evaluation for traumatic injury.

PENILE INJURIES

Penile injury may result from penetrating or blunt trauma.[58] Prompt surgical exploration without initial imaging is usually required for penetrating injuries.[59] Blunt traumatic injuries are often evaluated with imaging to determine clinical management. Similar to the scrotum, sonography is the preferred technique for penile imaging because it is well tolerated and widely available. Furthermore, penile blood flow is rapidly evaluated with color and spectral Doppler ultrasound. As MR imaging has become more accessible, this modality has gained acceptance for imaging of penile trauma. MR imaging is able to demonstrate the architecture of the fascial layers of the penis with high tissue conspicuity and sensitivity for injury. Given the dramatic degloving nature of surgical exploration, patients often refuse this mode of management. The MR imaging results can help counsel and persuade the patient toward surgical intervention when truly needed, while sparing others an unneeded exploration.

Anatomically, the penis[60] is composed of paired corpora cavernosa along the dorsal aspect of the penis and one midline corpus spongiosum along the ventral surface. The crura of the corpora cavernosa attach to the ischial rami proximally. The corpora cavernosa are composed of venous

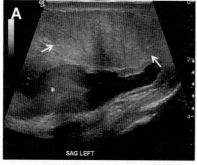
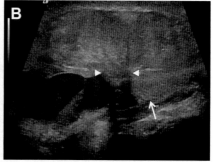

Fig. 13. Testicular fracture. (A) Sagittal image of the left testicle (white arrows) demonstrates a heterogeneous echotexture. Within the scrotum there is intermediate mixed echogenicity fluid (asterisk) consistent with a hematocele. (B) Sagittal image through a different portion of the testicle demonstrates rupture of the tunica albuginea visualized as discontinuity of the echogenic line surrounding the testicle with blood and testicular parenchyma seen extruding through the defect (arrowheads). Hematocele (arrow) is again noted. These findings were confirmed at surgery and a repair of the tunica albuginea was performed.

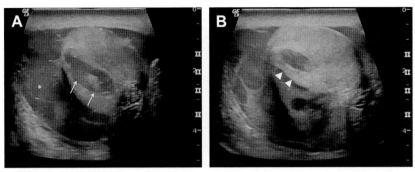

Fig. 14. Testicular fracture. (*A*) Transverse image of the left testicle demonstrates an oval defect extending into the testicular parenchyma consistent with a laceration with resultant hematoma (*arrows*). Within the scrotum there is intermediate mixed echogenic fluid (*asterisk*) consistent with a hematocele. (*B*) Transverse image more superiorly demonstrates the large volume of blood within the scrotum causing mass effect on the underlying testicle (*white arrowheads*). Immediate hematocele evacuation and tunica albuginea repair were performed.

sinusoids that engorge with blood during erection. The corpus spongiosum surrounds the urethra and forms the glans penis distally. The tunica albuginea is a strong fascial sheath that individually surrounds the 2 corpora cavernosa and forms a septum (the intercavernous septum) between them. A tunica albuginea also surrounds the corpus spongiosum. All 3 erectile bodies contribute to the firmness of erection; however, the corpora cavernosa becomes firmer than the corpus spongiosum.[61]

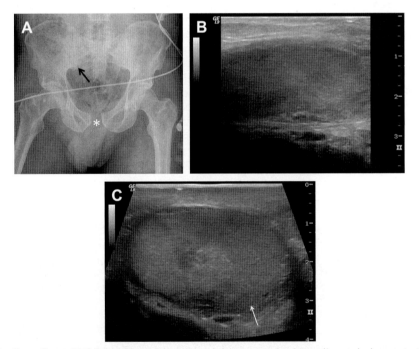

Fig. 15. Pelvic disruption with bilateral testicular injury. (*A*) Anteroposterior radiograph demonstrates an "open book" pelvic injury with diastasis of the symphysis pubis (*asterisk*) and widening of the right sacroiliac joint (*arrow*). (*B*) Sagittal image of the right testicle demonstrates heterogeneous echotexture filling the hemiscrotum without definable margins to indicate the tunica albuginea. Complete avulsion of the tunica albuginea was found at surgery with extrusion of the seminiferous tubules. The testicle was deemed nonviable and an orchiectomy was performed. (*C*) Sagittal image of the left testicle demonstrates heterogeneous echotexture consistent with intratesticular hematoma and poor tunica albuginea definition posteriorly (*arrow*). The testicular contour was grossly maintained. On surgical exploration, the left testicle was found to be "bruised with hematoma" but viable. Orchiopexy was performed.

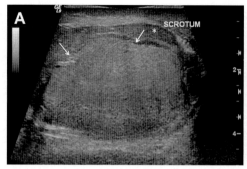
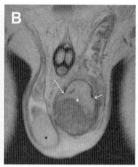

Fig. 16. Progressive avulsion of the tunica albuginea evaluated with ultrasound and subsequently with MR imaging. (*A*) Sagittal gray-scale ultrasound image of the left testicle demonstrates a mildly heterogeneous echotexture with a focal contour abnormality ventrally (*arrows*). A hematocele is also noted (*asterisk*). The patient refused immediate surgical exploration. (*B*) Two hours later, scrotal MR imaging was performed. T2-weighted coronal image demonstrates the normal right testis (*black asterisk*). Evaluation of the left testicle demonstrates retraction of the low-signal tunica albuginea (*edges are indicated with arrows*) and extrusion of the seminiferous tubules and blood into the inferior portion of the hemiscrotum (*white asterisk*). The progression of the avulsion and hemorrhage is attributed to the 2-hour delay.

Superficial to the tunica albuginea is a loose connective tissue called Buck fascia, also known as the deep fascia of the penis.

Ultrasound evaluation of the penis[62,63] is performed with a high-frequency (7.5- to 10-MHz) linear transducer (**Fig. 17**). Anatomic positioning and plentiful gel allow for high-quality images. Sonographically, the 3 corporal bodies are well demarcated. The corpus spongiosum generally appears mildly hypoechoic compared with the corpora cavernosa. The corpora cavernosa have a homogeneous mixed echogenicity appearance because of the innumerable interfaces created by its complex system of vascular sinusoids. There is commonly a region of shadowing between the corpora cavernosa that extends over the expected location of the urethra. Color and spectral Doppler examinations may be used to demonstrate patency and the character of flow within the penile arteries and veins.[64] The patent dorsal veins of the penis should be easily compressible by the transducer and color Doppler flow should be detectable.

MR imaging of the penis is best performed with the penis in anatomic position, lying on the abdomen (**Fig. 18**).[65,66] At our institution, the same protocol programmed for evaluation of the female pelvis is used. The protocol focuses on a small field of view with triplane high-resolution T2 non–fat-saturated sequences and T1-weighted

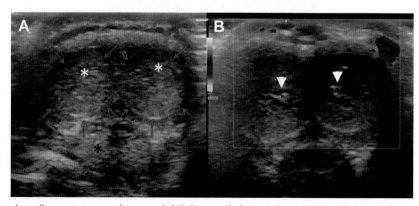

Fig. 17. Normal penile anatomy on ultrasound. (*A*) Gray-scale image demonstrates the corpora cavernosa (*white asterisks*) and corpora spongiosum (*black asterisk*). The tunica albuginea, best seen ventrally, is indicated with red arrows. (*B*) Color-scale image demonstrates small areas of color flow in the central arteries of each corpus cavernosum (*arrowheads*).

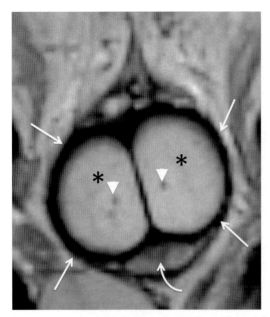

Fig. 18. Normal penile anatomy on MR imaging. Axial T2-weighted MR image through the penis demonstrates the paired high-signal corpora cavernosa (*asterisks*) surrounded by the dark-signal tunica albuginea (*straight arrows*). Flow voids from the central artery of each corpus cavernosum (*arrowheads*) and the flattened urethra (*curved arrow*) within the corpus spongiosum are indicated.

images in the sagittal and coronal planes. On T1-weighted images, the 3 corpora are of intermediate signal and there is poor tissue contrast. T1 hyperintense blood products may be well visualized. On T2-weighted images, the substance of the corpora is of high signal and is well differentiated from the enveloping low-signal tunica albuginea. Direct visualization of tunica discontinuity is best seen on T2-weighted images. The tunica albuginea and Buck fascia are indistinguishable from one another on T1- and T2-weighted images because of their similar low signal.

The penis is most vulnerable to injury when erect, frequently as a result of sudden lateral bending.[67] A penile fracture is a rupture of one or both corpora cavernosa because of a tear of the tunica albuginea, which is one of the strongest fascias in the human body.[68] One reason for the increased risk of penile fracture in the erect state is that the cavernosal tunica albuginea is markedly stretched and thinned during erection.[68] Clinically, penile fracture results in rapid loss of erection, pain, swelling, and penile hematoma. Concomitant injury to the penile urethra is estimated to occur in 10% to 20% of penile fractures and should be suspected if there is associated blood at the urethral meatus or in the setting of bilateral cavernosal injury.[69,70]

Ultrasound, if tolerated, can accurately depict the normal anatomy and delineate the nature and extent of penile injury.[71,72] Sonography can detect the exact site of the fracture as an interruption of the thin echogenic line of the tunica albuginea with extruding hematoma, which may be seen deep to the Buck fascia or the skin (Fig. 19).[63,71] Evaluation of the urethra with ultrasound is limited, and when there is concern for urethral injury, RUG is necessary.[31] The presence of echogenic air within the injured cavernosa suggests communication with the urethra and urethral injury.[72]

Where and when available, MR imaging may be used in the evaluation of a penile injury.[73,74] MR imaging offers superb soft tissue definition and directly demonstrates interruption of the cavernosal tunica albuginea (Fig. 20). Similar to ultrasound, foci of air, seen as susceptibility artifact, may indicate urethral injury. Fluid signal within the corpus spongiosum can indicate urine extravasation in the setting of urethral injury (Fig. 21).

Currently, the vast majority of authors favor immediate surgical repair of blunt penile injuries.[75] The "degloving" nature of the surgery is often unwelcomed by the patient; proper preoperative imaging diagnosis is therefore helpful in convincing the patient of the need for surgery. Complications of conservative management include plaque or nodule formation at the fracture site, missed urethral injury and subsequent stricture development, penile abscess, penile deformity, painful erection, and erectile dysfunction.[76]

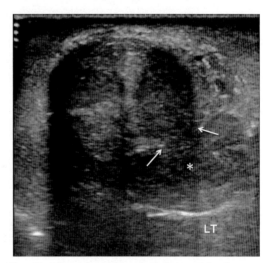

Fig. 19. Ultrasound demonstrating penile fracture. (*A*) Transverse gray-scale image of the penis demonstrates lack of definition of the ventral aspect of the left corpus cavernosum consistent with fracture (*arrows*). Blood products and extruded corpus cavernosal tissue is seen ventrolaterally (*white asterisk*).

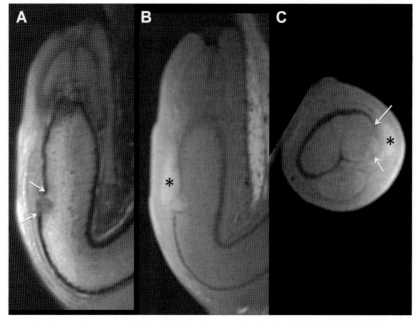

Fig. 20. MR imaging of penile fracture. (*A*) Sagittal T2-weighted image demonstrates focal interruption of the tunica albuginea consistent with tunica albuginea rupture (*arrows*). (*B*) T1-weighted image demonstrates high signal blood products in the overlying Buck fascia (*asterisk*). (*C*) Axial T1-weighted image demonstrates fracture of the cavernosum with discontinuity of the T1-weighted hypointense tunica albuginea on the left lateral side (*arrows*). High-signal overlying hematoma is again seen (*black asterisk*).

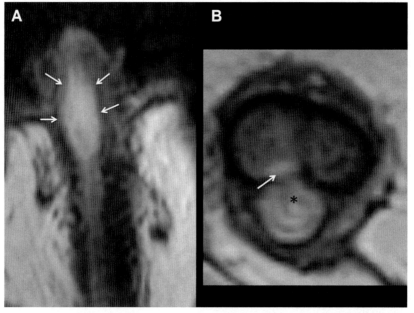

Fig. 21. MR imaging of penile fracture with injury of the urethra. (*A*) Long-axis T2-weighted image demonstrates expansion and increased T2 signal within the corpus spongiosum (*arrows*) concerning for urine extravasation and edema. (*B*) Axial image demonstrates fluid signal within the substance of the corpus spongiosum (*black asterisk*) extending into the right corpus cavernosum (*white arrow*). The tunica albuginea at this level is ill defined. A penile fracture with urethral injury was suspected. Surgical exploration and cystoscopic urethral visualization confirmed this diagnosis.

SUMMARY

Male genital trauma is uncommon and therefore requires the radiologist and trauma team to recognize the clinical signs of injury. In the context of high clinical suspicion, the radiologist must be familiar with the role of imaging and the specific imaging findings found in these diagnoses. Ultrasound is frequently the first-line imaging tool for genital evaluation, with MR imaging, CT, and RUG playing important roles in troubleshooting. Confident identification of normal and abnormal imaging appearances of the bladder, urethra, scrotum, and penis will allow the radiologist to efficiently direct either prompt urologic repair or conservative management.

REFERENCES

1. McCormack R, Strauss EJ, Alwattar BJ, et al. Diagnosis and management of pelvic fractures. Bull NYU Hosp Jt Dis 2010;68(4):281–91.

2. Slater SJ, Barron DA. Pelvic fractures: a guide to classification and management. Eur J Radiol 2010; 74(1):16–23.

3. Yoon W, Kim JK, Jeong YY, et al. Pelvic arterial hemorrhage in patients with pelvic fractures: detection with contrast-enhanced CT. Radiographics 2004;24(6):1591–605.

4. Kertesz JL, Anderson SW, Murakami AM, et al. Detection of vascular injuries in patients with blunt pelvic trauma by using 64-channel multidetector CT. Radiographics 2009;29(1):151–64.

5. Frevert S, Dahl B, Lönn L. Update on the roles of angiography and embolisation in pelvic fracture. Injury 2008;39(11):1290–4.

6. Vaccaro JP, Brody JM. CT cystography in the evaluation of major bladder trauma. Radiographics 2000; 20(5):1373–81.

7. Carroll PR, McAninch JW. Major bladder trauma: mechanisms of injury and a unified method of diagnosis and repair. J Urol 1984;132:254–7.

8. Cass AS. The multiple injured patient with bladder trauma. J Trauma 1984;24(8):731–4.

9. Hochberg E, Stone NN. Bladder rupture associated with pelvic fracture due to blunt trauma. Urology 1993;41(6):531–3.

10. Morey AF, Iverson AJ, Swan A, et al. Bladder rupture after blunt trauma: guidelines for diagnostic imaging. J Trauma 2001;51(4):683–6.

11. Gomez RG, Ceballos L, Coburn M, et al. Consensus statement on bladder injuries. BJU Int 2004;94(1): 27–32.

12. Chan DP, Abujudeh HH, Cushing GL Jr, et al. CT cystography with multiplanar reformation for suspected bladder rupture: experience in 234 cases. AJR Am J Roentgenol 2006;187(5):1296–302.

13. Peng MY, Parisky YR, Cornwell EE, et al. CT cystography versus conventional cystography in evaluation of bladder injury. AJR Am J Roentgenol 1999;173: 1269–72.

14. Newport JP, Dusseault BN, Butler C, et al. Gadolinium-enhanced computed tomography cystogram to diagnose bladder augment rupture in patients with iodine sensitivity. Urology 2008;71(5): 984.e9–984.e11.

15. Mee SL, McAninch JW, Federle MP. Computerized tomography in bladder rupture: diagnostic limitations. J Urol 1987;137(2):207–9.

16. Horstman WG, McClennan BL, Heiken JP. Comparison of computed tomography and conventional cystography for detection of traumatic bladder rupture. Urol Radiol 1991;12(4):188–93.

17. Wolk DJ, Sandler CM, Corriere JN Jr. Extraperitoneal bladder rupture without pelvic fracture. J Urol 1985; 134(6):1199–201.

18. Ambos MA, Bosniak MA, Lefleur RS, et al. The pear-shaped bladder. Radiology 1977;122(1):85–8.

19. Hagiwara A, Nishi K, Ito K, et al. Extraperitoneal bladder rupture with severe lacerations of the urogenital diaphragm: a case report. Cases J 2009;2(1):56.

20. Corriere JN Jr, Sandler CM. Management of the ruptured bladder: seven years of experience with 111 cases. J Trauma 1986;26(9):830–3.

21. Kotkin L, Koch MO. Morbidity associated with nonoperative management of extraperitoneal bladder injuries. J Trauma 1995;38(6):895–8.

22. Kong JP, Bultitude MF, Royce P, et al. Lower urinary tract injuries following blunt trauma: a review of contemporary management. Rev Urol 2011;13(3):119–30.

23. Wirth GJ, Peter R, Poletti PA, et al. Advances in the management of blunt traumatic bladder rupture: experience with 36 cases. BJU Int 2010;106(9): 1344–9.

24. Brereton RJ, Philp N, Buyukpamukcu N. Rupture of the urinary bladder in children. The importance of the double lesion. Br J Urol 1980;52(1):15–20.

25. Kim FJ, Chammas MF Jr, Gewehr EV, et al. Laparoscopic management of intraperitoneal bladder rupture secondary to blunt abdominal trauma using intracorporeal single layer suturing technique. J Trauma 2008;65(1):234–6.

26. Lima E, Rolanda C, Osório L, et al. Endoscopic closure of transmural bladder wall perforations. Eur Urol 2009;56(1):151–7.

27. Bartlett CS, Ali A, Helfet DL. Bladder incarceration in a traumatic symphysis pubis diastasis treated with external fixation: a case report and review of the literature. J Orthop Trauma 1998;12(1):64–7.

28. Seckiner I, Keser S, Bayar A, et al. Successful repair of a bladder herniation after old traumatic pubic symphysis diastasis using bone graft and hernia mesh. Arch Orthop Trauma Surg 2007;127(8):655–7.

29. Geracci JJ, Morey AF. Bladder entrapment after external fixation of traumatic pubic diastasis: importance of follow-up computed tomography in establishing prompt diagnosis. Mil Med 2000;165(6):492–3.

30. Kohler TS, Yadven M, Manvar A, et al. The length of the male urethra. Int Braz J Urol 2008;34(4):451–4.

31. Kawashima A, Sandler CM, Wasserman NF, et al. Imaging of urethral disease: a pictorial review. Radiographics 2004;24(Suppl 1):S195–216.

32. Steiner MS. The puboprostatic ligament and the male urethral suspensory mechanism: an anatomic study. Urology 1994;44(4):530–4.

33. Mundy AR, Andrich DE. Urethral trauma. Part I: introduction, history, anatomy, pathology, assessment and emergency management. BJU Int 2011;108(3):310–27.

34. Assimos DG, Patterson LC, Taylor CL. Changing incidence and etiology of iatrogenic ureteral injuries. J Urol 1994;152(6 Pt 2):2240–6.

35. Kashefi C, Messer K, Barden R, et al. Incidence and prevention of iatrogenic urethral injuries. J Urol 2008;179(6):2254–7.

36. Mundy AR, Andrich DE. Urethral trauma. Part II: types of injury and their management. BJU Int 2011;108(5):630–50.

37. Andrich DE, Mundy AR. The nature of urethral injury in cases of pelvic fracture urethral trauma. J Urol 2001;165(5):1492–5.

38. Rosenstein DI, Alsikafi NF. Diagnosis and classification of urethral injuries. Urol Clin North Am 2006;33(1):73–85.

39. Goldman SM, Sandler CM, Corriere JN Jr, et al. Blunt urethral trauma: a unified, anatomical mechanical classification. J Urol 1997;157:85–9.

40. Kommu SS, Illahi I, Mumtaz F. Patterns of urethral injury and immediate management. Curr Opin Urol 2007;17(6):383–9.

41. Elliott DS, Barrett DM. Long-term followup and evaluation of primary realignment of posterior urethral disruptions. J Urol 1997;157(3):814–6.

42. Mouraviev VB, Coburn M, Santucci RA. The treatment of posterior urethral disruption associated with pelvic fractures: comparative experience of early realignment versus delayed urethroplasty. J Urol 2005;173(3):873–6.

43. Singh BP, Andankar MG, Swain SK, et al. Impact of prior urethral manipulation on outcome of anastomotic urethroplasty for post-traumatic urethral stricture. Urology 2010;75(1):179–82.

44. Elgammal MA. Straddle injuries to the bulbar urethra: management and outcome in 53 patients. Int Braz J Urol 2009;35(4):450–8.

45. Deurdulian C, Mittelstaedt CA, Chong WK, et al. US of acute scrotal trauma: optimal technique, imaging findings, and management. Radiographics 2007;27(2):357–69.

46. Rao KG. Traumatic rupture of testis. Urology 1982;20(6):624–5.

47. Bhatt S, Dogra VS. Role of US in testicular and scrotal trauma. Radiographics 2008;28(6):1617–29.

48. Ragheb D, Higgins JL Jr. Ultrasonography of the scrotum: technique, anatomy, and pathologic entities. J Ultrasound Med 2002;21(2):171–85.

49. Woodward PJ, Schwab CM, Sesterhenn IA. From the archives of the AFIP: extratesticular scrotal masses: radiologic-pathologic correlation. Radiographics 2003;23(1):215–40.

50. Cassidy FH, Ishioka KM, McMahon CJ, et al. MR imaging of scrotal tumors and pseudotumors. Radiographics 2010;30(3):665–83.

51. Guichard G, El Ammari J, Del Coro C, et al. Accuracy of ultrasonography in diagnosis of testicular rupture after blunt scrotal trauma. Urology 2008;71(1):52–6.

52. Buckley JC, McAninch JW. Use of ultrasonography for the diagnosis of testicular injuries in blunt scrotal trauma. J Urol 2006;175(1):175–8.

53. Buckley JC, McAninch JW. Diagnosis and management of testicular ruptures. Urol Clin North Am 2006;33(1):111–6.

54. Jeffrey RB, Laing FC, Hricak H, et al. Sonography of testicular trauma. AJR Am J Roentgenol 1983;141(5):993–5.

55. Kim W, Rosen MA, Langer JE, et al. US MR imaging correlation in pathologic conditions of the scrotum. Radiographics 2007;27(5):1239–53.

56. Cramer BM, Schlegel EA, Thueroff JW. MR imaging in the differential diagnosis of scrotal and testicular disease. Radiographics 1991;11(1):9–21.

57. Kubik-Huch RA, Hailemariam S, Hamm B. CT and MRI of the male genital tract: radiologic-pathologic correlation. Eur Radiol 1999;9(1):16–28.

58. Mydlo JH, Harris CF, Brown JG. Blunt, penetrating and ischemic injuries to the penis. J Urol 2002;168(4 Pt 1):1433–5.

59. Wessells H, Long L. Penile and genital injuries. Urol Clin North Am 2006;33(1):117–26.

60. Healy JC. Penis. In: Standing S, editor. Gray's anatomy. London: Elsevier; 2005. p. 1315–7.

61. Lee J, Singh B, Kravets FG, et al. Sexually acquired vascular injuries of the penis: a review. J Trauma 2000;49(2):351–8.

62. Older RA, Watson LR. Ultrasound anatomy of the normal male reproductive tract. J Clin Ultrasound 1996;24(8):389–404.

63. Wilkins CJ, Sriprasad S, Sidhu PS. Colour Doppler ultrasound of the penis. Clin Radiol 2003;58(7):514–23.

64. Roy C, Saussine C, Tuchmann C, et al. Duplex Doppler sonography of the flaccid penis: potential role in the evaluation of impotence. J Clin Ultrasound 2000;28(6):290–4.

65. Pretorius ES, Siegelman ES, Ramchandani P, et al. MR imaging of the penis. Radiographics 2001;21(Spec No):S283–98.

66. Vossough A, Pretorius ES, Siegelman ES, et al. Magnetic resonance imaging of the penis. Abdom Imaging 2002;27(6):640–59.

67. Sawh SL, O'Leary MP, Ferreira MD, et al. Fractured penis: a review. Int J Impot Res 2008; 20(4):366–9.

68. Bitsch M, Kromann-Andersen B, Schou J, et al. The elasticity and the tensile strength of tunica albuginea of the corpora cavernosa. J Urol 1990;143(3): 642–5.

69. El-Bahnasawy MS, Gomha MA. Penile fractures: the successful outcome of immediate surgical intervention. Int J Impot Res 2000;12(5):273–7.

70. Hoag NA, Hennessey K, So A. Penile fracture with bilateral corporeal rupture and complete urethral disruption: case report and literature review. Can Urol Assoc J 2011;5(2):E23–6.

71. Nomura JT, Sierzenski PR. Ultrasound diagnosis of penile fracture. J Emerg Med 2010;38(3):362–5.

72. Bertolotto M, Mucelli RP. Nonpenetrating penile traumas: sonographic and Doppler features. AJR Am J Roentgenol 2004;183(4):1085–9.

73. Narumi Y, Hricak H, Armenakas NA, et al. MR imaging of traumatic posterior urethral injury. Radiology 1993;188(2):439–43.

74. Boudghene F, Chhem R, Wallays C, et al. MR imaging in acute fracture of the penis. Urol Radiol 1992;14(3):202–4.

75. Shenfeld OZ, Gnessin E. Management of urogenital trauma: state of the art. Curr Opin Urol 2011;21(6): 449–54.

76. Yapanoglu T, Aksoy Y, Adanur S, et al. Seventeen years' experience of penile fracture: conservative vs. surgical treatment. J Sex Med 2009;6(7):2058–63.

Index

Note: Page numbers of article titles are in **boldface** type.

Radiol Clin N Am 50 (2012) 1219–1225
http://dx.doi.org/10.1016/S0033-8389(12)00193-5
0033-8389/12/$ – see front matter

United States Postal Service

Statement of Ownership, Management, and Circulation
(All Periodicals Publications Except Requestor Publications)

1. Publication Title
Radiologic Clinics of North America

2. Publication Number
5 9 6 – 5 1 0

3. Filing Date
9/14/12

4. Issue Frequency
Jan, Mar, May, Jul, Sep, Nov

5. Number of Issues Published Annually
6

6. Annual Subscription Price
$421.00

7. Complete Mailing Address of Known Office of Publication *(Not printer) (Street, city, county, state, and ZIP+4®)*
Elsevier Inc.
360 Park Avenue South
New York, NY 10010-1710

Contact Person
Stephen Bushing

Telephone *(Include area code)*
215-239-3688

8. Complete Mailing Address of Headquarters or General Business Office of Publisher *(Not printer)*
Elsevier Inc., 360 Park Avenue South, New York, NY 10010-1710

9. Full Names and Complete Mailing Addresses of Publisher, Editor, and Managing Editor *(Do not leave blank)*

Publisher *(Name and complete mailing address)*
Kim Murphy, Elsevier, Inc., 1600 John F. Kennedy Blvd. Suite 1800, Philadelphia, PA 19103-2899

Editor *(Name and complete mailing address)*
Adrianne Brigido, Elsevier, Inc., 1600 John F. Kennedy Blvd. Suite 1800, Philadelphia, PA 19103-2899

Managing Editor *(Name and complete mailing address)*
Adrianne Brigido, Elsevier, Inc., 1600 John F. Kennedy Blvd. Suite 1800, Philadelphia, PA 19103-2899

10. Owner *(Do not leave blank. If the publication is owned by a corporation, give the name and address of the corporation immediately followed by the names and addresses of all stockholders owning or holding 1 percent or more of the total amount of stock. If not owned by a corporation, give the names and addresses of the individual owners. If owned by a partnership or other unincorporated firm, give its name and address as well as those of each individual owner. If the publication is published by a nonprofit organization, give its name and address.)*

Full Name	Complete Mailing Address
Wholly owned subsidiary of	1600 John F. Kennedy Blvd., Ste. 1800
Reed/Elsevier, US holdings	Philadelphia, PA 19103-2899

11. Known Bondholders, Mortgagees, and Other Security Holders Owning or Holding 1 Percent or More of Total Amount of Bonds, Mortgages, or Other Securities. If none, check box ☐ None

Full Name	Complete Mailing Address
N/A	

12. Tax Status *(For completion by nonprofit organizations authorized to mail at nonprofit rates) (Check one)*
The purpose, function, and nonprofit status of this organization and the exempt status for federal income tax purposes:
☐ Has Not Changed During Preceding 12 Months
☐ Has Changed During Preceding 12 Months *(Publisher must submit explanation of change with this statement)*

PS Form **3526**, September 2007 (Page 1 of 3 (Instructions Page 3)) PSN 7530-01-000-9931 **PRIVACY NOTICE** See our Privacy policy in www.usps.com

---

13. Publication Title
Radiologic Clinics of North America

14. Issue Date for Circulation Data Below
July 2012

15. Extent and Nature of Circulation

		Average No. Copies Each Issue During Preceding 12 Months	No. Copies of Single Issue Published Nearest to Filing Date
a. Total Number of Copies *(Net press run)*		3250	2808
b. Paid Circulation (By Mail and Outside the Mail)	(1) Mailed Outside-County Paid Subscriptions Stated on PS Form 3541. *(Include paid distribution above nominal rate, advertiser's proof copies, and exchange copies)*	1783	1607
	(2) Mailed In-County Paid Subscriptions Stated on PS Form 3541 *(Include paid distribution above nominal rate, advertiser's proof copies, and exchange copies)*		
	(3) Paid Distribution Outside the Mails Including Sales Through Dealers and Carriers, Street Vendors, Counter Sales, and Other Paid Distribution Outside USPS®	782	751
	(4) Paid Distribution by Other Classes Mailed Through the USPS (e.g. First-Class Mail®)		
c. Total Paid Distribution *(Sum of 15b (1), (2), (3), and (4))*		2565	2358
d. Free or Nominal Rate Distribution (By Mail and Outside the Mail)	(1) Free or Nominal Rate Outside-County Copies Included on PS Form 3541	95	77
	(2) Free or Nominal Rate In-County Copies Included on PS Form 3541		
	(3) Free or Nominal Rate Copies Mailed at Other Classes Through the USPS (e.g. First-Class Mail)		
	(4) Free or Nominal Rate Distribution Outside the Mail (Carriers or other means)		
e. Total Free or Nominal Rate Distribution *(Sum of 15d (1), (2), (3) and (4))*		95	77
f. Total Distribution *(Sum of 15c and 15e)*		2660	2435
g. Copies not Distributed *(See instructions to publishers #4 (page #3))*		590	373
h. Total *(Sum of 15f and g)*		3250	2808
i. Percent Paid *(15c divided by 15f times 100)*		96.43%	96.84%

16. Publication of Statement of Ownership
☒ If the publication is a general publication, publication of this statement is required. Will be printed in the **November** 2012 issue of this publication.
☐ Publication not required.

17. Signature and Title of Editor, Publisher, Business Manager, or Owner

[signature] Stephen R. Bushing – Inventory Distribution Coordinator

Date September 14, 2012

I certify that all information furnished on this form is true and complete. I understand that anyone who furnishes false or misleading information on this form or who omits material or information requested on the form may be subject to criminal sanctions (including fines and imprisonment) and/or civil sanctions (including civil penalties).

PS Form **3526**, September 2007 (Page 2 of 3)

Moving?

Make sure your subscription moves with you!

To notify us of your new address, find your **Clinics Account Number** (located on your mailing label above your name), and contact customer service at:

Email: journalscustomerservice-usa@elsevier.com

800-654-2452 (subscribers in the U.S. & Canada)
314-447-8871 (subscribers outside of the U.S. & Canada)

Fax number: 314-447-8029

Elsevier Health Sciences Division
Subscription Customer Service
3251 Riverport Lane
Maryland Heights, MO 63043

*To ensure uninterrupted delivery of your subscription, please notify us at least 4 weeks in advance of move.

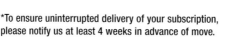
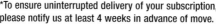